LASERS IN GYNAECOLOGY

Lasers in Medicine and Surgery Series

General Editors

Mr J. A. S. Carruth,
Department of Otolaryngology,
Royal South Hants Hospital,
Southampton, UK.

Professor S. N. Joffe,
College of Medicine,
University of Cincinnati Medical Center,
Cincinnati,
Ohio, USA.

Lasers are finding increasing uses in many branches of medicine and surgery. This new series will review the applications in various specialities, and will provide authoritative and up to date accounts of current practice. Each editor will select an international team of contributors chosen for their particular expertise. Little background knowledge of lasers will be assumed, and the books should therefore appeal to all physicians and surgeons in the relevant speciality.

1. Lasers in Otolaryngology
   Edited by J. A. S. Carruth and G. T. Simpson
2. Lasers in Gastroenterology
   Edited by N. Krasner
3. Lasers in Neurosurgery
   Edited by R. V. Jeffreys
4. Lasers in Gynaecology
   Edited by C. Sutton

LASERS IN GYNAECOLOGY

Edited by

Chris Sutton

Consultant Obstetrician and Gynaecologist,
Royal Surrey County Hospital,
Guildford, Surrey, UK

CHAPMAN & HALL MEDICAL
London · New York · Tokyo · Melbourne · Madras

Published by Chapman & Hall, 2–6 Boundary Row, London SE1 8HN

Chapman & Hall, 2–6 Boundary Row, London SE1 8HN, UK

Chapman & Hall Japan, Thomson Publishing Japan, Hirakawacho Nemoto Building, 7F, 1-7-11 Hirakawa-cho, Chiyoda-ku, Tokyo 102, Japan

Chapman & Hall Australia, Thomas Nelson Australia, 102 Dodds Street, South Melbourne, Victoria 3205, Australia

Chapman & Hall India, R. Seshadri, 32 Second Main Road, CIT East, Madras 600 035, India

---

First edition 1992

Typeset in 10/12pt Palatino by Graphicraft Typesetters Ltd., Hong Kong

Printed in Great Britain at The University Press, Cambridge

ISBN 0 412 32360 5

A catalogue record for this book is available from the British Library

Contents

Colour plates appear between pages 112 and 113

Contributors xi

Preface xv

1. **The physics of light and lasers** 1
GREGORY T. ABSTEN
1.1 Introduction 1
1.2 Laser 2
1.3 Light waves 2
1.4 Light emission 5
1.5 Special properties of laser light 8
1.6 The laser medium 11
1.7 Energy concepts 13
1.8 Pulsing concepts and nonlinear effects 15
1.9 Biophysics and tissue interaction 16
1.10 Conclusions 22
References 23

2. **Gynaecological microsurgery using the CO_2 laser** 25
JOSEPH FESTE
2.1 Introduction 25
2.2 Instrumentation 26
2.3 Laser surgery for endometriosis 28
2.4 Adhesiolysis 33
2.5 Clinical techniques 36
2.6 Laser surgery of the Fallopian tube 38
2.7 Ovarian cystectomies 46
2.8 Laser treatment of polycystic ovarian disease 46
2.9 Myomectomy 47
2.10 Metroplasty 49
2.11 Conclusions 51
References 52

3.		**Assessment of results of laparoscopic laser surgery** MICHAEL P. DIAMOND	55
	3.1	Introduction	55
	3.2	Therapeutic alternatives: incision, coagulation, haemostasis	56
	3.3	Procedures performed at laparoscopy	59
	3.4	Revived procedures	63
	3.5	Efficacy	65
	3.6	Alternatives of assisted reproduction technology	66
	3.7	Concerns in endoscopic surgery	66
	3.8	The future	67
		References	68
4.		**CO_2 laser laparoscopy in endometriosis** J. DONNEZ	73
	4.1	Introduction	73
	4.2	Advantages	73
	4.3	Equipment	74
	4.4	Methods	77
	4.5	Results	81
	4.6	Conclusion: the future	88
		References	91
5.		**Adhesions and laser laparoscopic adhesiolysis** RUSSELL MACDONALD and CHRIS SUTTON	95
	5.1	Introduction	95
	5.2	What is the mechanism of adhesion formation?	95
	5.3	What are the clinical implications of adhesions?	98
	5.4	Adhesions and abdominal pain	98
	5.5	Laparoscopic adhesiolysis for abdominal pain	100
	5.6	Adhesions and infertility	102
	5.7	How should adhesiolysis be performed?	103
	5.8	Does adjuvant therapy improve the effectiveness of adhesiolysis?	109
	5.9	Conclusions	112
		References	113
		Advanced operative laser laparoscopy JAMES F. DANIELL	119
	6.1	Introduction	119
	6.2	History of the development of visible light lasers for laparoscopy	119

6.3 Physics and tissue interaction of the argon and KTP lasers 120
6.4 Advantages and disadvantages of visible light laser energy for laparoscopy 120
6.5 Delivery techniques 122
6.6 Specific procedures performed laparoscopically 126
6.7 Future possibilities for visible light lasers for advanced operative laparoscopic techniques 137
6.8 Safety in advanced laser laparoscopy 137
6.9 Conclusions 138
References 139

7. **Neodymium-YAG laser laparoscopy** 141
STEPHEN L. CORSON
7.1 Basic science 141
7.2 The sapphire probe 142
7.3 CO_2 vs YAG contact probe lasers 143
7.4 Laboratory experiments 148
7.5 Clinical applications 150
7.6 Description of technique 151
7.7 Additional laparoscopic techniques 152
References 154

8. **Ectopic pregnancy** 155
JÖRG KECKSTEIN
8.1 Introduction 155
8.2 Technical aspects 158
8.3 Experimental and clinical studies 163
8.4 Results and discussion 164
8.5 Conclusion 170
References 171

9. **Neodymium-YAG laser hysteroscopy: total endometrial ablation** 175
MILTON H. GOLDRATH
9.1 Introduction 175
9.2 Methods 176
9.3 Results 178
9.4 Complications 179
9.5 Conclusion 180
References 181

10. **Laser hysteroscopic surgery and focal ablation of the endometrium** 183
JACQUES DEQUESNE
10.1 Introduction 183
10.2 Focal ablation of the endometrium 184
10.3 Practical aspects of the procedure 186
10.4 Results 187
10.5 Alternatives to the Nd-YAG laser in hysteroscopic surgery 190
10.6 Complications and side effects 192
10.7 Conclusion 193
References 193

11. **Laser treatment of cervical and vaginal intraepithelial neoplasia** 195
NIGEL SAUNDERS, FRANK SHARP and JOSEPH A. JORDAN
11.1 Historical aspects of cervical intraepithelial neoplasia 195
11.2 Conservative trends in management 198
11.3 Available treatment methods 199
11.4 Techniques of laser vaporization and excisional conization 204
11.5 Problems of vaginal intraepithelial neoplasia 205
11.6 Advantages of laser 206
11.7 Organization of a colposcopic laser service 206
References 207

12. **Laser surgery on the vulva** 211
RICHARD REID
12.1 Basic treatment philosophy 211
12.2 Principles of effective laser surgery 213
12.3 Depth control during vulvar laser surgery 221
12.4 The role of extended laser ablation 227
12.5 Adjuvant regimens 231
12.6 Conclusion 234
References 235

13. **Laser safety: hazards and precautions** 237
E. J. KERSHAW and M. J. VAN BOVEN
13.1 Laser safety 237
13.2 Anaesthetic hazards 238
References 246

14.	**Education and credentialling in gynaecologic laser surgery**	249
	JAMES H. DORSEY	
14.1	Introduction	249
14.2	Education and training	249
14.3	Specific credentialling procedures	250
14.4	Criteria for evaluating laser surgery	251
14.5	Endoscopic laser surgery	253
14.6	Conclusion	255
	References	256
15.	**The future of laser surgery**	257
	WILLIAM R. KEYE	
15.1	Introduction	257
15.2	Current status and future needs	258
15.3	Development of new delivery systems	259
15.4	Controlled tissue destruction	260
15.5	Techniques for development of tissue sensitization to laser energy (photodynamic therapy)	261
15.6	Diagnostic techniques using lasers	265
15.7	Miniaturization of laser systems	266
15.8	Conclusion	266
	References	267
	Index	269

Contributors

G. T. ABSTEN
President, Advanced Laser Services Corporation, P.O. Box 99, Grove City, OH 43123, USA

M. J. VAN BOVEN
Consultant Anaesthetist, Catholic University of Louvain, Cliniques Universitaires Saint-Luc, Avenue Hippocrate 10, B-1200 Brussels, Belgium

S. L. CORSON MD
Clinical Professor, Department of Obstetrics and Gynaecology, University of Pennsylvania School of Medicine, Philadelphia Fertility Institute, 330 South 8th Street, Philadelphia, PA 1907-6096, USA

J. F. DANIELL MD
The Women's Health Group, 2222 State Street, Nashville, TN 37203-1870, USA

J. DEQUESNE
Department of Gynaecology and Obstetrics, Croix-Rouges 16, 1007 Lausanne, Switzerland

M. D. DIAMOND MD
Assistant Professor, Department of Obstetrics and Gynaecology, Yale University School of Medicine, 339 Farnam Memorial Building, P.O. Box 3333, New Haven, CT 06510, USA

J. DONNEZ MD, PhD
Head of Department of Gynaecology, Catholic University of Louvain, Cliniques Universitaires Saint-Luc, Avenue Hippocrate 10, B-1200 Brussels, Belgium

J. H. DORSEY MD
Department of Gynaecology, Greater Baltimore Medical Center, 6701 N. Charles Street, Baltimore, MD 21204, USA

Contributors

J. FESTE MD
Associate Clinical Professor, Department of Obstetrics and Gynaecology, Baylor College of Medicine, 7550 Fannin, Houston, TX 77054-1989, USA

M. H. GOLDRATH MD
Chairman, Department of Obstetrics and Gynaecology, Sinai Hospital of Detroit, 6767 West Outer Drive, Detroit, MI 48235-2899, USA

J. A. JORDAN
Consultant Gynaecologist, Birmingham & Midland Hospital for Women, Showell Green Lane, Sparkhill, Birmingham B11 4HI, UK

J. KECKSTEIN MD
Senior Lecturer, Department of Gynaecology and Obstetrics of the University of Ulm, Prittwitzstrasse 43, 7900 Ulm, Germany

E. J. KERSHAW
Consultant Anaesthetist, Department of Anaesthetics, Royal Surrey County Hospital, Guildford, Surrey, UK

W. R. KEYE JR MD
Associate Professor, Chief, Division of Reproductive Endocrinology, University of Utah School of Medicine, Salt Lake City, UT 84132, USA

R. MACDONALD FRCS, FRCOG
BP Research Fellow, Department of Obstetrics and Gynaecology, Royal Northern Hospital, London N1, UK

R. REID MD
Director, Cervical and Vulvar Dysplasia Clinic, Sinai Hospital of Detroit, 6767 West Outer Drive, Detroit, M1 48235-2899 USA

N. SAUNDERS
Department of Obstetrics and Gynaecology, Clinical Sciences Centre, Northern General Hospital, Sheffield S5 7AU, UK

F. SHARP
Department of Obstetrics and Gynaecology, Clinical Sciences Centre, Northern General Hospital, Sheffield S5 7AU, UK

C. J. G. SUTTON MA, MB, BCh, FRCOG
Consultant Gynaecologist, Department of Obstetrics and Gynaecology, Royal Surrey County Hospital, Guildford, Surrey, UK; Chairman, Gynaecological Section, British Medical Laser Association; Secretary, British Society for Gynaecological Endoscopy.

Preface

The past decade has been an exciting time for those of us involved in laser surgery. In gynaecology the CO_2 laser has become firmly established as the treatment of choice for pre-malignant disease of the cervix. The association of this condition with the human papilloma virus and its spread as a sexually transmitted disease has produced an increase of cases of almost epidemic proportions which is doubling in incidence every 3 years. Some cytology clinics in central London are finding an abnormal smear in every five patients and it is against this background that a colposcopy and laser unit are no longer the provenance of a few elite units but are now to be found in most district general hospitals. To this end I have included some essentially practical chapters on laser surgery of the cervix and also the vulva, which increasingly is involved in HPV infections and presents an area that is uniquely suited to laser surgery. Laser skinning vulvectomy is an operation that is technically difficult to perform but the excellent healing and lack of scarring represents a beautiful example of the advantages of the laser over the traditional cold-knife or electrodiathermy.

Although they are present in all textbooks of laser surgery I have deliberately included chapters on basic laser physics, laser–tissue interactions and laser safety since these are essential for any surgeon to understand before he or she is allowed access to a surgical laser. I make no apology for this because failure to adhere to strict safety precautions can result in dire consequences, even blindness from the backscatter of Nd-YAG laser radiation, whilst a blast from a ruby laser could pass straight through a human being turning the operating theatre into a scene from Star Wars.

Potentially the most exciting development of recent years has been the explosion of interest in endoscopic laser operations, culminating in the general surgeons at long last recognizing the value of laparoscopy by removing the gall-bladder by this route. Laparoscopy has been used increasingly in gynaecology for the diagnosis of pelvic pain and infertility, and the introduction of lasers of differing wavelengths offers a very real possibility of being able to perform corrective surgery at the same time. The fact that over 500 laser laparoscopy sets were sold last year in the United States alone bears witness to the growing popularity of this procedure. We have included chapters from both sides of the Atlantic describing the development of laser laparoscopy, its present and future applications and the possible role of Nd-YAG, argon, KTP and CO_2 lasers in the treatment of gynaecological diseases. Since this is essentially a practical textbook we have included detailed descriptions of several laparoscopic operations ranging from laparoscopic drilling of polycystic ovaries to excision of ovarian endometriomas and from the removal of sub-serous fibroids to the conservative treatment of ectopic pregnancy.

Certain laser surgical procedures are beginning to challenge traditional methods and this is particularly true of laser photovaporization of the endometrium. Here Nd-YAG laser energy is passed down a flexible fibre and the entire endometrium is destroyed under hysteroscopic control as a new way of treating patients with menorrhagia. Although the procedure is difficult and tedious the advantage for the patient is considerable and she is able to go home the following day with little more discomfort than that experienced after a dilatation and curettage. More important, she can return immediately to active life and work rather than put up with a 7-day hospital stay and a couple of months out of action which is the norm for an abdominal hysterectomy. Bearing in mind that some 700 000 hysterectomies are performed annually in the United States alone and that about half of these could be treated by laser obliteration of the endometrium, the benefits in terms of health economics are enormous.

Another area of recent technological advance has been the treatment of infertility, particularly with increasing use of *in-vitro* fertilization (IVF) and gamete intrafallopian transfer (GIFT). We have therefore included several chapters on laser tubal surgery, both open and laparoscopic, and the use of laser laparoscopy to prepare the pelvis for these new fertility techniques.

Finally, realizing that this type of surgery requires high standards of training we end with practical considerations on learning laser surgery and an overview of the new types of laser that may soon be placed at our disposal.

It has been my intention in compiling this book to bring together the foremost experts in the field of gynaecological laser surgery from the United States and Europe. I sincerely hope that this wealth of combined talent will be of practical help to those gynaecologists who are about to embark on these new and very exciting surgical techniques.

Chris Sutton

1 *The physics of light and lasers*

GREGORY T. ABSTEN

1.1 Introduction

Lasers are devices that produce intense beams of light energy. Electricity is converted into light which is further intensified to cut, vaporize, or coagulate tissue. The key mechanism of action, first described by Albert Einstein in the early 1900s, is the stimulated emission of radiation (Einstein, 1917). In the context of laser, radiation merely means light, not ionizing radiation which is associated with X-rays. A radiant body shines, or emits light.

Through stimulated emission, atoms and molecules may be energized and manipulated to produce this unique type of light called laser light. Lasing action occurs in a resonator tube which is capped at each end with mirrors that face each other. As waves of laser light produced by stimulated emission travel down the tube, they reflect back and forth between the mirrors, creating a cascading effect of growing light energy through stimulated emission of radiation in the material. This results in a tremendously bright beam of light which exits the tube through a partially reflective mirror. This is the emitted laser beam. So, just as a stereo amplifier can amplify and emit electrical signals as music, lasers amplify light.

The surgical effects of most medical lasers are due to localized heating when the slender beam of light is absorbed by tissue. As tissue begins to heat it first blanches white as it coagulates, shrivels as it dessicates, and finally turns to steam and vapour when it is vaporized by heating above 100°C. This vaporization may be made to occur instantaneously. There are also ways to produce small 'shock waves' and sparks with lasers that see applications in ophthalmology and urology.

We can further discuss these principles of physics and biophysics from a physician's point of view. As physicians, it is unneccessary to learn the detailed electronics and physics of lasers on a technical level. However, to derive the maximum benefit of these technologies for patients, and to develop 'finesse' in surgical laser use, it is useful to

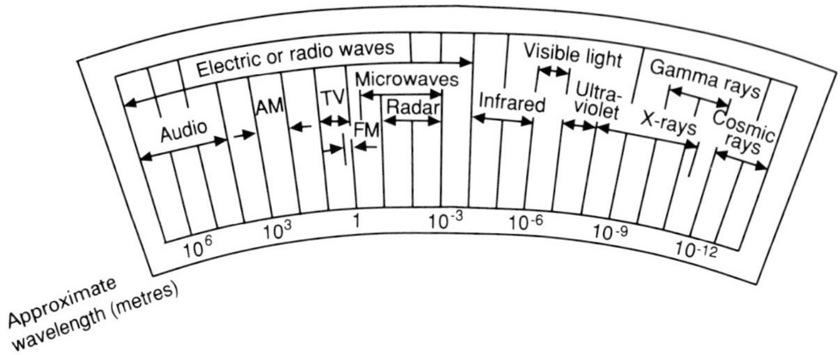

Figure 1.1 The electromagnetic spectrum, showing the wide range of wavelengths from the very short cosmic rays to the very long radio waves.

acquire a conceptual perspective of laser physics and understand the physical parameters of laser application that govern surgical control (Absten, 1985).

1.2 Laser

Laser is an acronym which stands for Light Amplification by the Stimulated Emission of Radiation. The theory of stimulated emission was first proposed by Albert Einstein in the early 1900s to explain how photovoltaic cells are able to generate electricity from sunlight (Einstein, 1917). In the 1950s Arthur Schawlow and Charles Townes coauthored a paper, for which they later received the Nobel prize, which basically explained how this process could be used to generate and amplify visible light (Schawlow and Townes, 1958). This work was simultaneously achieved by Nikolai Basov and Aleksandr Prokhorov in the Soviet Union. Theodore Maiman produced the first working laser in 1960 and coined the term 'Laser' (Maiman, 1960).

Visible light is only one small portion of the electromagnetic spectrum (Figure 1.1) which spans a very large wavelength range from the long waves of radio to the very short waves of X-ray and beyond. Lasers can theoretically produce light at any point on this spectrum, though the common lasers in use today are infra-red, visible or ultraviolet. Masers, amplifying microwaves, existed in the 1950s. Before Maiman coined the term 'Laser' they were called optical masers.

1.3 Light waves

The nature of light is somewhat dichotomous. It displays characteristics of discrete particles (photons) seen as the straight beam of sunlight

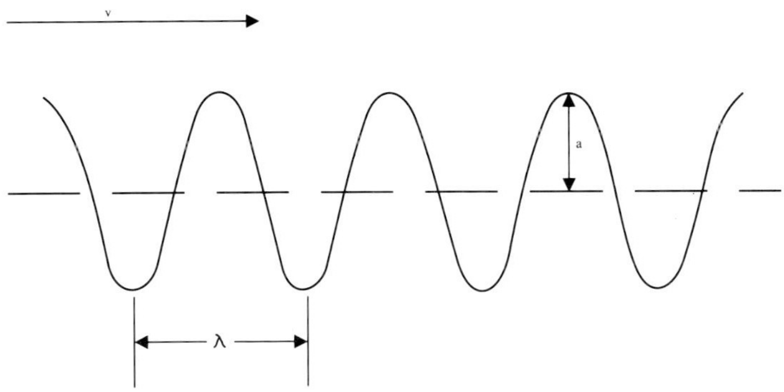

Figure 1.2 The basic properties of a wave. The diagram shows a wave of velocity v, wavelength λ and amplitude a.

projecting through a break in the clouds, or sometimes wave characteristics like differing colours of light. The ancient Greek philosophers speculated about the physical nature of light and vision but, lacking the experimental method, made little progress in understanding light. The first substantial contribution to the understanding of the visual process was made by Alhazen in the 11th century. He deduced that light coming from various portions of an illuminated object forms a visual image in the eye. The 17th century saw the development of wave and particle theories of light. René Descartes and Pierre Fermat were both proponents of a corpuscular (particle) theory of light, though they differed on specifics. Christian Huygens, whose Treatise on Light was published in 1690, considered light a wave disturbance rather than a stream of particles.

We will look at light primarily in terms of its wave characteristics to discuss lasers. Four quantities characterize any wave: (1) wavelength, (2) amplitude, (3) frequency and (4) velocity. In our discussion these characteristics of the wave nature of light can be likened to waves of water in the ocean (Figure 1.2). An understanding of these concepts allows us to see the difference between laser light and regular light.

1.3.1 WAVELENGTH

The wavelength is the distance between two successive crests of the wave. The colour of light is determined by its wavelength measured in nanometers (nm). One nanometer is equal to one one-billionth (10^{-9}) of a metre. We perceive only visible light which spans the narrow range from about 385 to 760 nm. More energy is required to produce shorter wavelengths (ultraviolet) than the longer wavelengths (infra-red). It is important for the physician to know the specific wavelength laser with which he or she is working because laser safety eyeglasses are labelled according to the wavelengths for which they offer protection.

1.3.2 AMPLITUDE

Amplitude is power, or brightness. It is the height of a wave and, like the ocean wave, determines the power in the wave.

1.3.3 VELOCITY

A unique characteristic of a light wave is that its velocity is constant in all frames of reference, equal to approximately 186 000 miles/s or 300 000 km/s in a vacuum. Nothing is known to travel faster than the speed of light. Because this speed is constant, any change in frequency is also a change in wavelength (colour). This principle is employed in certain frequency doubling crystals such as KTP (potassium titanyl phosphate) which, for instance, changes the 1064 nm infra-red output of a Nd-YAG laser to the 532 nm green light of the KTP.

1.3.4 FREQUENCY

Frequency is expressed in cycles per second, or hertz (Hz), and is the number of waves passing a given point per second. Because velocity is constant, the shorter the wavelength the higher the frequency, since more waves will be able to pass a given point in a certain time. This is a critical concept for communications technologies since the amount of information a wave may carry (i.e. number of phone calls carried by one signal) is proportional to the frequency of the wave. This gives rise to technologies such as telephone communications via fibreoptically delivered laser light.

The relationship of one wave to another is also important and is described by phase and coherence.

1.3.5 PHASE

Waves of the same length (colour) are in phase when their troughs or peaks align. The peak of each wave begins at the same 'time'. When waves phase in this manner a reinforced wave results which is increased in amplitude (brightness). Waves have an additive effect when in phase. Conversely, if troughs and peaks of the two waves do not

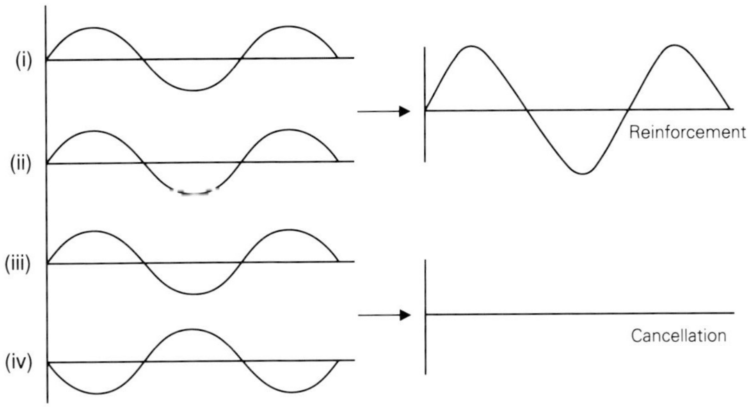

Figure 1.3 Phase. Waves (i) and (ii) are 'in phase' since all the troughs and all the peaks are opposite each other. The result is a reinforced wave of double the amplitude. Waves (iii) and (iv) and 'out of phase' since the troughs are opposite the peaks. The result is a complete cancellation.

coincide, then the wave 'disappears' by flattening out. Waves cancel each other when out of phase (Figure 1.3).

1.3.6 COHERENT LIGHT

When the waves of light are in phase, and travelling in the same direction (path through space), the light is said to be coherent in both time and space (temporal and spatial coherence). Coherent light simply consists of waves of light that have perfectly superimposed upon one another. Lasers are sources of coherent light.

1.4 Light emission

Light results from either an accelerating electric charge or a nuclear fusion or fission reaction. With the exception of sunlight and starlight, however, light usually is the result of changes in the electronic structure of atoms and molecules as they absorb and emit energy.

In an atom, electrons are found to occupy certain discrete energy levels or orbits. Each atom is characterized by a unique set of energy levels in which it may exist. When the energy of an atom is changed, the electrons must move up or down to the next orbital level. This determines the transition energy (TE) involved.

According to quantum mechanics, the atom interacts (absorbs or emits) light of a frequency n (frequency is related to wavelength and colour), this frequency being determined by the equation $n = TE/h$, where h is Planck's constant, equal to 6.62×10^{-34} Joule-seconds. In effect, this makes atoms and molecules electronic 'instruments' that may be tuned to 'play' certain colours of light on demand.

Three kinds of interaction are possible: absorption, stimulated emission and spontaneous emission. An atom in the lower state can absorb light and be excited to the upper state; an atom in the upper state can fall spontaneously to the lower state, emitting light in the process; or the atom can be stimulated by the presence of light to jump down to the lower state and emit additional light while doing so. Spontaneous emission is unaffected by the presence of light. This process occurs at random, emitting multiple colours of light travelling in all directions and out of phase (Figure 1.4).

In stimulated emission the additional light that is emitted will have the same frequency and directional characteristics as the light that stimulates it. This is the crucial feature on which the properties of the laser are based, and, for the laser to work effectively, stimulated emission must predominate over both absorption and spontaneous emission.

The probabilities of occurrence of stimulated emission and absorption are both proportional to the light intensity; stimulated emission, however, can happen only to upper-state atoms, whereas absorption can happen only to lower-state atoms. For stimulated emission to dominate absorption, therefore, more atoms must be in the upper state than in the lower state. This unusual situation is called population inversion and can be achieved by supplying energy ('pumping' the laser) and carefully selecting the active medium.

Stimulated emission may then occur when a photon from an initial spontaneous decay stimulates each excited atom in its path to emit an identical photon, in phase, of the same colour and travelling in the same direction. These photons actually fuse together in time and space producing a coherent output. A photon cascade of growing energy sweeps through the medium (Figure 1.5) and is reflected back and forth many times by the mirrors at each end of the laser resonator (Figure 1.6). The mirrors are perfectly aligned to face each other, creating a type of 'infinity' tunnel in which the trapped light waves ricochet back and forth at the speed of light, increasing the brightness of the beam with each pass. The output mirror is partially reflective (like a two-way mirror) which allows some of this light to 'leak out'. This emits the beam of laser light.

Once the beam is emitted it is delivered to the surgical field. The various attachments and delivery systems determine the utility of any laser. Fibres or articulated arms deliver the beam and lenses or probes focus or intensify the energy.

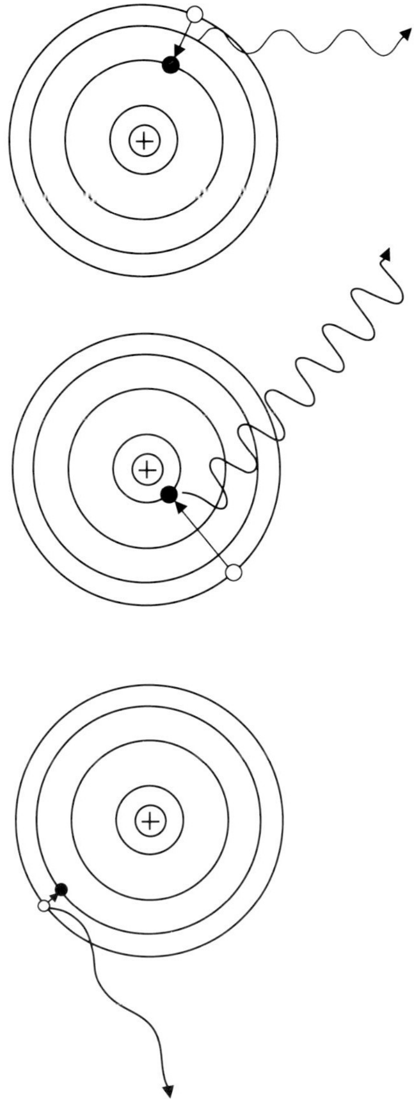

Figure 1.4 Spontaneous emission. The diagrams show energized electrons in three atoms decaying back to their original orbits with the spontaneous production of a photon of light. The wavelength and amplitude of the emitted light varies according to the magnitude of the energy change, and is distributed in random directions. The overall light output is incoherent.

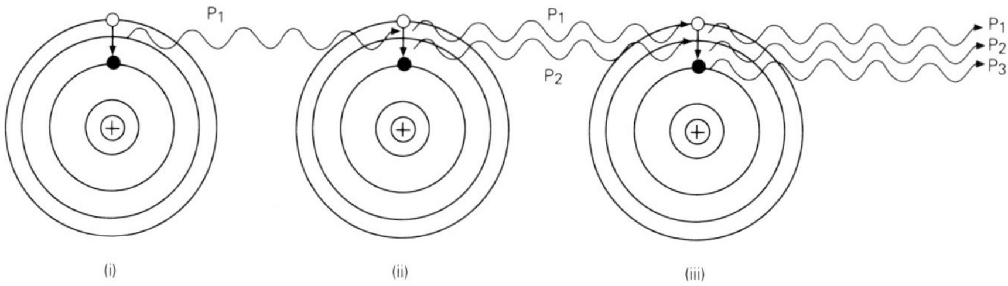

Figure 1.5 Stimulated emission. The diagrams show energized electrons in three atoms in a substance which has undergone a population inversion, so that many of the atoms are in an excited state. The first atom (i) undergoes a spontaneous decay and emits a photon, P_1. This interacts with a second energized atom (ii), and stimulates the emission of a second photon, P_2, with precisely the same wave characteristics, and in perfect phase with P_1. Each of these identical photons can then further stimulate energized atoms to produce additional identical photons, as P_3, etc.

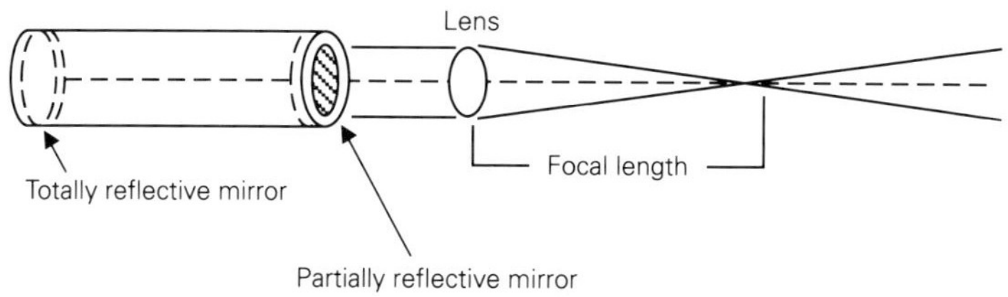

Figure 1.6 Schematic diagram of laser chamber. The growing cascade of light produced by the stimulated emission is reflected back and forth between the mirrors at either end of the laser chamber until the beam leaves the chamber through the partially reflective mirror. It can then be focused by a lens, and pass into a suitable delivery system.

1.5 Special properties of laser light

Laser light differs from ordinary light in much the same way that music differs from noise. Three particular properties are responsible for this difference: coherence, collimation and monochromaticity.

1.5.1 COHERENCE

Ordinary light, from a lamp or fire, is 'incoherent', and consists of light waves radiating (shining) in all directions out of phase with one another. Since multiple wavelengths (colours) are produced, it is not even possible to phase the waves. When a handful of stones is thrown into a pool of water, the choppy wave pattern this creates on the

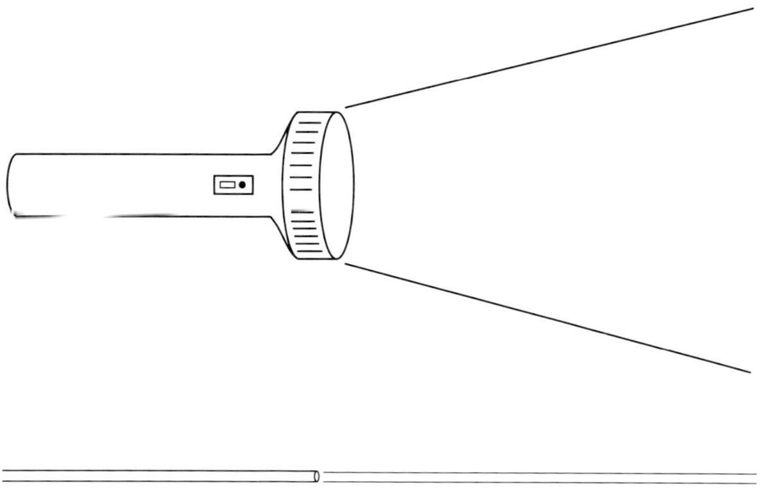

Figure 1.7 Collimation. The light from a flash light (torch) is not collimated and will spread out along the lenght of the beam. In contrast, the light from a laser is highly collimated, and has an insignificant spread along the length of the beam.

surface is 'incoherent' because the ripples produced by each individual stone are out of phase with one another.

Laser light is 'coherent'. It is also of one wavelength (colour) which allows the waves to 'synchronize' when they are phased together. When a piano tuner strikes his tuning fork, he phases the piano string to the tuning fork. The surf breaking onto the beach is also a phased wave pattern. When the peaks and troughs align, they are in phase.

1.5.2 COLLIMATION

A collimated beam is parallel and does not diverge, in contrast to the light from, say, a flashlight (torch) which will spread out as it travels further and further away (Figure 1.7). Laser light is practically parallel, so that a laser pulse fired at the moon produces a spot a half a mile wide, at a distance of 240 000 miles. For practical everyday purposes this spread is insignificant. This means two things for us in medicine: (1) that there is a minimum loss of power along the beam, and (2) that it can be focused to intensify its effect or couple it into a slender single fibre. A laser beam can be a billion times brighter than sunlight.

1.5.3 MONOCHROMATICITY

Monochromaticity indicates that the light is all of the same wavelength (colour). Ordinary light sources produce light from a 'hot body'

Table 1.1 Characteristic wavelengths of light from some lasers in current or developing medical use

Laser	*Colour*	*Wavelength (nm)*
CO_2	Infrared	10 600
Erbium-YAG	Infrared	2 940
Holmium-YAG	Infrared	2 060
Nd-YAG	Infrared (tissue fusion)	1 300
Nd-YAG	Infrared (primary Nd-YAG in medicine)	1 064
Ruby	Red	694
Dye laser	(Variable with dyes)	
	Red	632
	Yellow	577
	Green	504
Krypton	Red	647
	Yellow	568
	Green	531
Helium–neon	Red	632
Gold vapour	Red	632
Copper vapour	Yellow	578
KTP	Green	532
Argon	Blue	488
	Green	515
Excimers	Ultraviolet	
Argon fluoride		193
Krypton fluoride		248
Xenon chloride		308
Xenon fluoride		351
Free electron laser		Variable

process. Like the glowing filament in a lamp, the light usually consists of a mixture of all possible colours in a broad range. This results in white light. All the light of the laser is concentrated in a few discrete wavelengths (frequently one) (Table 1.1). Lasers produce pure colours of light. Different materials emit characteristic colours.

One area of medicine that is evolving, photodynamic therapy (PDT), utilizes the pure colour output and brightness of the laser to chemically activate certain drugs in target cells. At present this work is focused on cancer therapy and treatment of atherosclerosis, but its potential applications are very broad. The laser light is not hot and it is not used as a surgical instrument. The light is bright and causes a photochemical reaction to occur within the specific target cell. Other cells are unharmed by the bright laser light.

1.6 The laser medium

A laser is usually named after its active medium (Table 1.1), the substance which exhibits the lasing action. This can be a liquid, solid, or a gas. Substances which have found the widest applications in medicine at the moment are those based on CO_2, argon, Nd–YAG, krypton and various dyes. All of these substances need to be energized into a state of population inversion. Solid and liquid lasers tend to be energized optically, usually by flash lamps or another laser, and gas lasers tend to be energized electrically by direct current, or radiofrequency (RF).

1.6.1 WHAT ARE SEALED TUBE LASERS? CO_2

When the CO_2 gas mixture is energized and stimulated to emit its light, there is a disassociation of the molecule into carbon monoxide and a free oxygen radical, unlike argon or neodymium atoms which do not break apart (Figure 1.8). The resulting molecule is no longer able to produce light. Complicating this is the fact that the electrodes in the laser tube give off contaminants which further degrades the gas mixture. In medicine, three basic configurations of CO_2 lasers have resulted.

(a) *Flowing gas systems*

Because of the disassociation of the molecule, and electrode contamination, a flowing gas system is used to purge the tube and replenish the gas. This requires cylinders of replacement gas, pressure regulators, and a vacuum pump to draw the gas through the system. All of this adds to the maintenance, noise, and expense of operating the laser. On the other hand, flowing gas systems produce a reliable, steady output, and easily generate high powers (for medicine) of 50–100 W. They also produce stable, low-power outputs of around 1 W.

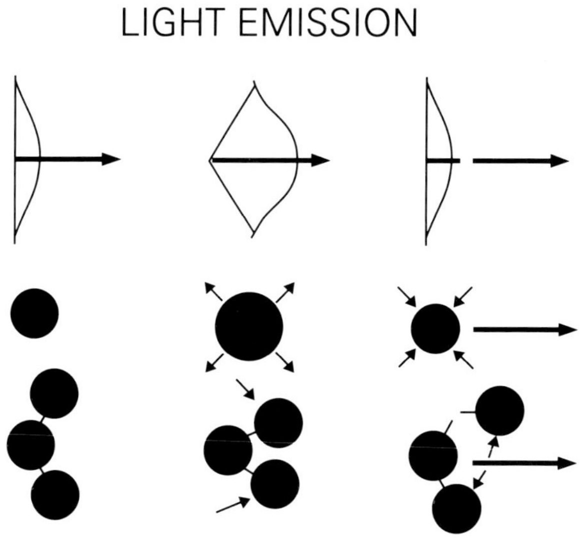

Figure 1.8 Disassociation of the CO_2 molecule.

(b) Free space, sealed tube lasers

These are a newer generation laser tube that eliminates the need for replacement laser gas mixture, regulators and vacuum pumps. They can produce power levels comparable to flowing gas systems up to about 100 W.

This sealed tube laser uses direct current (DC) excitation as do the flowing gas systems. The electrodes are specially treated, and catalysts and inhibitors are added to the self-contained gas mixture to retard breakdown of the gas. This allows for a sealed tube type of laser system. After several years the tubes will need to be recharged as the power begins to gradually fall from the high end.

(c) Radio-frequency waveguides

These are also sealed tube systems but instead of using DC applied through electrodes to energize the gas they utilize a radio-frequency that is transmitted transversely across the tube to excite the gas molecules, which eliminates the electrode problems. The ceramic tube of the laser is also impregnated with catalysts and inhibitors to retard breakdown of the gas. The radio-frequency is contained within a 'waveguide' structure of the laser (not to be confused with a waveguide delivery system for the CO_2 laser that we shall discuss later). There is no interference with monitors or electrical equipment. Radio-frequency waveguide lasers have typically produced lower power of

25 W and under, though newer technology systems are producing outputs of up to 120 W.

Sealed tube systems of both varieties are generally simpler to operate, quieter, and require less routine maintenance than flowing gas systems.

Both flowing gas and sealed tube systems each have their own advantages.

1.7 Energy concepts

Power is simply a measure of the rate of energy delivery in Joules/second, and is expressed in watts.

Of greater importance is the amount of power which can be focused into a spot. This power density, or irradiance (sometimes called spot brightness), of a laser is the number of W/cm^2 of a spot, and is the single most important factor in the effective application of a laser. The surface area of the spot (spot size, controlled by the surgeon in the field), and the total power in watts (set at the laser by the operator) determine the power density as

$$\frac{\text{watts} \times 100}{\text{Pi} \times r^2} = \text{watts/cm}^2$$

Power density determines the rate of tissue removal and eye–hand co-ordination on the part of the surgeon. A common misconception is that the laser power determines the co-ordination required.

Power density over a spot determines the rate of tissue removal within that spot. One can effectively change the size of the 'paintbrush' (spot size) with which one is working without changing the overall rate of tissue removal (power density) within that spot by varying the spot sizes and power. The larger the spot, the greater the power required to maintain the same power density, shown as

	0.6 mm spot	2.0 mm spot
1900 W/cm^2:	10 W	60 W

The total energy within the beam is expressed in joules. Power multiplied by delivery time equals the number of joules. Ten watts delivered for 3 s is 30 J of energy. Joules describes the total energy delivered but does not by itself indicate how concentrated this dose of light is. Most of the medical Nd-YAG lasers in use will have a 'delivered joules' readout, though other laser types usually do not. This number, in absolute terms, is not important in determining how much laser energy to apply since it is the visual result that determines the treatment. Pulsed applications however, such as for ophthalmology and for laser lithotripsy, use a millijoules 'dosage' as a treatment parameter.

Fluence combines the concepts of power density (spot brightness) and dosage (joules), and is expressed in J/cm^2. Though the specific numbers are usually unimportant in most applications, it is critical to understand this concept. Since lasers are used to cause tissue heating, it is very important to keep this heat localized to only the intended target.

Fluence describes how the 'dosage' of light is delivered. As an illustration, 100 J of energy may be delivered as either a 'bolus' of light at 100 W for 1 s, or as a 'drip' of light at 1 W for 100 s. Utilizing higher powers (rate of energy delivery) for shorter times will always result in more thermal precision and less damage to adjacent tissue. This may be unimportant in applications such as Nd-YAG laser ablation of the endometrium for menorrhagia, but is very important for CO_2 laser work on the cervix or vulva.

This critical concept is easily understood intuitively. Suppose one has an electric hotplate and wants to determine whether or not the surface is hot. If one licks (ones) finger to make it moist and 'taps' the surface quickly it will not be burned if the surface is hot. However, if one leaves (ones) finger in contact with the surface for a few seconds a third degree burn may result. The temperature of the hotplate did not change, only the time of application which allowed for a conduction heat burn. The longer the laser is left in place, even at low power, the more extensive is the thermal conduction to adjacent tissues. It is very important to visualize this spread of heat during any laser procedure.

The benefit of utilizing high fluence rates is most pronounced with the CO_2 laser. When vaporizing or ablating tissue (not cutting) the best results are always obtained at the maximum power setting of that particular laser (assuming the spot size may be varied such as with a handpiece or on a colposcope). The tendency to avoid maximum power use for ablation with a CO_2 laser stems again from the misconception that high power is uncontrollable. Surgical control is maintained by two methods.

1. Broadening the spot sufficiently to maintain a controllable power density, i.e. adjusting the size of the 'paintbrush'. The correct spot size for any given power of a focused CO_2 laser beam may be seen by the shape of the crater formed by test firing. Use of maximum power through laparoscopes does not work since the spot size is fixed.
2. Pulsing the laser in short bursts of around 0.1 s, in combination

with use of the correct spot size. This makes even 100 W lasers perfectly controllable and results in a cleaner ablation. This pulsed technique is much slower than using the laser in the continuous mode and, as one's experience allows, continuous mode will decrease the procedure time. A repeat pulse mode is more convenient than pumping the foot pedal for each pulse.

1.8 Pulsing concepts and nonlinear effects

Most medical lasers offer a choice of operating modes to include continuous and pulsed modes. Many CO_2 lasers additionally offer a superpulse mode. It is important to remember that these terms, such as 'pulsing' are used loosely and often do not fit the correct technical definition. A brief summary of these modes and relative time scales will help present a clearer picture of how lasers may be manipulated to achieve different effects (Table 1.2).

Continuous wave (CW) refers to a steady-state power output from the laser. Most medical laser systems work in this CW mode, even when set to a 'pulse' of around 0.1 s. This term also sometimes refers to a mode in which the laser beam is emitted the entire time the foot pedal is depressed. Technically the latter is incorrect since a series of true pulses may also be emitted in this manner, but it is a common expression for laser operation and should be noted.

Table 1.2 Relative time scales as they relate to pulsing of laser energy

Term	*Time*	*Fraction*	*Exponent*
Second	1.0	Full second	
continuous wave (CW) operation			
Millisecond	0.001	Thousandths	10^{-3}
(gated pulse – still primarily in a CW mode, just timed)			
Microsecond	0.000001	Millionths	10^{-6}
(pulsed, frequently causing induced shock wave effects such as for laser lithotripsy)			
Nanosecond	0.000000001	Billionths	10^{-9}
Picosecond	0.000000000001	Trillionths	10^{-12}
(both are pulsed, such as Q-switched or mode-locked, to cause direct shock wave effects primarily used by ophthalmologists as a 'cold cutting' laser)			
Femtosecond			
Attosecond			

Gated pulse is most commonly referred to as simply 'pulse'. This is merely a timer for a CW beam and is seen most often on CO_2 lasers. True laser pulses, which are different, may also be emitted in this timed fashion. The differentiating characteristic on a gated pulse is that the peak power output of the 'pulses' are no higher than they would be if the laser were emitted in a continuous fashion.

Most of the CO_2 lasers offer an option for a repeat pulse. This is simply the gated pulse that continues to be emitted at short intervals as long as the foot pedal is depressed. This is a very useful feature on CO_2 lasers and models that allow for varying the speed of the repeat rate are the best.

A true laser pulse is able to compress the power output of the laser tube and deliver very high peak powers of energy during the pulse but cannot maintain these high powers in a steady state. A 504 nm dye laser may be pulsed in microseconds to deliver 40 kW of peak power to fragment kidney stones in laser lithotripsy. Even though the peak power is very high, it is not sustained and the total delivered energy will only amount to 10–60 mJ.

Q-switching and mode-locking are terms used to describe pulsing techniques that produce peak powers on the order of tens of millions of watts, for pulse durations of only a few nanoseconds. Total delivered energy is again very low, 3–10 mJ, because of the short pulse width. This is commonly employed in the ophthalmic Nd-YAG lasers to achieve the 'cold cutting' sonic effect.

Superpulse is found on many CO_2 lasers and is called various names by manufacturers, such as superpulse, varipulse, megapulse, etc. This is a true pulse on CO_2 lasers, usually producing a train of pulses from 250 to 500 W maximum per pulse at a rate of 300–1000 times per second (Hz). This rate is so fast that it looks continuous but the pulsing may be picked up as an audible 'buzz' as the focused beam hits its target. Again, the total delivered energy is not as high as the 500 W pulses might imply. On CO_2 lasers this will be read out as the 'average power' of the beam rather than joules of energy, and the maximum average power in superpulse will always be substantially lower than the maximum power available in continuous mode. Superpulse allows for cleaner cutting of tissues with less resulting charring.

1.9 Biophysics and tissue interaction

The effects created by surgical lasers – cutting, vaporizing and coagulation – are all caused by heating of the tissue. Table 1.3 describes the effects on soft tissue as temperatures increase, from laser or any other source of heat. The wavelength (colour) of the laser is important only

Table 1.3 Laser effects on tissue by absorptive heating

Temperature (°C)	*Visual change*	*Biological change*
100	Smoke plume	Vaporization, carbonization
90–100	Puckering	Desiccation
65–90	White/grey	Protein denaturization
60–65	Blanching	Coagulation
37–60	None	Warming, welding

in determining how efficiently this heat transfer occurs, and over what volume of tissue.

Several parameters control the delivery of laser energy to tissue. These include the power (watts), total energy delivered (watts and time), power density (how small the focused spot used to intensify the light), the colour of the light and the colour and vascularity of tissue.

In some ways these concepts are intuitive. An analogy is the use of a magnifying glass to focus sunlight and create a burn. The brighter the sun (power), the more it burns. The smaller the spot created with the lens (power density), the 'hotter' it burns. The longer the sun is focused in one place (total energy), the more extensively it burns. The wetter the target you are trying to burn (vascularity), the longer it takes to create the same effect. The surgeon has control over a combination of three parameters – power, time and spot size – to create the desired effect.

The nature of interaction of all laser light with biological tissue can be described in terms of reflection, transmission, scattering or absorption (Figure 1.9).

In order for light to heat tissue it must be absorbed. If it is reflected from, or transmitted through tissue no effect will occur. If the light is scattered, it will be absorbed over a larger volume so that its effects will be more diffuse.

Figure 1.10 compares the relative effects of CO_2, argon (or KTP) and Nd-YAG lasers, and shows the relative spread of thermal damage from just the raw beams and ignores other important factors such as delivery systems, power densities, powers and pulse times.

As indicated, the CO_2 laser is the most highly absorbed, only 30–90 microns in water, and causes the most intense heating effects – cutting and vaporization. It will coagulate tissue, but only superficially.

The Nd-YAG laser scatters its light over a broad volume of tissue, causing coagulation as deep as 4–6 mm if desired. This can be controlled to very minimal depths by lowering total power and pulse time. At higher power densities it will vaporize, but leaves the underlying

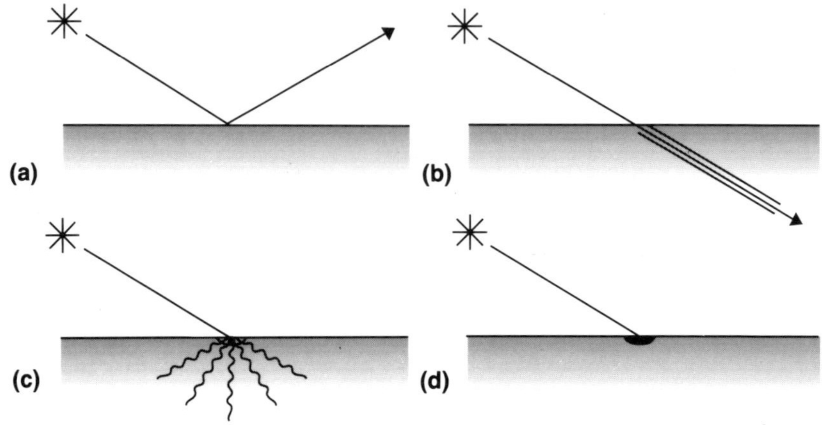

Figure 1.9 (a) Reflection. A laser beam is reflected from the surface of a tissue, and has no effect. (b) Transmission. A laser beam is transmitted through a tissue, and has no, or only very minimal, effect. (c) Scattering. A laser beam is scattered by a tissue, and absorbed over a large area. Its effects are diffuse and weakened. (d) Absorption. A laser beam is absorbed by a small volume of tissue, and exerts its effects within this volume.

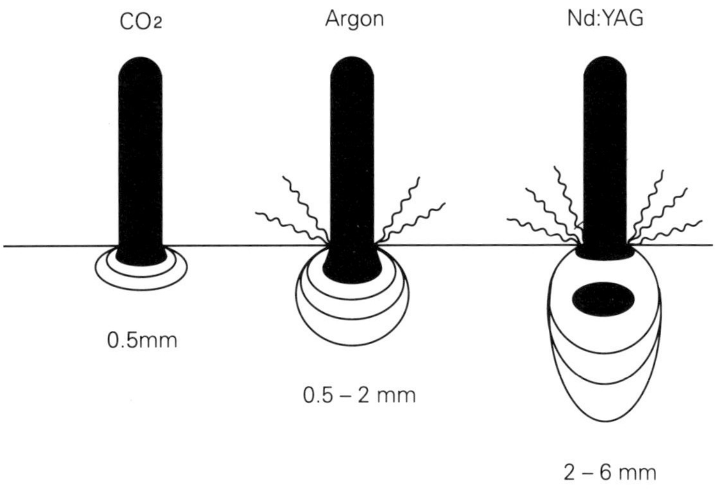

Figure 1.10 Tissue absorption with the CO_2, argon and Nd-YAG lasers. (From Absten, G. T., *Fundamentals of Laser Surgery*. © 1985.)

deep coagulation beneath the base of the crater. Sapphire probes can completely change these characteristics since the laser fibre heats the probe to very high temperatures and causes hot cutting, vaporization or coagulation of tissue with the hot sapphire probes themselves.

The argon (488 and 515 nm) and the KTP (532 nm) lasers produce very similar, if not identical, tissue effects from a clinical perspective. They are generally considered as superficial coagulators, cooking 0.5–2.0 mm deep. At smaller spots and higher power densities they can also be used for very fine cutting, although they proceed very slowly because of their relatively low powers of around 15 W. There are some differences in absorption peaks of argon and KTP, as well as the high-frequency pulsing of the KTP, but for a general understanding of tissue effects they are considered equivalent. These fibreoptic lasers may cut nicely by placing the fibre tip in tissue and dragging it tangentially to make the haemostatic cut. Even though high-power densities at the tip create much of the cutting effect, much also results from the high tip temperatures of the slender quartz fibre. Fibres will eventually burn with this technique, but they are easily recleaved for continued use.

Vaporization of tissue (cutting or ablation) occurs when cellular fluid is heated to its boiling point. The rapid rise in intracellular temperature and pressure causes an explosion of the cell, throwing off steam and cellular debris (Figure 1.11).

Soft tissue vaporizes at 100°C. If the remnant carbon is allowed to build, and lasing is attempted through this carbon, the lasing point will begin to incandesce to an orange glow as tissue heats to over 1500°C. This would cause extensive thermal damage resulting in a branding iron type burn and concomitant scarring. It is usually created by lasing at too low power densities for excessive lengths of time.

There are three classic physics mistakes to avoid when using the CO_2 laser. The first is the use of more power (actually power density) than the surgeon's experience allows control over. This results in penetrating tissue or cutting too deeply. One avoids this by starting at low powers and working up as experience dictates, provided that no charring is allowed to occur. The second mistake is exactly the opposite – spending excessive time on tissue because of very low powers. When used in delicate areas this creates significant spread of heat damage and destruction of adjacent tissue. It is avoided by using higher powers and pulsing on short pulses. The short pulses avoid excessive damage from the power, and allow for cooling of tissue in between pulses. The third mistake involves relasing over char created by the laser. This increases the surface temperatures from just over 100°C for the first pass, to over 1500°C when lasing through the char. On skin this would cause significant heat spread and scarring. It is avoided by using power

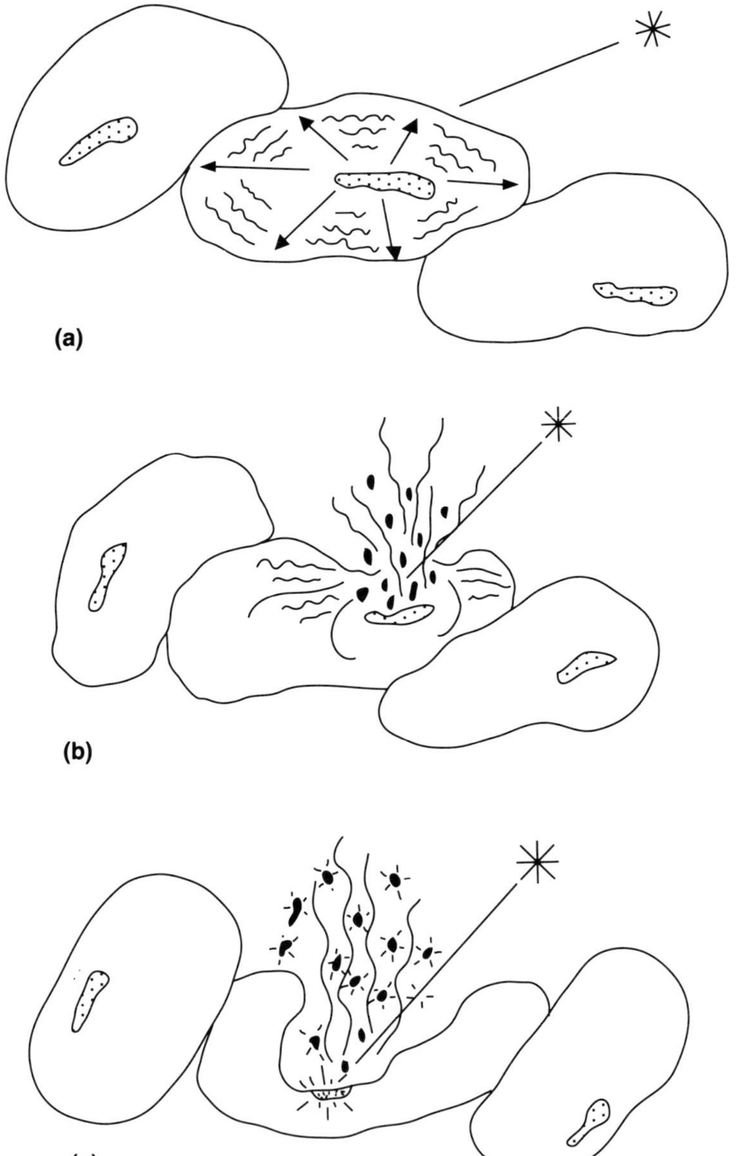

Figure 1.11 Tissue vaporization. (a) A cell has absorbed laser light and is heated to boiling point. The cell is destroyed. (b) The cell explodes, throwing off steam and cellular debris. (c) The steam and debris rise from the site of impact and are carbonized in the laser beam.

densities sufficient enough to preclude buildup of char. One may also wipe away any accumulated char with a moist sponge before lasing the same area. Lasing through char does offer excellent haemostasis because of the heat spread and in some situations it may be warranted when debulking a vascular tumour, or cutting a vascular organ. However, heat damage to adjacent tissue may be substantial.

Cutting is simply vaporizing tissue along a line, using very small spot sizes of 0.1–0.5 mm. Defocusing the beam slightly, using higher power to maintain power density, and cutting with this broader beam, results in less precision but better haemostasis for vascular areas. This is primarily done with the CO_2 laser, though the argon and KTP lasers cut nicely with the tip of the fibre and the Nd-YAG laser is used with sapphire probes.

Coagulation of tissue with laser has a broader meaning than simply achieving haemostasis. The laser has the ability to destroy cells by denaturing the protein without necessarily vaporizing it. This would be like heating egg white and seeing it turn white as it coagulates. Deep coagulation may sometimes be desirable, as when treating bladder tumours. The Nd-YAG laser has the deepest coagulating abilities, followed by the argon. Haemostasis, or cautery, is achieved by sealing the ends of the capillaries or vessels with the laser heat secondary to cutting or vaporizing. The greater the blood flow through a vessel, the more it acts as a heat sink, and the greater the difficulty in achieving haemostasis. Applying pressure to slow the blood flow helps to achieve better haemostasis when possible.

Haemostasis achieved with a laser may be similar to spray coagulation achieved with electrosurgery, with the laser being more controllable and predictable, and able to work in a non-contact mode. However, laser does not eliminate the need for electrosurgery and in many cases the advantages of laser over electrosurgical coagulation have been vastly overstated. Electrosurgery may take many different forms, from delicate coagulation with bipolar forceps, fine cutting with a micro-needle, to the charring and burning in the spray coagulation mode. Laser cannot perform tissue excavation or snaring as can electrosurgery. These modalities complement one another.

Since bone and cartilage contain relatively little water, they vaporize differently from soft tissue. Bone has a tendency to heat as does carbon, and conducts heat into the adjacent soft tissue. To protect these tissues and limit the thermal damage, a superpulse mode is preferred on the CO_2 lasers. As previously discussed, this appears as a continuous beam, but is actually cycling on and off from 250 to 1000 times per second with high peak powers (250–500 W) on each spike. This allows a 'cooler' cutting of the bone or cartilage. Most CO_2 lasers offer some variety of superpulse. Though this modality is useful, commercial claims of the usefulness of varying different superpulse parameters are exaggerated. Bone may also need to be continuously irrigated to prevent flaming. It must be said that cutting of bone with a CO_2 laser is not entirely satisfactory. The mid-infrared lasers at around 2900 nm produce a superb bone cut more precisely than a bone saw and with no lateral heat damage. These devices are investigational in medicine at present.

1.10 Conclusions

Because most laser procedures utilize the heating effect of the laser, and given the number of parameters that may be varied, such as power density, power, pulsing and heating of fibre tips and probes, significant overlap in applications of the various lasers can result. This is readily apparent in the conflicting claims of laser manufacturers as seen in promotional material. In spite of this, each type has its strengths.

The CO_2 laser is a specialty instrument, particularly for microscopic applications in neurosurgery, otolaryngology and gynaecology. Its haemostasis and vaporizing abilities allow its use in dermatology, and general surgery for tumour resection and haemostasis. In gynaecology it seems best for colposcopy (cervix and vagina), and through a micromanipulator for laparotomy. The beam is focused and delivered by handpieces and micromanipulators on microscopes. Through the laparoscope it requires the use of a special laser coupler on a special laser laparoscope to allow for line of sight delivery of the beam through the operating channel. Recently, waveguide delivery systems have been introduced for CO_2 laser laparoscopy using standard laparoscopes. These function as hollow, slender tubes through which the beam is transmitted via hundreds of glancing internal reflections in the tube which emits the beam at its tip. This eliminates many of the alignment problems of coupler cube type systems and allows the beam to be delivered in close proximity to the target.

The Nd-YAG laser is the primary endoscopic instrument in pulmonary, gastroenterology and urology. The use of contact tips, though not a panacea, will increase its applications, particularly in general surgery. Its primary use in gynaecology is for endometrial ablation with bare fibres for deep coagulation. Its use for laparoscopy with contact probes is quickly growing.

Green light lasers (argon and KTP) are colour-selective photocoagulators. In some configurations they may be used to cut tissue and are fibreoptically delivered. Their best use in gynaecology appears to be for laparoscopic treatment of endometriosis and lysis of adhesions.

References

Absten, G. T. (1985), Laser physics for the non-specialist. In *Lasers in Medicine. An Introductory Guide* (eds G. T. Absten and S. N. Joffe), Chapman & Hall, London, pp. 1–13.

Einstein, A. (1917), Zur quantentheorie der strahlung. *Physio. Z.*, **18**, 121–8.

Gordon, J. P., Townes, C. H. and Zeigler, H. J. (1955), The maser – a new type of amplifier, frequency standard and spectrometer. *Physiol. Rev.*, **99**, 1264–74.

Maiman, T. (1960), Stimulated optical radiation in ruby. *Nature*, **187**, 493.

Schawlow, A. L. and Townes, C. H. (1958), Infrared and optical masers. *Physiol. Rev.*, **112**, 1940.

2 *Gynaecological microsurgery using the CO_2 laser*

JOSEPH FESTE

2.1 Introduction

The CO_2 laser produces a highly directional, collimated beam of light that may be focused to a precise point. Laser microsurgery involves use of the laser as a light scalpel with a spot size ranging from 200 to 2000 μm in diameter. With this small spot size, fine dissection is easily accomplished. The laser beam is also used to vaporize and thus physically remove tissue while small vessels are sealed with little damage to neighbouring cells. A minimum amount of suture material is thus required and scar formation is kept to a minimum as compared with conventional surgery. Although the laser has been utilized in recent years to treat lower genital tract pathology, its application to intra-abdominal surgery is in its formative phases. Special adaptation of the operative microscope with special accessory instruments is necessary for use of the laser within the abdominal cavity. The range of procedures amenable to CO_2 laser treatment includes wedge resection of ovaries, ovarian cystectomy, myomectomy, metroplasty, endometriosis, adhesiolysis, tubal pregnancy, and tubal repair.

Surgeons treating infertile patients arc obligated to restore normal anatomy and thus increase or enhance the chances for a successful pregnancy. As in most surgical procedures, the first attempt is usually the most important. As a microsurgical tool the laser should be used in accordance with the guidelines established for conventional microsurgery (Gomel, 1980). In addition, the following rules of good reproductive surgery should be observed. Atraumatic techniques and special instruments should be utilized with avoidance of gauze sponges (Raj and Hulka, 1982). Haemostasis should be as complete as possible since active bleeding is known to contribute significantly to formation of adhesions. Even minute blood vessels that cease bleeding and the need to be recauterized may provide additional necrotic tissue for adhesion formation (Tulandi, 1987). Complete excision of pathological tissue is important, particularly in salpingitis isthmica nodosum (SIN) and in endometriosis. Precise alignment of tissue planes and reperitonealization should be attempted whenever possible (Kistner, 1975). Magnification should be used as it allows for the use of fine suture material and helps to delineate borders of pathology to facilitate removal (Chong and Baggish, 1984). Pelvic lavage may be achieved with heparinized Ringer's lactate.

The laser, which is essentially a light scalpel, can, if properly used, offer several advantages over conventional surgery. The advantages which have been clearly demonstrated include (1) reduction in operating time, (2) attainment of excellent haemostasis and thus the possible reduction of post-operative formation of adhesions, and (3) the capability, with use of a flat-surfaced rhodium silver mirror, of reaching operative sites that would otherwise be inaccessible. Despite the advantages that the laser offers, it is not a panacea, and is no better than the surgeon using it. When other techniques would provide better results, they should be used instead.

Because the use of the laser in microsurgery is relatively new, its efficacy will not be apparent for several years. As of yet, significantly increased pregnancy rates have not been reported. However, many second-look laparoscopies following laser surgery have shown the remaining adhesions to be filmy and the degree of the adhesion formation to be decreased (Raj and Hulka, 1982; Tulandi, 1987).

2.2 Instrumentation

The major requirements for microsurgery are a laser, a microscope with micromanipulator, or hand-held instrument, titanium rods, atraumatic forceps, a front-surfaced rhodium mirror, and fine 6-0 to 8-0 sutures (Vicry 1 or PDS).

2.2.1 HANDPIECE

Most hand-held pieces used have a focal length of 125 mm with a spot size of 0.20 mm and will deliver a power density of 26 000 W/cm^2. The handpiece, like a scalpel, may be easily manipulated. However, the depth of the insertion into the pelvis is limited not only because of the obstruction of the view of the lower pelvis by the surgeon's hand, but also the instrument itself. The fact that the laser may be focused and defocused rapidly gives it a wide range of power density changes that may be taken advantage of in the mid pelvis. Loupes may be used to aid in more precise surgery. Control is adequate for ablation, incision, or coagulation, but because a change of a few millimetres in the focusing point will cause significant change in the power density, extra caution is required to prevent unnecessary tissue damage. In contrast, with the microscope, spot size change is controlled by a special adaptor on the micromanipulator and requires a separate adjustment.

The temptation to use the mirror in conjuction with the hand-held unit should be avoided because of the steadiness required to keep the mirror and handpiece from moving in different directions and thus the resulting difficulty in controlling the precise point of impact of the laser beam.

A recommended precaution is the use of backstops to prevent the laser from penetrating into unintended areas. Backstops commonly in use include soaked sponges, irrigating solutions, and/or titanium rods. The tissue itself may be used as a backstop during lysis of adhesions. Since the adhesions are excised rather than incised, there will be a lased area on both ends of the attachments of the adhesions. Where there are vessels under 1.2–1.5 mm in diameter, the CO_2 laser generally will control bleeding. However, instead of defocusing to decrease the power density and possibly causing more fibrosis and necrosis, it is preferable to use bipolar microcautery to control the bleeding from larger vessels.

2.2.2 MICROMANIPULATORS (MICROSCOPE)

The microscope equipped with a micromanipulator and variable spot size adaptor provides greater depth of field and better cutting control to achieve sharper and more precise incisions than with the hand-held instrument. It is less easily defocused and thus is less likely to cause increased areas of necrosis because of unintentional decreases in power density. Additionally, the micromanipulators and joysticks provide a variable focus and greater control of the aiming beam and are safer to use than hand-held units.

The main disadvantage of using the microscope is that the entire field is not visible at all times. The resulting difficulty in maintaining orientation requires that the surgeon be familiar with the techniques of conventional microsurgery before attempting to use the laser. Safety precautions are the same as those for use of the hand-held laser.

2.2.3 MIRRORS

Used in conjunction with the microscope, the front-surfaced silver rhodium mirrors are very helpful in dealing with inaccessible areas deep in the pelvis. However, several precautions should be noted. The mirrors will crack very easily if they are not kept free of moisture or debris. In either case, the moisture or debris will overheat the surface of the mirror causing it to crack or be pitted. They will also crack if superpulse laser energy rather than continuous or repeated single pulses are used. Moreover, special care must be taken to prevent other organs, hands, or instruments of the operating surgeon from migrating into the field between the mirror and the point of impact.

2.2.4 TITANIUM RODS

During the process of vaporizing diseased or abnormal tissue, a backstop is required to prevent damage to adjacent normal tissue. In the past, quartz rods have been used. However, because of their limited tolerance of heat and inherently poor tensile strength, they frequently have cracked or have broken during use. To prevent this problem, titanium rods, 3–6 mm in diameter, have been used to absorb the energy of the CO_2 laser. They also offer the advantage that tissue does not readily adhere to them as it will to quartz rods. Both round and flat surface rods are available.

2.3 Laser surgery for endometriosis

Endometriosis is thought to account for approximately 25–30% of women undergoing laparoscopy and up to 15–20% of those undergoing laparotomy because of infertility (Kistner, 1975). With the development of advanced techniques by laparoscopy, most cases of stage 1 or 2 endometriosis and some selected stage 3, can now be treated by laparoscopy as an out-patient.

Endometriosis is a condition particularly amenable to laser surgery because it develops on the surface of the peritoneum. It is possible to vaporize the surface of the lesion, laser into deeper tissues where the endometriosis is embedded and safely penetrate through to normal tissue. Since there is a very thin layer of retroperitoneal fat throughout the pelvic cavity, the water vapour created by vaporization of this thin layer is an indication of complete removal of the lesion. In treatment of the endometriotic implants, the vaporized glandular layer has a brownish appearance while the deeper stromal layer is white and appears curdy. It is important to vaporize a margin of 1–2 mm around each lesion to eradicate any remaining foci of microscopic disease.

Prior to laser surgery for endometriosis, preparation of the patient is important. Patients who have endometriomas of more than 3 cm in diameter should receive a GnRH agonist, (Lupron) or Danocrine (Danazol) to reduce the endometrioma to its minimum size. There are still questions as to whether the endometriomas should be drained of the chocolate material prior to the commencement of medical therapy. This theoretically would allow a shorter time for the endometrioma to regress. Vaporization is thus made easier and it is possible to preserve a greater amount of normal ovarian tissue. The duration of medical treatment depends upon the size and response of the lesion. Treatment for 3 months is adequate to suppress most endometriomas. In those cases where this technique is chosen, it would be recommended that the peritoneal disease be treated first at the time of the diagnostic laparoscopy, for the medical therapy may suppress the disease significantly enough to cause difficulty in recognizing deposits after several months of medical therapy. Yet, 3–6 months after medical therapy, it is very likely that those suppressed implants not sufficiently treated would become active. If Danocrine or Lupron suppression is not needed, surgery is scheduled in the proliferative phase of the patient's cycle to avoid operating around a newly formed corpus luteum.

The laser beam may either be controlled by a hand-held instrument or delivered through the microscope. Magnification, whether with loupes or with the microscope, assures the surgeon complete vaporization of the endometriosis. Probably because the degree of magnification may be increased to outline the margins of each lesion as well as allow the surgeon to see 20–30% more lesions, preference has been shown for use of the microscope.

The treatment for endometriosis varies according to its location.

2.3.1 PERITONEAL ENDOMETRIOSIS

Endometrial implants along the uterosacral ligaments, lateral pelvic wall and bladder peritoneum can be vaporized with continuous or repeat pulse modes. In areas where there are no vital structures, a continuous mode can be used with safety. Power densities between 4000 and 7000 W/cm^2 with a spot size of 0.8–1.2 mm are adequate to debulk these lesions. While moving the joystick rapidly, one can easily vaporize the lesion off the surface of the peritoneum down to normal retroperitoneal fat (Figure 2.1). However, during vaporization over ureters, bladder, and blood vessels, it may become necessary to switch to single or repeat pulse modes, to limit the amount of penetration of the laser beam through the peritoneum. Single or repeat pulse modes vaporize the lesion 100–300 μm at a time. Defects created over 1–2 cm in diameter may be closed with fine sutures of 6-10 Vicryl or PDS. Experience has shown that if two lased or traumatized areas are not in close proximity to each other, adhesion formation is unlikely. Haemostasis is excellent and blood loss is almost non-existent.

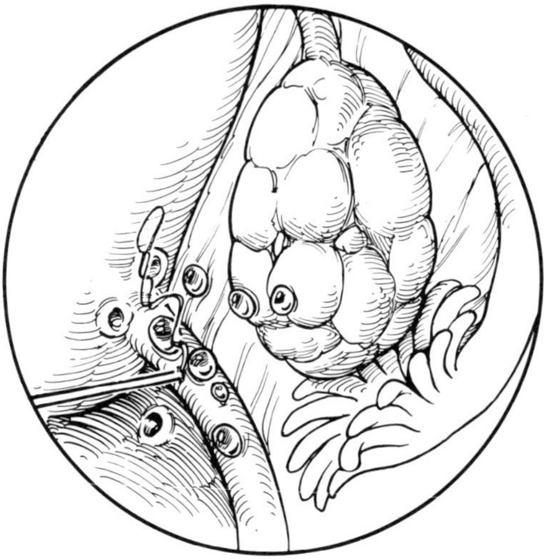

Figure 2.1 Laser vaporization of endometriosis on parietal peritoneum.

2.3.2 TUBAL ENDOMETRIOSIS

When lesions involving the Fallopian tubes are vaporized, it is necessary to use a much smaller spot size, rapid exposure time of 1/20–1/10 of a second, and a power density in the range of 2000–3000 W/cm^2. In this way, penetration through the delicate muscularis of the tube is prevented and more precise control of the laser is provided. Frequent irrigation is important following vaporization to provide a cooling effect and thus to decrease thermal damage to adjacent tissue. Defects in the tube, particularly if they are in close proximity to another lasered area, should be closed with 6-0 or 8-0 interrupted Vicryl or PDS suture.

2.3.3 OVARIAN ENDOMETRIOSIS

Laser vaporization of the ovaries may vary according to the size of the endometrioma and the presence or absence of adhesions. Periovarian adhesions are best vaporized with a single pulse mode, particularly when a front-surfaced rhodium mirror is used to visualize the adhesions. Since many adhesions are inaccessible to direct vision, they may be vaporized by reflecting the beam off the surface of the mirror. Whenever possible, titanium rods are interphased between the adhesion and pelvic wall to prevent any vaporization of normal tissue. After the ovary is brought into position from its attachment, there are three

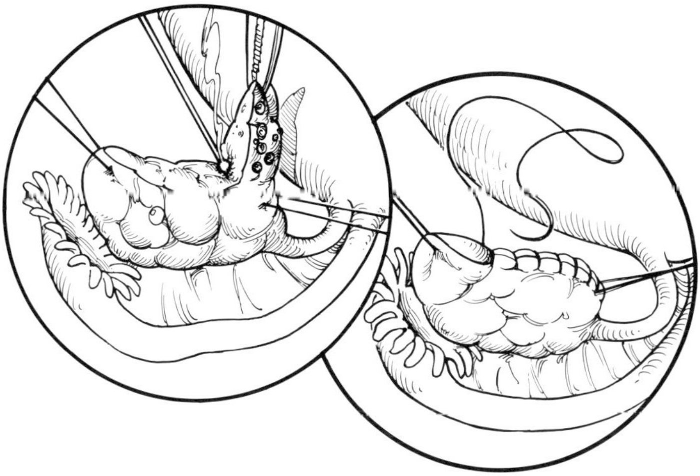

Figure 2.2 Laser excision of an ovarian endometrioma.

techniques used to treat the endometriomas. (1) Endometriomas of less than 3 cm in diameter may be vaporized with the continuous mode with the ovary istself used as its own backstop. (2) Larger endometriomas of more than 3 cm in diameter are opened by excising an elliptical portion of the ovarian cortex with a continuous pulse mode of 3000–4000 W/cm^2. The chocolate material is drained from the endometrioma, and the cyst lining is thoroughly irrigated. With a defocused beam of 1.5–2 mm and a power setting of 20–30 W, the entire lining of the endometrioma is vaporized down to normal ovarian tissue. Unless the glandular and stromal components are completely removed, recurrence of the endometrioma is possible. (3) Another option for these larger endometriomas is to enter the capsule of the ovary and enucleate the entire cyst wall. In all of these techniques, the deep layer of the defect is closed with interrupted suture of 3-0 Vicryl, and the capsule carefully approximated with 6-0 PDS suture (Figure 2.2). All of these procedures will preserve most of the ovarian cortex and will result in minimal loss of ovarian function and tissue.

2.3.4 ENDOMETRIOSIS ON THE COLON

Small endometriomas involving the serosa and muscularis of the colon may be vaporized with repeat or single pulse modes using a defocused beam of 0.8–2.0 mm in diameter to limit the degree of penetration of the laser. Use of 1/20–1/10 of a second exposure times or a 5–7 W average power superpulse allows removal of endometriomas at the rate of 100–200 μm down through the lesion to the normal muscularis or mucosa. All patients with colonic disease should have a bowel preparation in case of inadvertent entry into the colon or the unforeseen presence of extensive lesions. Following complete vaporization of the lesion, the muscularis and serosal surfaces may be approximated loosely with interrupted suture of a 2 to 3-0 non-absorbable suture. Treatment of small lesions in this way may eliminate the need for wedge or segmental resection of the colon or rectum. However, in cases of large endometriomas, involving the mucosa or lying circumferentially around the rectum, wedge or segmental resection is mandatory. In these cases, it is important that haemostasis be achieved following resection and that all peritoneal defects be closed without tension along the suture closure line.

2.3.5 ADJUNCTIVE THERAPY

In all patients treated for endometriosis, heparinized Ringer's lactate (5000 U/litre) is used as an irrigating solution, and an optional 100 ml of 32% Dextran-70 (Hyskon) is instilled into the pelvic cavity prior to closure of the abdomen. The rationale to use pre-operative vs post-operative medical therapy has yet to be resolved. All the patients reported in this chapter had 6–8 weeks of pre-operative medical therapy followed by an additional 3–6 months depending upon the amount of disease present at the time of major surgery. It appears more efficacious for a longer post-operative than pre-operative medical therapy so as not to mask the lesions at laparotomy with the medical therapy.

2.3.6 FOLLOW-UP AND RESULTS

Over the past 5 years, few publications have reported pregnancy rates following major laser surgery. Chong and Baggish (1984) reported a pregnancy rate of 50% in patients with stage 1 to stage 3 endometriosis. The duration of follow-up had been less than 1 year in 45 infertile women treated for endometriosis. Friedlander (1975) reported that reduction of pelvic pain and visible amelioration of endometriosis may be expected in 40% of patients treated with Danocrine. Dmowski and Cohen (1975) and Greenblatt and Tzingounis (1979) reported a 50% response rate. Regression of disease following conservative surgery has been reported in 30–94% of patients following conservative surgery using a combination of sharp dissection and needle cautery. Buttram (1979), correlating success of surgical treatment with severity of disease, reported an 84% pregnancy rate for mild stages of endometriosis and 75 and 56%, respectively, with moderate or severe endometriosis.

Since December 1981, the author has treated 147 patients for stages 2, 3 and 4 endometriosis by laparotomy (Feste, Whitworth and Guerani, submitted). The stage 2 cases were treated by laparotomy until 1985. After this time most of these cases were treated by laparoscopy. Table 2.1 reveals the pregnancy rates calculated by all available methods. The most significant method for comparison is by the life table analysis at 24 months and the monthly fecundity rates. Those patients with endometriosis alone had cumulative pregnancy rates of 75, 67 and 74% for stages 2, 3 and 4, respectively. The increased results in stage 4 may be accounted for by the liberal use of the second-look laparoscopy in these patients. The fecundity rates at 6 months were 0.087, 0.068 and 0.049 for those patients with endometriosis only. If all patients in the series are considered, the pregnancy rates are decreased in almost all categories. The life table analyses for all three stages are illustrated in Figure 2.3.

In summary, the CO_2 laser offers some strategic advantages over conventional operative methods for conservative management of endometriosis. Good haemostasis and surgical precision are two major benefits. The ability of the laser beam to reach into recessed or otherwise poorly visible areas such as an ovarian endometrioma densely adherent to the pelvic side wall represents a significant technological advance. The follow-up period is as yet too brief to allow meaningful comparisons between results of laser treatment and of treatment by conventional methods. Second-look laparoscopy should be performed in most, if not all, patients with stage 4 endometriosis to assess the results of conservative surgery as well as to provide the opportunity to treat any residual adhesions.

2.4 Adhesiolysis

Over the last several years, little clinical information has been gathered concerning the results of CO_2 laser in the treatment of post-operative or post-infective pelvic adhesions. Initial studies in animals have shown no significant difference in adhesion formation when results of laser surgery were compared with those of conventional electrosurgery (Pittaway, Maxson and Daniell, 1983; Filmar, Gomel and McComb, 1986). Many papers have described the ideal techniques for vaporizing pelvic adhesions (Kelly and Roberts, 1983; Diamond *et al.*, 1984), but the efficacy of laser surgery in preventing formation of new adhesions post-operatively and the pregnancy rates achieved subsequent to surgery are being presently evaluated. Potentially, evaluation of results may be complicated by variations in the skill of surgeons, in the techniques used, in the degree of tubal damage and/or in the interpretation

Table 2.1 Laparotomy results (147 patients)

Crude	*Corrected by factors (%)*	*Corrected 24 mo f.u. endo only (%)*	*Corrected 24 mo f.u. all patients (%)*	*Life table analysis* 24 mo	60 mo	*Fecundity at 6 mo*
				* *endo only (%)* ○ *all patients (%)*		* *endo only* ○ *all patients*
Stage 2 (56) 62%	36	83	76	* 75 ○ 66	* 88 ○ 79	* 0.0873 ○ 0.073
Stage 3 (53) 58%	58	78	73	* 67 ○ 54	* 90 ○ 74	* 0.068 ○ 0.044
Stage 4 (38) 47%	47	29	72	* 74 ○ 65	* 74 ○ 65	* 0.049 ○ 0.049

f.u., follow up; endo, endometriosis.

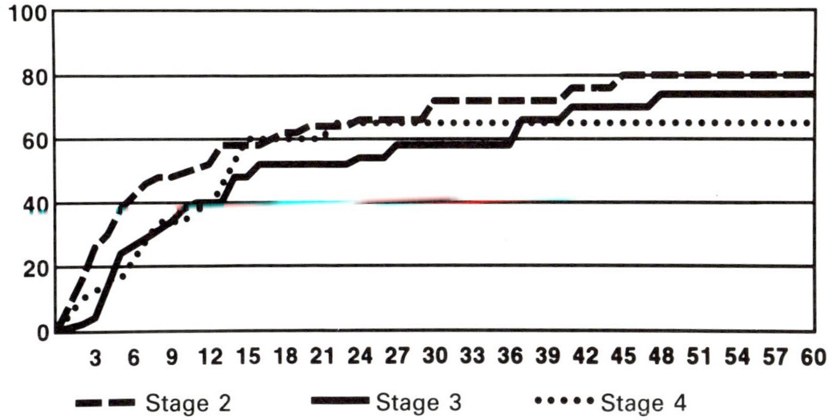

Figure 2.3 Life table analysis: all patients with stage 2, 3 and 4 endometriosis following laparotomy. Total patients = 147.

of findings. In one of the few studies published, Kelly and Roberts (1983) reported five (24%) pregnancies in 21 patients. The majority of the pregnancies occurred in those with stage 1a and 2a adhesions. After 1 year, there was a pregnancy rate of 46.2% with 32.6% of these carrying to term.

An article by Diamond *et al.* (1984) showed no significant difference between post-operative formation of adhesions in patients who had laser surgery and those who were treated with micro-electrosurgery. The 106 patients evaluated showed no significant decrease in adhesions except in areas over the colon and the cul-de-sac. There appeared to be increased tubal patency at the time of second-look laparoscopy in patients who had laser neosalpingostomies. However, the number of adhesions at second-look laparoscopy was shown to be similar to the number in the group treated with micro-electrocautery.

In another series, Bellina (1983) reported 26 patients treated for adhesions with laser surgery and followed for two or more years. Ten of 26 patients (38.5%) conceived. Several other authors have reported that pregnancy rates did not differ significantly between those patients treated with laser and those treated with electrosurgical techniques (Tulandi, 1986, 1987; Barbot *et al.*, 1987).

Laser surgery, however, offers several advantages over standard micro-electrocautery for the treatment of post-operative adhesions.

1. The laser may be reflected through front-surfaced silver rhodium mirrors to vaporize adhesions between the ovaries and tubes that

are not accessible under direct vision and thus are also inaccessible with the microelectrode needle.

2. Adhesions developed after laser surgery have been shown to be finer and much easier to treat at second-look laparoscopy. This suggests that the amount of thermal damage to surrounding tissues is less with laser than with the microelectrode needle.
3. If the laser is used in conjunction with the microscope, very precise control of surgical dissection is possible.
4. Since the laser beam is focused from a distance, it does not occupy additional space and thereby allows for an unobstructed view of the surgical field.
5. There may be a shorter time from surgery to conception with the use of the CO_2 laser (Bellina, 1983).

2.5 Clinical techniques

When dense adhesions between the ovary and tube are vaporized, the development of a plane between these two structures may be carefully performed with the CO_2 laser. With single pulse, repeat pulse or low-power superpulse modes, small segments of adhesions can be vaporized slowly and directly. This separates the two structures with little change of anatomy. The amount of thermal damage at the higher power densities (more that 4000–5000 W/cm^2) will give as little as 100 μm irreversible thermal effect to the tube or ovarian surface. Higher magnifications will allow performance of this procedure with precise control, thus the tube and ovary can be virtually dissected with minimal thermal effect on either structure. If vessels are more than 1.2–1.5 mm in diameter they must be sealed with microbipolar cautery.

In cases of adhesions between the ovary or tube and lateral pelvic wall, a tube holder is used to grasp the tube or ovary and put tension between these structures. Adhesions may be vaporized using a front-surfaced rhodium mirror to reflect the beam (Figure 2.4). Single pulse modes or repeat pulse modes, and occasional continuous pulse modes, should be used for this technique. Problems encountered include difficulty in learning to move the mirror in the correct direction while looking through the microscope. This may create difficulty in controlling the point of laser beam impact. Because the ovary or tube usually is densely adhered to the pelvic wall, it is feasible only occasionally to insert a titanium rod behind an adhesion. In these instances, mirror vaporization of adhesions themselves will free the ovary or tube and leave an area of thermal effect of not more than 100 μm in depth. Once the ovary and tube are freed of their adhesions, the pelvic cavity may

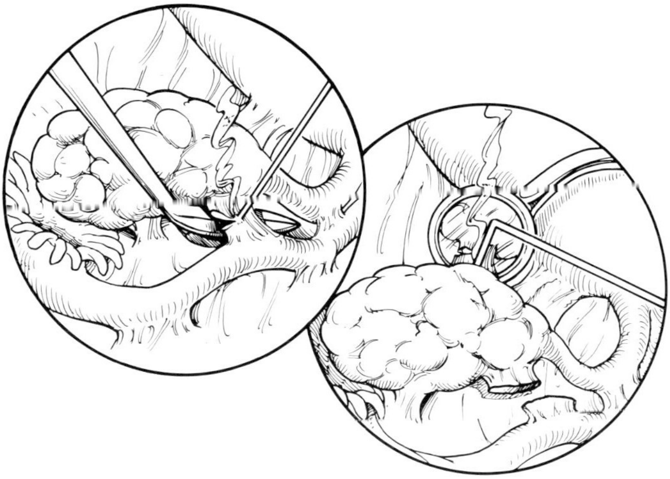

Figure 2.4 Laser vaporization of adhesions with a titanium rod as a backstop and with a front-surfaced rhodium mirror to reflect the laser beam.

be packed with a lint-free Kerlex pack, and the adhesions 'picked' off the ovary and tube with higher magnification and single pulse modes. This technique of adhesion removal is preferred over the 'painting' of the entire ovarian surface with a defocused beam.

Adhesions overlying the bladder, ureter, rectum or even large vessels are best removed by vaporization with single pulse, repeat pulse or superpulse modes. This prevents penetration of the laser beam to more than 100–200 μm and makes it possible for the attachment of the adhesions to be vaporized rather than incised.

Many techniques are used to prevent recurrence after vaporization of adhesions. Hyskon, heparinized Ringer's lactate, and biodegradable peritoneal grafts have been used. An important element in irrigation with heparinized Ringer's lactate is removal of the greatest amount possible of carbon and of fibrin, which is a contributor to post-operative adhesions. It is best not to remove the carbon with a cotton pledget because some microscopic bleeding may result and thus defeat the purpose of using the laser as a sealing light scalpel. Proper haemostasis and proper irrigation are the two of the most important factors in successful laser vaporization of post-operative or post-infective adhesions.

Confirmation of the hypothesized advantages of laser over the microelectrode needle will require further studies that include superpulse. It is important to note that many cases of pelvic adhesive disease treated by laser surgery have been severe. Many of the cases chosen might otherwise have been neglected or treated by hysterectomy in the past. Therefore, it is important in comparing results to stage adhesions in the manner described by Raj and Hulka (1982) or the Classification of Adhesions as set forth by the American Fertility Society (1988) to evaluate effects of surgery by second-look laparoscopy.

2.6 Laser surgery of the Fallopian tube

Although endometriosis accounts for 25–30% of infertility, tubal disease is equally responsible. Tubal disease is most commonly associated with infection, particularly with gonorrhoea and chlamydia as causative agents. Tubal surgery is also frequently performed for reversal of sterilization requested because of separation, divorce, or death of an infant. Whether the tubal procedure is performed by laser or conventional technique, careful pre-operative evaluation of the patient is extremely important.

2.6.1 ISTHMIC AND AMPULLARY DISEASE

Over the past 6 years, a significant amount of experience has been accumulated in use of the CO_2 laser in tubal reanastomosis. Animal studies have shown no difference in adhesion rates, patency rates or pregnancy rates when comparing results of the CO_2 laser with those of conventional electrosurgical techniques (Badaway, El Bakay and Baggish, 1987). Numerous reports have suggested that the laser incision of the tube in preparation for anastomosis requires significantly less time and achieves greater haemostasis than standard techniques of microsurgery. However, other studies have shown neither decrease in operating time nor a measurable reduced amount of blood loss. Within the realm of presently available technology (10 000–200 000 W/cm^2 and the TEM_{00} mode with a 0.2 mm spot size), the results of anastomosis are comparable to those achieved by other microsurgical techniques.

Apparently the preparation of the tubes for reanastomosis may be performed equally well by either laser or microelectrode. Advocates of the use of the unipolar microelectrode state that in the hands of experienced surgeons it decreases operating time. The transection can be precise with tissue surrounding the tubal lumen showing neither combustion nor charred debris. For these surgeons, handling the microelectrode is easier and probably safer than using the laser. However, advocates of the use of the laser consider it equally safe and expedient.

The process of preparation of the tube (using the laser technique) consists of three steps: (1) the serosal layer is vaporized with a power density over 10 000 W/cm^2 with a very small spot size, range 0.2–0.5 mm; (2) the muscular layer is then incised to the mucosa with a power density of 20 000 W/cm^2 with a repeat pulse mode of 0.05 a second exposure time; (3) the mucosa is divided with a knife or iris scissors. In some instances, it has been reported that the tube may be prepared by laser incision through its full thickness and the mucosa can be freshened with a pair of scissors or a sharp knife. This may eliminate the problem of post-operative fibrosis. Pregnancy rates with this technique have been as good as those with the microelectrode, and in the hands of a competent surgeon, the operating time has been reduced significantly. Kelly and Roberts (1983) reported use of the CO_2 laser in treatment of 20 patients with tubal anastomosis. Twelve of these patients were post-tubal ligation and after anastomosis, a pregnancy rate of 71.4% was reported. Baggish and Chong (1981) reported that from 52 cases, there were 17 pregnancies of which five were terminated as abortions or ectopic pregnancies. Twenty-nine of the 52 showed tubal patency in post-operative hysterosalpingography. This series included both unipolar and bipolar as well as diseased tubes with no differentiation made between the diseased tubes and the unipolar or bipolar post-tubal ligation anastomosis.

2.6.2 INTERSTITIAL OR CORNUAL OBSTRUCTION

The most significant utilization of the laser for an anastomosis is for a cornual or interstitial anastomosis. A technique borrowed from lower genital tract surgery provides haemostasis as an adjunct to laser surgery. A 1:20 vasopressor solution injected via a 1 ml tuberculin syringe through a 27-gauge needle produces considerable vasoconstriction. This technique takes advantage of the laser's excellent haemostatic properties and leaves mucosal architecture normal at 500 μm from the laser impact zone. The vasoconstriction causes larger vessels (>1 mm) that would otherwise be severed to go into spasm. The transversing laser beam may then seal these larger vessels. As the cornu is opened, small oozing vessels may be sealed by focusing the beam. Use of the laser precludes the need for clamping vessels and applying ligature and/or cautery coagulation. The laser may be used to outline the tube at the serosal area and incise down through the interstitial portion of the tube if necessary to within 2 mm of the endometrial cavity. This haemostatic technique provides a 'lip' on which to place sutures making the anastomosis less difficult (Figure 2.5).

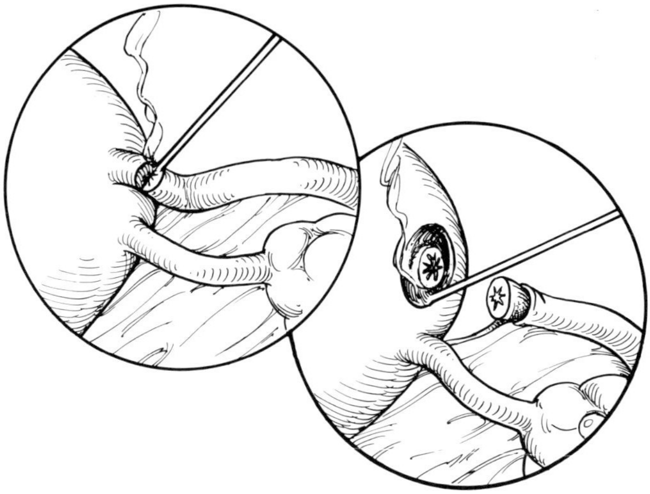

Figure 2.5 Vaporization around interstitial portion of the Fallopian tube in preparation for an interstitial anastomosis.

2.6.3 TUBAL RECONSTRUCTION: DISTAL OCCLUSION OF THE FALLOPIAN TUBE

Distal tubal reconstruction may be achieved by two different procedures: fimbrioplasty and neosalpingostomy. Fimbrioplasty includes those procedures in which the tubal fimbria are agglutinated or adhered but not completely closed, i.e. clubbed. This pathology usually results from post-operative adhesions, endometriosis, and sometimes from mild tubal infections. In contrast to the techniques used for saccular hydrosalpinges which result from gonoccocal endosalpingitis or other overt infections of the tube, the techniques used to treat these cases are basically comparable to those used with the microelectrode. In the last 3 years, reports of patency rates have been few but the pregnancy rates have been as good with the CO_2 laser. Initial studies in animals showed no significant differences between the use of the conventional (Baggish and Chong, 1981) micro-electrosurgical technique and microlaser techniques. Bruhat and Magee (1983) reported salpingostomies in 30 patients treated with electro-microsurgery and 28 patients treated with CO_2 laser surgery. He reported a term pregnancy rate of 16.6% in the electrosurgical group and 23.7% in the laser microsurgical group. Similar results were reported by several investigators (Fayez, McComb and Harper, 1983; Tulandi *et al.*, 1984; Tulandi and Vilos, 1985; Daniell *et al.*, 1986). Tulandi *et al.* (1984) reported that 23 patients treated with CO_2 lasers for hydrosalpinx showed a

21.7% pregnancy rate as compared to 22.7% with conventional microdiathermy. In my series of 24 patients followed for a period of 24 months, 16 had a post-operative second-look laparoscopy or hysterosalpingogram with 27 tubes evaluated for patency. There were two closed tubes and 25 open tubes resulting in a patency rate of 93%. This is similar to those reported with the micro-electrocautery techniques. The term pregnancy rate in this patient group was 23%.

The technique of fimbrioplasty by laser surgery consists of use of magnification with single pulse or repeat pulse modes to vaporize the adhesions between the fimbriae. It is best to use a titanium rod inside the ostium of the fimbria as a backstop and to transilluminate the hydrosalpinx whenever possible. Transillumination with the fibreoptic bundle provides a clear view of the adhesions between the mucosal folds. With a small spot size of 0.2 and 0.5 mm, the adhesions may be vaporized to create normal fimbrial architecture.

Laser neosalpingostomy with a completely distended hydrosalpinx is accomplished by injecting the tube with indigo carmine dye to distend its distal portion. The point of 'puckering' is then noted. The locations of the incisions for the laser are outlined with single or repeat pulse modes so as not to penetrate into the lumen of the hydrosalpinx until the markings are completed. In this way, when the hydrosalpinx is entered and the fluid within is released, boundaries for creating the four flaps may be easily identified. When the hydrosalpinx is entered, a 3 mm titanium rod is placed into the lumen. With continuous or superpulse mode at a high-power density (20 000 W/cm^2), four flaps are created by incising through the serosa, muscularis, and mucosa for a distance of approximately 1.5 cm. Any bleeding encountered is treated with bipolar microcautery.

Following the development of the four flaps, the technique as described by Bruhat and Mage (1983) (or flowering technique) is performed with a power density in the range of 200–300 W/cm^2. Moving this defocused 2 mm beam rapidly across the peritoneal surface will coagulate serosal tissue and retract the edges of the peritoneum folding the tube towards the proximal ampulla (Figure 2.6). Fine suture of 7 or 8–0 Vicryl usually is preferred to stabilize the edges and to prevent retraction at a later date.

In the case of a much thicker hydrosalpinx, these flaps are more difficult to create and the flowering technique is nearly impossible. Yet the pregnancy rate usually is higher with this type of tube because there is less damage to the tubal mucosa. The size of the hydrosalpinx, presence or absence of mucosal folds or adhesions, and the thickness of the tubal wall are important factors to evaluate in determining the success of the repair. These criteria have been published by the

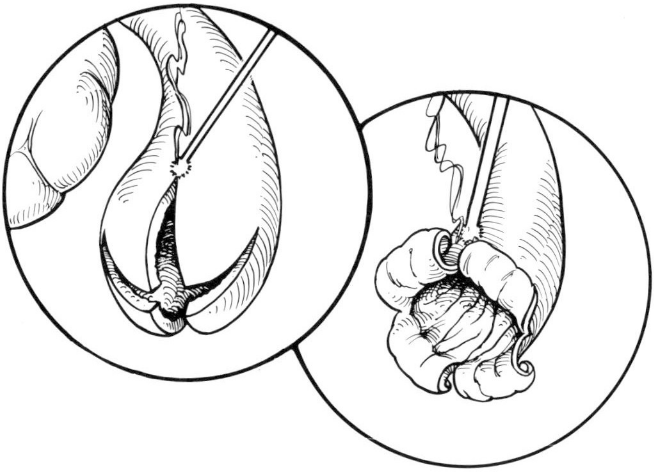

Figure 2.6 Incision of a hydrosalpinx with the CO_2 laser and 'Bruhat manoeuvre' to evert the edges.

American Fertility Society (1988) for proper classification of distal tubal disease. Kelly and Roberts (1983) reported a pregnancy rate of 11% in 28 patients with neosalpingostomies followed for a period of 1 year. The pregnancy rates reported by others have ranged from 13.8 to 29% (Kelly and Roberts, 1983; Tulandi *et al.*, 1984). Follow-up of at least 3–5 years will be required for comparison of pregnancy rates following neosalpingostomy with laser and pregnancy rates achieved with standard microsurgical techniques. Assuming that the mucosa is the limiting factor, use of the laser might be expected to improve the outcome significantly over standard microsurgery by leading to a higher tubal patency rate and fewer post-operative adhesions.

2.6.4 TUBAL IMPLANTATION

Tubal implantation is rarely performed because the preferred technique, interstitial isthmic anastomosis, is associated with a better prognosis for pregnancy. However, it may be indicated when there is no remaining interstitial tube. If this procedure is undertaken, the following steps can be followed. After injection of a dilute solution of Pitressin (1:20) into myometrium, a defocused beam at the controllable high-power density can be used to quickly and rapidly drill a hole into the endometrial cavity (Figure 2.7). To prevent damage to the opposite side of the intrauterine cavity, it is important that dye distend the cavity while laser vaporization is being performed. The size of the opening can easily be adjusted according to the size of the tube to be

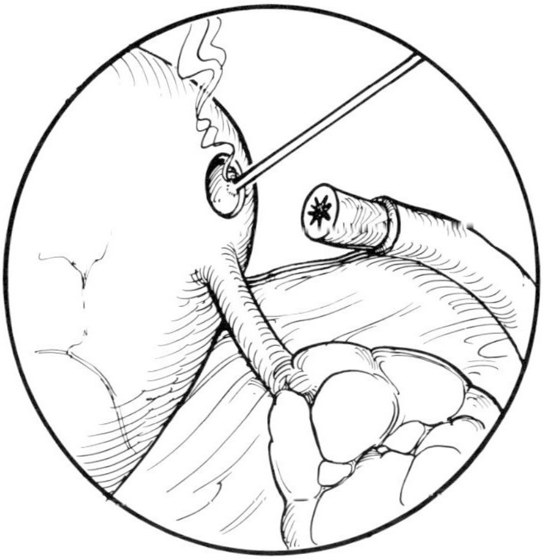

Figure 2.7 Preparation of the uterus with the CO_2 laser for tubal implantation.

implanted. The only disadvantage in this technique is that when a blood vessel larger than 1.5 mm is encountered with the laser, there will be an obvious welling up of blood which will absorb the laser energy and prevent adequate penetration. In most instances, however, this can be prevented by the use of Pitressin as a vasoconstrictor.

Following the preparation of the orifice, the isthmic portion of the tube is prepared by either bivalving the distal isthmic portion of the tube or by splitting the antimesenteric border as described by Gomel (1980).

2.6.5 CORNUAL POLYPS

Cornual polyps have been reported as the cause of infertility for several years. The first reports were those by Phillip and Huber (1939). The incidence of polyps as diagnosed by hysterosalpingogram varies from 1.2 to 2.77%. Among the findings with hysterosalpingography have been intraluminal cornual densities within the cornua of the Fallopian tube (Strangel, Chervenak and Mouradian-Davidian, 1981). Polyps of various sizes have been described but most commonly are approximately 5 mm in diameter. They can appear unilaterally as well as bilaterally. The success of treatment with medication has been extremely limited in the past (David, Ben-Zwi and Langer, 1981). In most instances surgeons have elected to correct the problem with excision of the polyps and a uterotubal implantation. However, experience with implantations suggests a poor prognosis.

The first to report microsurgical tubal implantation after excision of cornual polyps were Boeck *et al.* (1978). They reported no pregnancies in their series. Others have suggested microsurgical linear salpingostomies to preserve the integrity and physiology of the uterotubal junction as well as to maximize tubal length. McLaughlin (1984) reported a successful outcome following removal of bilateral cornual polyps by microsurgical linear salpingostomy with the aid of the CO_2 laser. This technique appears to be the most efficacious for dealing with such tubal disease.

The usual technique includes injection of dilute Pitressin (1:20) into the cornua as well as into the base of the polyps. With a small spot size of 0.2 mm and power density of approximately 15 000 W/cm^2, a linear incision is made into the cornua. The polyps are excised at their bases with single repeat pulse modes. The tubal muscularis is reapproximated with 8-0 Vicryl or PDS suture and the serosa with suture material.

Significant benefits of linear salpingostomy are that a waiting period is not required before pregnancy is attempted and if pregnancy is achieved, a Caesarean section is not mandatory. Therefore until new techniques are developed, salpingostomy as performed by McLaughlin (1984) appears to be the most effective means of dealing with this unusual problem.

2.6.6 SALPINGOSTOMY FOR ECTOPIC PREGNANCY

With the early use of ultrasound and quantitative beta-HCGs, early, unruptured, ectopic pregnancies may now be diagnosed. If possible, the oviduct may be saved. Laparoscopic linear salpingostomy or salpingectomy is preferable to laparotomy. Laparotomy is necessary, however, if the ectopic pregnancy is too large for a laparoscopic procedure to be performed safely or if bleeding is a problem. A laser linear salpingostomy can usually be performed as a bloodless procedure. A small 27-gauge needle is used to inject the serosa and mesosalpinx of the tube with dilute Pitressin (1:20). The larger vessels are constricted and the cushion of fluid absorbs the heat of the laser beam and protects the surrounding oviductal tissue. The operative microscope with micromanipulator is used to direct the beam with power densities ranging from 10 000 to 20 000 W/cm^2 using a continuous mode. The products of conception can then be easily teased out through this small defect (Figure 2.8). Generally, the edges of the incision are adequately sealed because of the coagulating properties of the laser. Should bleeding occur, a microbipolar coagulator may be applied. Generally, it is not necessary to close the salpingostomy incision and it may be allowed to heal by secondary intention. Cropp, Cowell and Rock (1987) reported one case of

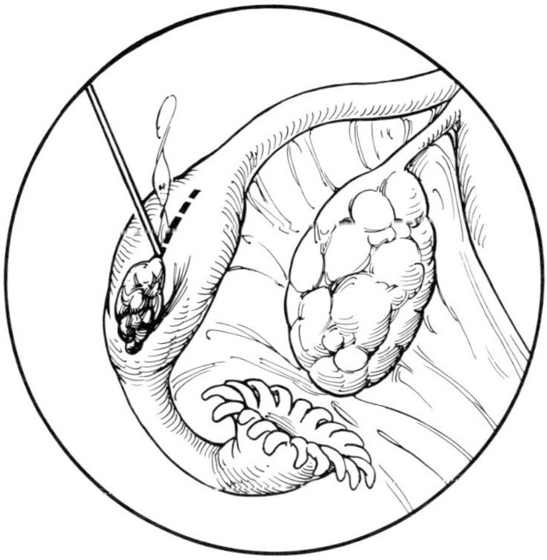

Figure 2.8 Salpingostomy for ectopic pregnancy with the CO_2 laser.

failure of tubal closure following laser salpingostomy for an ampullatory tubal ectopic pregnancy.

Baggish and Chong (1983) reported six cases treated by this technique, and patency of the surgically treated tube was demonstrated post-operatively in all patients. Voros *et al.* (1984) also cited six ectopic pregnancies managed conservatively with the CO_2 laser. Within 6 months after surgery, 33% of the patients had conceived with intra-uterine pregnancies.

2.6.7 WEDGE RESECTION OF THE OVARIES

In those cases where an ovarian wedge resection is desired, the CO_2 laser provides an excellent method because of its ability to give good haemostasis and precise cutting. With a 0.2 mm spot size using the hand-held unit or a 0.5 mm spot size with the micromanipulator, a wedge of ovary can be removed effectively by using a high-power density over 15 000 – 20 000 W/cm^2. This high-power density is necessary due to the presence of fluid in follicles that would abort the energy rapidly at lower levels and prevent efficient cutting. When vessels of more than 1.5 mm in diameter are noted, a microbipolar cautery should be used to coagulate the vessel prior to being cut. Vessels over this size can usually be incised with the laser without experiencing uncontrollable bleeding. With the exception of less post-operative oozing, this technique does not appear to have any significant advantage over a microneedle electrocautery.

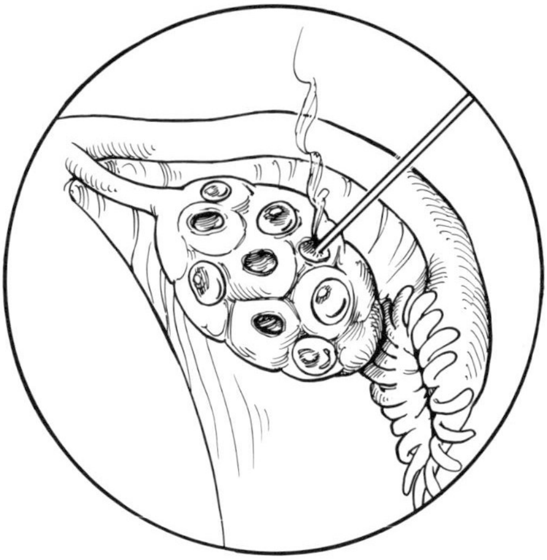

Figure 2.9 Drilling polycystic ovaries with the CO_2 laser.

2.7 Ovarian cystectomies

The technique of ovarian cystectomy with the CO_2 laser requires extreme caution in order to prevent penetration through the capsule of the cyst. The ovarian capsule must first be entered with a single pulse mode to prevent entering the cyst. A flat titanium rod inserted between the cyst and the capsule of the ovary will act as a backstop, preventing penetration of the laser beam through the cyst wall. When excising large endometriomas, a larger spot size and high-power density can prevent unnecessary blood loss as the endometrioma is shelled out. On few occasions, the base or vascular attachment of the endometrioma must be clamped and tied with absorbable suture to maintain better haemostasis. Following removal of the endometrioma, the deep layer is approximated with 3-0 PDS or Vicryl and then the cortex with continuous running sutures of 6-0 PDS.

2.8 Laser treatment of polycystic ovarian disease

Polycystic ovaries have been treated in the past by wedge resection. However, the significant occurrence of post-operative adhesions has made this technique less desirable. In the last few years, there have been reports of treating these ovaries laparoscopically with a cautery or drilling multiple holes in the ovarian stroma for those patients not responding to Clomiphene therapy and who will not or cannot undergo gonatrophin stimulation (Figure 2.9) (Gjonnaess, 1984; Daniell and

Miller, 1989). The CO_2, Nd-YAG argon and KTP lasers have been used to treat polycystic ovaries by drilling multiple holes in the ovary to decrease androgen production by destruction of ovarian cysts. The results have been excellent with spontaneous ovulation occurring in 60% of the patients and the other 40% responding to Clomiphene. Although these data have been reported from laparoscopic operations, the same procedure could be performed at laparotomy using any one of the above lasers. This procedure, though unlikely to be done often, would decrease the possibility of post-operative adhesions compared with routine wedge resection.

2.9 Myomectomy

The rationale for myomectomy in infertility patients is primarily due to the potential interference of fibromyomata with implantation, causing uterine contractions, obstruction of the tubal ostium or interference with sperm transportation.

Buttram and Reiter (1981) discussed myomectomy for primary infertility after reviewing 4773 cases recorded in the literature from 1931 to 1980. Forty per cent conceived after myomectomy, and the fetal wastage was reduced pre-operatively from 41 to 19% post-operatively. They found that less than 10% of those women undergoing myomectomy had distorted uterine cavities. They hypothesized that uterine fibroids caused venous dilatation and congestion, thus preventing implantation and/or impairing placental blood flow during embryo development. They recommended myomectomy for those symptomatic patients experiencing infertility, menorrhagia, or pelvic pain. Myomectomy was also recommended if the fibroid was 2 cm or greater, and if it was located submucosally, intramurally, or subserosally adjacent to the uterotubal junction.

For asymptomatic females who desired conception, they suggested a waiting period of 6–12 months providing the uterus was not greater than 10 weeks in size. If the uterus remained less than 10 weeks in size, those patients who then underwent myomectomy conceived 100% of the time. However, they noted that if the fibroids were greater than 10 weeks in size, even if conception was not desired immediately, myomectomy was recommended because those patients appeared to have a less favourable prognosis for future fertility. Their technique employed one vertical incision anteriorly away from the cornua to minimize bleeding with no vasopressin or tourniquet used. They did not prefer an omental graft.

McLaughlin (1982) described microlaser myomectomy as a technique to enhance reproductive potential. Eight patients were reported, with five desiring conception. Three patients conceived during the 12-month follow-up with two intrauterine pregnancies and one ectopic pregnancy. The marked haemostatic property of the CO_2 laser, as well as the ability to preserve more normal tissue, was reported.

McLaughlin (1985) later published an expanded report comparing 18 microlaser myomectomies with nine myomectomies done conventionally. The laser group averaged 200 ml blood loss per patient vs 311 per patient in the conventional surgery group – a 35% reduction in blood loss. One-third of the laser group conceived with an average of 10.4 months of unprotected intercourse.

There have been several articles written in the last 3 years on the use of GnRN analogues to reduce the size of the fibroids prior to their removal (Friedman *et al.*, 1988; Kessel *et al.*, 1988; Maheux, Lemay and Turcot-Lemay, 1988). This would facilitate the removal by virtue of reducing the tumors from 40 to 50% of their pre-treatment size. There was also noted a decrease in amount of bleeding in those cases reported. These two facts would allow preservation of more normal myometrium and less blood loss which, in turn, would probably decrease the amount of adhesion formation.

2.9.1 TECHNIQUE

One may use the operating microscope with the joystick on the microslad for small (<2 cm) fibroids, but the hand-held laser for larger fibroids is preferred (Figure 2.10). It is important to use moistened non-woven gauze laparotomy sponges to prevent accidental reflection of the laser beam to other intra-abdominal vital structures. Dilute Pitressin (10 units in 200 ml saline) is injected into the base and capsule of the fibroid. The laser is used in the continuous mode at 18 000 W/cm^2 or greater and slightly defocused to provide a larger surface area with which to operate. After the base of the fibroid is injected with Pitressin, a small fibroid may be directly vaporized using a circular technique; the serosal area is closed with interrupted 4-10 Vicryl or PDS. For medium and large fibroids, an elliptical incision is made around the top of the fibroid using traction and countertraction (a towel clip or suture in the fibroid) to directly incise the base of the fibroid. The myometrium is approximated with 2-0 Vicryl or PDS and the serosa closed with continuous 4-0 PDS. If the myoma extends entirely through the wall of the uterus, care is taken to approximate the musculature in two layers with 2-0 PDS without placing the suture through the endometrial cavity. The serosa is closed with 4-0 PDS. An omental graft is not used to prevent subsequent adhesion formation. It is generally considered appropriate to perform an early second-look

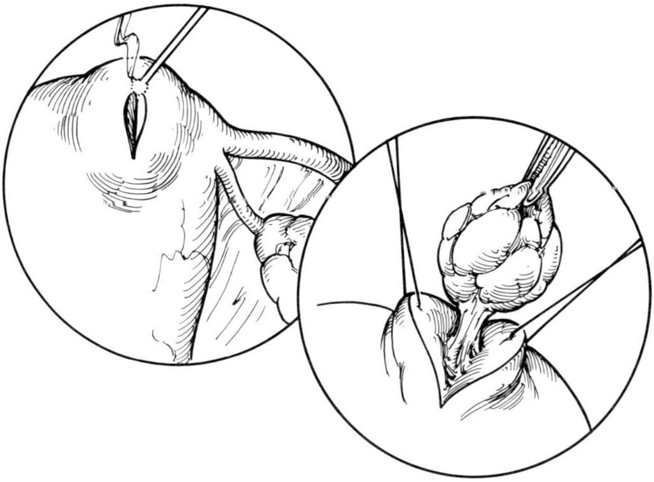

Figure 2.10 Myomectomy with the CO_2 laser.

laparoscopy if there are multiple incisions in the uterus due to a significant incidence of post-operative adhesion formation.

2.10 Metroplasty

For those cases of intra-uterine septa associated with a bicornuate or septate uterus that cannot be treated by hysteroscope incision, laparotomy procedures must be performed. Jones (1957) reported an 81% conception rate and delivery of a living child after metroplasty. The CO_2 laser has been used for uterine unification of the bicornuate and subseptate uterus. However, the technique of hysteroscopic incision of a septate uterus now eliminates the need for laparotomy in these cases. Improved haemostasis (183 ml per laser patient vs 350 ml per conventional patient) as well as the ability to preserve more normal uterine tissue are advantages of the CO_2 laser when surgically treating uterine anomalies. To date, there have been too few cases published to give an accurate assessment of its value in subsequent reproductive performance.

2.10.1 TECHNIQUE

The hand-held focusing piece is used to precisely make the incision with the CO_2 laser using approximately 18 000 W/cm^2 in a continuous mode. Two techniques are appropriate according to the size of the

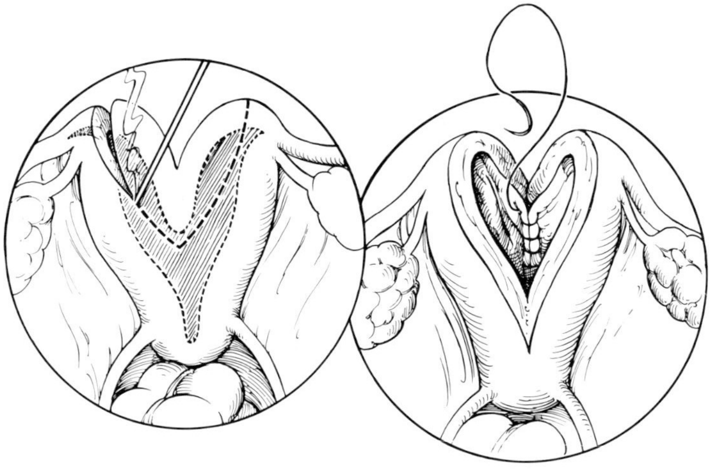

Figure 2.11 Jones procedure for unification of the uterus with the CO_2 laser.

septum. If one elects to remove the septum, the area to be removed in the subseptate uterus is outlined with a sterile marking pen, taking care to place the lateral edges of the triangle more medial to the full width of the septum. Dilute Pitressin (10 units in 200 ml of saline) is injected, and one traction suture 2-0 Vicryl is placed in the middle of the septum. The incision is made anteriorly to posteriorly over the triangular areas to be excised. When the triangular-shaped tissue is excised *in toto*, there should be a small opening into the uterine cavity at the level of the internal cervical os (Figure 2.11). Ninety-degree angled titanium rods are placed into each horn of the uterus and the remaining septum is vaporized over the titanium rods. Usually the endometrium will flower over the cut edges of the myometrium as the remaining vestige of the septum is removed. PDS (2-0) in continuous fashion anchoring one suture anteriorly and one suture posteriorly is utilized to close the myometrium in two layers. The anchor knot is tagged with a haemostat and both sutures are continued from anteriorly to posteriorly to anteriorly, first deep and then crossing to the superficial layer of the myometrium at the dorsum of the fundus and tied to the anchor knot of the other suture. The serosa is approximated with 4-0 Vicryl in continuous fashion. Care is taken to produce the best haemostasis possible in order to decrease the possibility of postoperative adhesions.

Another approach to a more narrow septum is to merely bivalve the uterus in half, through the centre of the septum, anterior to posterior. Titanium rods are placed in each horn and the remaining septum is

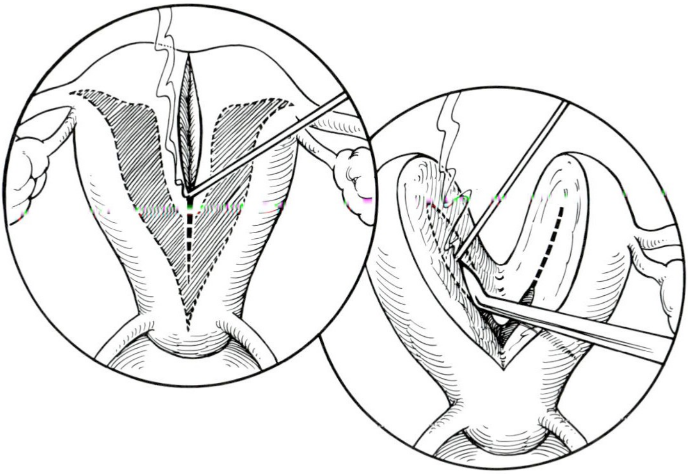

Figure 2.12 Tompkins unification with the CO_2 laser.

incised over the rod (Figure 2.12). The endometrium, myometrium and serosa are then closed as described above. For the true bicornuate uterus, the area to be incised on the uterine horns is marked with the sterile marking pen. The same Pitressin concentration and laser power densities are used to incise both cornua which are held by 2-0 PDS traction sutures. Two sutures of 2-0 PDS, one anteriorly and one posteriorly, are used continuously to approximate the uterine musculature. The serosa is closed with continuous 4-0 PDS, taking care to maximize haemostasis. As previously mentioned, no omental graft or peritoneal graft is used as it is rare to have subsequent adhesions to the uterine incision as seen on early second-look laparoscopy.

2.11 Conclusions

It is apparent that lasers are going to play an increasingly important role in the treatment of infertility-related disorders. As clinical experience and investigative protocols are reported, these important developments will almost surely validate the necessity for reproductive surgeons to become knowledgeable about laser surgery, if not proficient in its use. Even if the pregnancy rates do not surpass those achieved following conventional microsurgery, the other advantages of using the laser in microsurgery may not be ignored.

As newer wavelengths become applicable for surgical procedures, major advances may be expected in the treatment of endometriosis, adhesions and tubal disease.

References

American Fertility Society (1988), Classification of adnexal adhesions, distal tubal occlusion, tubal occlusion secondary to tubal ligation, tubal pregnancies, Mullerian anomalies, and intrauterine adhesions. *Fertil. Steril.*, **49**, 944.

Badaway, Z. A., El Bakay, M. and Baggish, M. S. (1987), Comparative study of continuous and pulsed CO_2 laser on tissue healing and fertility outcome in tubal anastomosis. *Fertil. Steril.*, **47**, 843.

Baggish, M. S. and Chong, A. P. (1981), Carbon dioxide laser microsurgery of the uterine tube. *Obstet. Gynecol.*, **58**, 111.

Baggish, M. L. and Chong, S. P. (1983), Intra-abdominal surgery with the CO_2 laser. *J. Reprod. Med.*, **28**, 269.

Barbot, J., Parent, B., Dubuisson J. and Aubriot, F. (1987), A clinical study of the CO_2 laser and electrosurgery for adhesiolysis in 172 cases followed by early second-look laparoscopy. *Fertil. Steril.*, **48**, 140.

Bellina, J. (1983), Microsurgery of the Fallopian tube with the carbon dioxide laser: analysis of 230 cases with two-year follow-up. *Laser Surg. Med.*, **3**, 255.

Boeck, W., Brosens, I., Gordts, S. and Vasquez, G. (1978), Tubal cornual polyps: microsurgical polypectomy and cornual anastomosis (Abstr.). Presented at the Fifth European Congress on Sterility, Venice, October 1978, p. 147.

Bruhat, M. A. and Mage, G. (1983), Pregnancy following salpingostomy: comparison between CO_2 laser and electrosurgery procedures. *Fertil. Steril.*, **40**, 472.

Buttram, V. C. Jr (1979), Surgical treatment of endometriosis in the infertile female: a modified approach. *Fertil. Steril.*, **32**, 635.

Buttram, V. C. Jr and Reiter, R. C. (1981), Uterine leiomyomata: etiology, symptomatology, and management. *Fertil. Steril.*, **36**, 433.

Chong, A. P. and Baggish, M. S. (1984), Management of pelvic endometriosis by means of intra-abdominal carbon dioxide laser. *Fertil. Steril.*, **41**, 14–19.

Cropp, C. S., Cowell, Pl. D. and Rock, J. A. (1987), Failure of tube closure following laser salpingostomy for ampullary tubal ectopic pregnancy. *Fertil. Steril.*, **48**, 887.

Daniell, J. F., Diamond, M. P., McLaughlin, D. S., Martin, D. C., Feste, J., Surrey, M. W., Friedman, S. and Vaughn, W. K. (1986), Clinical results of terminal neosalpingostomy with the use of CO_2 laser: report of the intra-abdominal laser study group. *Fertil. Steril.*, **45**, 175.

Daniell, J. F. and Miller, W. (1989), Polycystic ovaries treated by laparoscopic laser vaporization. *Fertil. Steril.*, **51**, 232.

David, M. P., Ben-Zwi, D. and Langer, L. (1981), Tubal intramural polyps and their relationship to infertility. *Fertil Steril.*, **35**, 526.

Diamond, M. *et al.* (1984), Pelvic adhesions at early second look laparoscopy following carbon dioxide laser surgical procedures. *Fertil. Steril.*, **7**, 39–44.

Dmowski, W. P. and Cohen, M. D. (1975), Treatment of endometriosis with an antigonadotropin, danazol: a laparoscopic and histologic evaluation. *Obstet. Gynecol.*, **46**, 147.

Fayez, J. A., McComb, J. S. and Harper, M. A. (1983), Comparison of tubal microsurgery with the CO_2 laser and the unipolar microelectrode. *Fertil. Steril.*, **40**, 476.

Filmar, S., Gomel, V. and McComb, P. F. (1986), The effectiveness of CO_2 laser and electromicrosurgery in adhesiolysis: a comparative study. *Fertil. Steril.*, **45**, 407.

Friedlander, R. L. (1975), The treatment of endometriosis with danazol. *J. Reprod. Med.*, **10**, 197.

Friedman, A. J., Barbieri, R. L., Doubilet, P. M., Fine, C. and Schiff, I. A. (1988), Randomized, double-blind trial of a gonadotropin releasing-hormone agonist (Leuprolide) with or without medroxyprogesterone acetate in the treatment of leiomyomata uteri. *Fertil. Steril.*, **49**, 404.

Gjonnaess, H. (1984), Polycystic ovarian syndrome treated by ovarian electrocautery through the laparoscope. *Fertil. Steril.*, **41**, 20.

Gomel, V. (1980), Clinical results of infertility microsurgery. In *Microsurgery in Female Infertility* (eds P. G. Crosisgnani and B. L. Rubin), Academic Press, London, p. 77.

Greenblatt, R. B. and Tzingounis, V. (1979), Danazol treatment of endometriosis: long term follow up. *Fertil. Steril.*, **32**, 518.

Jones, W. S. (1957), Obstetric significance of female genital abnormalities. *Obstet. Gynecol.*, **10**, 113–27.

Kelly, R. W. and Roberts, D. K. (1983), Experience with the carbon dioxide laser in gynecologic microsurgery. *Am. J. Obstet. Gynecol.*, **146**, 585.

Kessel, B., Lui, J., Mortola, J., Berga, S. and Yen, S. S. (1988), Treatment of uterine fibroids with analogs of gonadotropin-releasing hormone. *Fertil. Steril.*, **49**, 538.

Kistner, R. W. (1975), Endometriosis in infertility. In *Progress in Infertility*, 2nd edn (eds R. W. Kistner and S. J. Behrman), Brown & Co., Boston, pp. 345–64.

Maheux, R., Lemay, A. and Turcot-Lemay, L. (1988), Dose-related inhibition of acute luteinizing hormone response during luteinizing hormone-releasing hormone agonist treatment for uterine leiomyoma. *Am. J. Obstet. Gynecol.*, **158**, 361.

McLaughlin, D. S. (1982), Micro-laser myomectomy technique to enhance reproductive potential: a preliminary report. *Laser Surg. Med.*, **2**, 107.

McLaughlin, D. S. (1985), Metroplasty and myomectomy with the CO_2 laser for maximizing the preservation of normal tissue and minimizing blood loss. *J. Reprod. Med.*, **30**, 1.

McLaughlin, M. D. (1984), Successful pregnancy outcome following removal of bilateral cornual polyps by microsurgery linear salpingostomy with the aid of the CO_2 laser. *Fertil. Steril.*, **42**, 939.

Phillip, E. and Huber, H. (1939), Cause of endometriosis with contribution on the pathology of the interstitial portion of the tube. *Zentralbl Gynakol.*, **67**, 7.

Pittaway, D. E., Maxson, W. S. and Daniell, J. F. (1983), A comparison of the CO_2 laser and electrocautery on postoperative intraperitoneal adhesion formation in rabbits. *Fertil. Steril.*, **40**, 366.

Raj, S. G. and Hulka, H. F. (1982), Second look laparoscopy in infertility surgery: therapeutic and prognostic value. *Fertil. Steril.*, **38**, 325.

Strangel, J., Chervenak, F. A. and Mouradian-Davidian, M. (1981), Microsurgical resection of bilateral Fallopian tube polyps. *Fertil. Steril.*, **35**, 580.

Tulandi, T. (1986), Salpingo-ovariolysis: a comparison between laser surgery and electrosurgery. *Fertil. Steril.*, **45**, 489.

Tulandi, T. (1987), Adhesion reformation after reproductive surgery with and without the carbon dioxide laser. *Fertil. Steril.*, **47**, 704.

Tulandi, T., Farag, R., McInnes, R., Gelfand, M., Wright, C. and Vilos, G. (1984), Reconstructive surgery of hydrosalpinx with and without the carbon dioxide laser. *Fertil. Steril.*, **42**, 839.

Tulandi, T. and Vilos, G. (1985), A comparison between laser surgery and electrosurgery for bilateral hydrosalpinx: A 2-year follow-up. *Fertil. Steril.*, **44**, 841.

Voros, J. I., Bellina, J. H., Moorehead, M. E. and Hemmings, R. (1984), Management of ectopic pregnancy by carbon dioxide laser. *J. LA State Med. Soc.*, **135**, 9–11.

3 *Assessment of results of laparoscopic laser surgery*

MICHAEL P. DIAMOND

3.1 Introduction

Therapeutic laser laparoscopic surgery increasingly offers new potentials for a wide variety of intra-abdominal applications. Use of the laser *per se* represents one of several therapeutic modalities, others being electrocautery and sharp dissection. The diversity of procedures performed using these modalities now includes cholecystectomy, liver biopsies, appendectomies, retroperitoneal lymph node dissection, and 'laparoscopic hysterectomies'. However, the most frequent application is in the diagnosis and treatment of tubo-peritoneal disease, pelvic pain and infertility by gynaecologists experienced in advanced laparoscopic reproductive pelvic surgical procedures.

The progression in the use of laparoscopy from that of a diagnostic modality to that of a therapeutic modality has primarily been possible because of advances in technology and instrumentation. A partial list of these modalities is listed in Table 3.1. Possibly the greatest contribution to the performance of operative endoscopic procedures has been the introduction of lasers. The CO_2 laser was the initial laser introduced for use at the time of laparoscopy. Subsequently, the argon, KTP-532 and Nd-YAG lasers have also been made available for these purposes. In order to perform these operative procedures, a need developed for the use of multiple second puncture probes. Concomitant with the use of multiple punctures was the more rapid loss of pneumoperitoneum and the consequent need for greater insufflation than previously available. This need has been met by the introduction of high-flow insufflators which allow insufflation at a rate of 5–6 litres of gas per minute. Additionally, with the introduction of multiple punctures, it is no longer possible for a single physician to be able to manipulate all of the instruments in use in a given procedure. Consequently, many procedures now require the co-ordinated activities of two to three individuals. The ability to co-ordinate procedures has been

Table 3.1 Advances in laparoscopic technology and instrumentation

Lasers
Carbon dioxide (CO_2)
Argon
Potassium titanyl phosphate-532 (KTP-532)
Neodymium-yttrium aluminium garnet (Nd-YAG)
High flow insufflators
Video systems
Pelviscopic surgical equipment
Endocoagulation
Aquadissection
Tissue morcellators

greatly facilitated by the introduction of high-resolution video equipment. Additional equipment which has been of use in facilitating operative procedures includes endocoagulators (for haemostasis), aquapurators (for tissue dissection with irrigating fluids), and 'morcellators', multiple tissue punch instruments to allow for tissue removal. Additionally, the introduction of laparoscopic equipment has facilitated the performance of such procedures as oophorectomy and salpingectomy, as well as introducing the potential for endoscopic suturing. Associated with these changes in the equipment available for the performance of laparoscopic procedures has been the requirement for a changing attitude by the operating room staff. No longer can laparoscopies be considered to be short procedures. It has become not uncommon for procedures to last several hours, requiring a similar amount of time to equivalent procedures performed at laparotomy. Finally, the introduction of endoscopic procedures which can be performed on an out-patient basis have raised the potential for limiting hospital costs. Changes in this direction have been increasingly demanded by third-party payers in the United States. Yet there remains controversy as to whether insurance companies are consistently willing to recognize the performance of advanced endoscopic techniques as clinically appropriate surgery with appropriate reimbursement.

3.2 Therapeutic alternatives: incision, coagulation, haemostasis

The operative laparoscopist has a variety of modalities available for performing incisions at the time of laparoscopy. These are listed in

Table 3.2 Endoscopic modalities with incisional capability

Laser
CO_2
Argon
KTP-532
Nd-YAG with sapphire tips
Scalpel
Electrocautery
Scissors

Table 3.2. The traditional incisional instruments used at laparotomy, a scalpel and scissors, are also available for use at laparoscopy. These agents, however, are more likely to be associated with bleeding than with other modalities which have varying degrees of concomitant coagulative effects. Similarly, just as an electrodiathermy needle can be used at the time of laparotomy for incision, electrocautery can also be used at the time of laparoscopy for incision. The other alternative is the use of lasers. Among the lasers available, the CO_2 laser, when used at its focal point with a high-power density, has a great incisional capability. The incisional capability can be maximized by utilizing superpulse mode. Incisional capability is also possible with the argon and KTP-532 lasers; however, these tend to have a greater coagulative tissue effect. At times when there is greater propensity to bleeding, such as when making a linear salpingotomy incision for an ectopic pregnancy, such coagulative tissue effect may be of greater theoretical advantage. Utilization of sapphire tips on the Nd-YAG laser also allows the creation of an incisional effect.

Coagulative capability can be utilized at the time of laparoscopy for the achievement of haemostasis, incision of adhesions, and treatment of endometriosis. Modalities used for coagulative effects in laparoscopy are listed in Table 3.3. Most gynaecologists have experience using electrocautery for the performance of tubal ligations. Electrocautery can also be utilized for treatment of endometriosis; however, most are hesitant to apply current when the endometriosis overlies blood vessels, the bowel, bladder or ureter. Concern for spread of the current is greater with unipolar than with bipolar electrocautery. An alternative to electrocautery is the use of fibre lasers. The greatest coagulative effect is with the Nd-YAG laser. It is for this reason that the Nd-YAG laser has been used for endometrial ablation. The use of the bare Nd-YAG laser fibre at laparoscopy has been limited; however, there are reports of its use for the treatment of endometriosis and ectopic

Table 3.3 Endoscopic modalities with coagulative capability

Electrocautery
Bipolar
Unipolar
Laser
CO_2
Argon
KTP-532
Nd-YAG
Endocoagulation

Table 3.4 Endoscopic modalities with haemostasis capability

Electrocautery
Bipolar
Unipolar
Laser
CO_2
Argon
KTP-532
Nd-YAG
Endocoagulation
Suturing
Haemostatic adjuvants (e.g. gelfoam, thrombin, avitene, etc.)
Surgical clips

pregnancies. More commonly used for this purpose are the argon and the KTP-532 lasers. These allow coagulation of small vessels while also simultaneously allowing incision of these vessels. The size of vessels being incised can be increased by occluding the vessels prior to treatment with the laser. Although the CO_2 laser is primarily thought of as an incisional modality, defocusing of the laser beam allows it to be used for coagulation as well. Finally, the endocoagulator has been described as an instrument which can be utilized to coagulate even larger vessels, such as those in the infundibulopelvic ligament.

Haemostasis can be achieved at the time of endoscopic procedures using the coagulative modalities just described as well as additional modalities listed in Table 3.4. Vascular ligation is now possible at the time of laparoscopy. This could be accomplished either using pre-tied sutures, in the form of endoloops, or by actually suturing intra-abdominally. Currently, such procedures are in part limited by the needles able to be passed through the laparoscopic trocars and by the suture material available. However, this is an area where advances in the near future can be expected. Although rarely used at laparoscopy because of concern for initiation of adhesions, haemostatic adjuvants can be applied through the laparoscope. This would be of particular use with raw or oozing areas as opposed to brisk vascular bleeding. An area under intense investigation at this time is the potential for endoscopic application of surgical clips. These could be utilized to ligate blood vessels as well as to treat intra-abdominal bleeding.

3.3 Procedures performed at laparoscopy

Several reproductive pelvic surgical procedures are now routinely performed at the time of laparoscopy. These include linear salpingotomy for the treatment of ectopic pregnancy, vaporization or excision of endometriosis, and incision of moderate to severe adhesions. These procedures are performed at laparoscopy rather than at laparotomy, despite the fact that well-designed clinical trials demonstrating equal or superior efficacy of the endoscopic technique have yet to be demonstrated. Comparison of recent reports from the literature for therapy at laparotomy and laparoscopy show similar pregnancy rates; approximately 40–50% after an ectopic pregnancy (Table 3.5), 50–60% after treatment of endometriosis (Table 3.6), and 45–60% after adhesiolysis (Table 3.7). However, as recently reviewed (Diamond, 1988), when comparing outcome of large clinical reports describing these procedures at laparoscopy and at laparotomy, outcome appears to be equivalent although laparoscopy inevitably allows a reduction in post-operative morbidity and expense. While such retrospective clinical reviews are not the ideal alternative to a randomized, prospective, double-blind study, the latter may never be performed with a sufficiently large number of patients. Nevertheless until the results of such clinical trials are available, reports of other surgeons' experience can serve as a guide for counselling patients.

More controversial is the role of operative endoscopy for the performance of other reproductive pelvic surgical procedures performed at laparotomy. These include the treatment of bilateral distal tubal occlusion (complete or partial), and the treatment of extensive, cohesive pelvic adhesions. For such procedures, laparotomy probably still remains the gold standard. However, the question exists as to the appropriate therapy for this pathology if the surgeon is technically able

Table 3.5 Pregnancy outcome after radical and conservative treatment of tubal ectopic pregnancies

Reference	*Laparotomy/ laparoscopy*	*No. of patients*	*No. attempting conception*	*No. of term pregnancies (%)*	*Laparoscopic failures (%)*
Radical					
1	Laparotomy	50	–	21(42)	
2	Laparotomy	71	71	37(52)	
3	Laparotomy	558	–	184(33)	
Conservative					
1	Laparotomy	48	–	19(39)	
3	Laparotomy	185	–	48(26)	
4	Laparoscopy	321	118	76(64)	15(13)
5	Laparoscopy	79	69	29(4)	2(3)
6	Laparoscopy	27	8	5(63)	1(13)

From Diamond, M. P. (1988), Surgical aspects of infertility. In *Gynecology and Obstetrics*, Vol. 5, Ch. 61 (ed. J. W. Sciarra), Harper and Row, Philadelphia.
1. DeCherney and Kase (1979). 2. Nagami, London and St Amand (1984). 3. Timonen and Nieminen (1967). 4. Pouly *et al.* (1986). 5. DeCherney and Diamond (1987). 6. Cartwright, Herbert and Maxson (1986).

Table 3.6 Pregnancy outcome after surgical treatment of endometriosis at laparotomy and laparoscopy

Total			*Classification*		*Minimal–Mild*		*Moderate*		*Severe–Extensive*	
Reference	*Laparotomy/ laparoscopy*	*Laser +/–*	*Patients*	*Pregnant (%)*	*Patients*	*Pregnant (%)*	*Patients*	*Pregnant (%)*	*Patients*	*Pregnant (%)*
1	Laparotomy	–	[a] 107	49(46)	8	6(75)	60	30(50)	39	13(33)
2	Laparotomy	–	[b] 214	115(54)	45	28(62)	88	48(55)	81	39(48)
3	Laparotomy	–	[a] 245	148(60)	69	56(81)	92	54(59)	84	38(45)
4	Laparotomy	–	[b] 176	70(40)	20	8(40)	99	42(42)	57	20(35)
5	Laparotomy	–	[a] 71	23(32)	3	2(66)	19	7(37)	49	14(28)
6	Laparotomy	+	82	28(34)	8	1(13)	35	10(29)	39	17(44)
7	Laparoscopy	–	NG 60	34(57)	35	20(57)	25	14(56)		
8	Laparoscopy	+	[b] 10	6(60)	3	3(100)	7	3(43)		
9	Laparoscopy	+	[b] 115	55(48)	56	23(41)	45	22(49)	14	9(64)
10	Laparoscopy	+	[b] 282	150(53)	170	97(57)	112	53(47)		
11	Laparoscopy	+	[c] 140	82(59)	106	62(58)	31	18(58)	3	2(67)
12	Laparoscopy	+	[c] 65	37(57)	31	20(65)	26	15(58)	7	2(29)
13	Laparoscopy	+	[b] 102	62(61)	24	18(75)	51	32(63)	27	12(44)
14	Laparoscopy	–	[a] 20	12(60)						
15	Laparoscopy	+	[c] 104	40(38)	38	19(50)	25	12(48)	41	18(44)
16	Laparoscopy	+	[b] 243	126(42)	74	45(61)	105	55(52)	64	26(40)
17[†]	Laparoscopy	+	[c] 104	89(85)	76	65(86)	27	22(82)	2	2(100)
18[†]	Laparoscopy	+	[c] 56	45(80)	41	32(78)	13	11(85)	2	2(100)

Adapted from Diamond, M. P. (1988), Surgical aspects of infertility. In *Gynecology and Obstetrics*, Vol. 5, Ch. 61. (ed. S. W. Sciarra), Harper and Row, Philadelphia.

* Classification of endometriosis: [a] Acosta, [b] American Fertility Society (AFS), [c] Revised American Fertility (RAFS). [†] Endometriosis alone.

1. Acosta, Buttram and Besch (1973). 2. Rock, Guzick and Sengos (1987). 3. Buttram (1979). 4. Gordts, Boeckx and Brosens (1984). 5. Garcia and David (1977). 6. Diamond, Daniell and Martin (unpublished data). 7. Daniell (1987). 8. Kelly and Roberts (1983). 9. Martin (198[illegible]). 10. Paulson and Asnar (1986, personal communication). 11. Feste (1985a). 12. Davis (1986). 13. Nezhat, Crowgey and Garrison (1986). 14. Reicht and McGlynn (1986). 15. Bruhat *et al.* (1989). 16. Donnez (1989). 17. Feste (1989). 18. Sutton and Hill (1990).

Table 3.7 Pregnancy outcome following adhesiolysis at laparotomy and laparoscopy

Reference	*Laparotomy/laparoscopy*	*Macrosurgery/microsurgery*	*Laser*	*Total no. of patients*	*No. of term pregnancies (%)*
1	Laparotomy	Macrosurgery	–	94	43(46)
2	Laparotomy	Macrosurgery	–	64	26(41)
3	Laparotomy	Macrosurgery	–	41	16(42)
4	Laparotomy	Macrosurgery	–	29	20(69)
5	Laparotomy	Macrosurgery	–	268	94(35)
6	Laparotomy	Microsurgery	–	101	38(38)
7	Laparotomy	Macrosurgery	–	42	27(64)
8	Laparotomy	Macrosurgery	–	220	55(25)
	Laparotomy	Microsurgery	–	140	80(57)
	Laparotomy	Microsurgery	–	33	17(52)
9		Microsurgery	+	30	16(53)
10	Laparotomy	Microsurgery	–	49	20(41)
11	Laparoscopy		–	92	54(59)
12	Laparoscopy		–	50	23(46)

From Diamond, M. P. (1988), Surgical aspects of infertility. In *Gynecology and Obstetrics*, Vol. 5, Ch. 61 (ed. J. W. Sciarra), Harper and Row, Philadelphia.

1. Wallach, Manara and Eisenberg (1983). 2. Jansen (1980). 3. O'Brien, Arronet and Eduljee (1969). 4. Betz, Engel and Penney (1980). 5. Grant (1971). 6. Caspi, Halperin and Bukorsky (1979). 7. Donnez and Casanas-Roux (1986). 8. Diamond (1979). 9. Tulandi (1986). 10. Frantzen and Schlosser (1982). 11. Gomel (1983). 12. Fayez (1983).

to perform the procedure at laparoscopy. Some may argue that at laparoscopy, dissection may not be as thorough and there would be greater difficulty in controlling venous and capillary oozing. In contrast, others could claim that such patients represent a patient population with a poor pregnancy outcome and thus justify offering patients the less morbid procedure. At this time, an additional consideration to performance of procedures at laparoscopy or at laparotomy is the issue of the appropriate circumstances for referring for *in vitro* fertilization as an alternative to surgical therapy.

3.4 Revived procedures

There are two procedures which were previously performed at laparotomy which have gone out of vogue. These are the Doyle procedure or transection of the uterosacral ligaments and ovarian wedge resections. Modifications of these procedures have allowed them to be performed at the time of operative laparoscopy.

3.4.1 LAPAROSCOPIC UTERINE NERVE ABLATION

Transection of the uterosacral ligaments is thought to be of potential benefit in the reduction of pelvic pain (Feste, 1985; Lichten and Bombard, 1987; Sutton, 1989). In particular, this procedure has been used for women with midline lower pelvic pain. In theory, the procedure involves transecting the sensory nerve fibres as they leave the uterus on the way to the pelvic plexuses. Because of divergence of these nerve fibres in the uterosacral ligaments, it has been recommended that this procedure be performed as close to the uterus as possible. The procedure had initially been performed at laparotomy or vaginally (Doyle, 1954), but was later adapted to operative laparoscopy using electrocautery. However, there was concern about spread of the electric current in this area because of the close proximity of the uterine artery and the ureter. More recently, this procedure has also been performed utilizing one of several lasers. When performing this procedure, the surgeon should be aware of the presence of an artery in the medial aspect of the uterosacral ligament and some large thin-walled veins in order to avoid injury to these vessels.

Analysis of the results of this procedure has been limited by the potential placebo effect of telling an individual that the uterosacral ligaments had been transected. Nevertheless, Feste (1985b) has described an improvement rate in the reduction of pelvic pain in approximately 70% of over 300 subjects and Sutton (1989) has shown improvement in 86% of 100 women with endometriosis and 73% of 16 women with primary dysmenorrhoea. These results are consistent with those of Lichten and Bombard (1987), who performed a randomized prospective double-blind study to evaluate the efficacy of this procedure. They excluded all individuals with an abnormal psychological profile or with demonstrable pelvic pathology. Neither the patient nor the clinical psychologist who conducted the initial or follow-up interview were aware of the group to which the patient had been randomized. They noted improvement in symptoms 3 months post-operatively which persisted in approximately 70% of the treated subjects for at least 1 year later.

3.4.2 LAPAROSCOPY TREATMENT OF POLYCYSTIC OVARIAN SYNDROME

Prior to the availability of human menopausal gonadotrophins for ovulation induction, ovarian wedge resection was frequently employed for induction of ovulation in women with polycystic ovarian syndrome. An all too frequent complication of this procedure, however, was the development of post-operative ovarian adhesions which limited subsequent fertility (Toaff, Toaff and Peyser, 1976). The postulated mechanism by which this procedure resulted in subsequent ovulation was the reduction in ovarian androgen production. A laparoscopic alternative to ovarian wedge resection is the 'drilling' of ovarian follicles at the time of laparoscopy (Gjonnaess, 1984; Katz and Cohen, 1984; Daniell and Miller, 1989). This has been performed both using electrocautery and with lasers. The procedure has been to drain the multiple sub-capsular ovarian cysts, thereby reducing ovarian androgen levels and allowing resumption of ovulation. There have been several studies which evaluate hormonal profiles before and after these procedures and which are able to demonstrate a reduction in circulating androgen levels (Greenblatt and Casper, 1987; Gjonnaess and Norman, 1987; Keckstein, 1989). Some of these trials have also evaluated subsequent ovulatory function and pregnancy outcome. To date, however, no controlled comparative trial has been performed.

In contrast to classical ovarian wedge resection which tended to have a permanent effect when the large wedges of ovarian tissue were excised, the ovarian 'drilling' effects have been more temporary. The difference may lie in the mass ovarian tissue affected with these treatments. Particularly when the CO_2 laser is utilized there may be no destruction of ovarian stroma and thus long-term potential for ovarian androgen production may not be significantly reduced. It is for this reason that some investigators have suggested that the Nd-YAG laser, which will destroy a greater extent of ovarian tissue, may be more beneficial in this procedure. This remains, however, to be demonstrated.

3.5 Efficacy

The overriding impression that can be gathered from the above description of laparoscopic surgery is that the available data, for the most part, is based on clinical experience of individual investigators. Use of comparative trials in general and prospective randomized double-blinded surgical trials is almost non-existent in the reproductive pelvic surgery literature. Clearly, there remains a major need for well-designed clinical trials to evaluate the efficacy of endoscopic laser surgical procedures. Questions to be addressed include the value of operative endoscopy as opposed to procedures performed at laparotomy as well as the relative efficacy of the various modalities available for incision, coagulation and establishment of haemostasis.

An additional area for future evaluation is the concern with post-operative adhesion development. Reproductive pelvic surgical procedures performed at laparotomy are frequently complicated by adhesion formation, occurring in approximately 90% of subjects (Diamond, 1988). Luciano *et al.* (1987) examined the effect of creation of equivalent lesions (e.g. equivalent power densities) with the CO_2 laser and micro-electrocautery. Comparing these two modalities, they observed no difference in tissue injury at the time of surgery, or post-operative fibrosis and adhesion development at the ovary or on peritoneal surfaces. As pointed out by Diamond *et al.* (1987), post-operative adhesion development includes not only adhesion reformation but *de novo* adhesion formation as well. It has been postulated that the extent of post-operative adhesion development might be reduced when procedures are performed endoscopically as compared to a laparotomy. Theoretical reasons include less drying of tissue, the decreased likelihood of getting talc or other contaminants on pelvic tissues, the avoidance of packs and retractors used at laparotomy, and minimization of tissue handling at laparoscopy. Luciano (1988) has performed elegant studies in the rabbit addressing this issue. He has demonstrated, by creating the same lesions with the laser at laparotomy and laparoscopy, that the extent of adhesion formation is reduced following laparoscopy. Furthermore, by attempting to lyse adhesions formed at the time of laparotomy either at the time of a second laparotomy or at the time of a second laparoscopy, the extent of adhesion reformation noted at the time of a third procedure is reduced after laparoscopic adhesiolysis. To date, data in the human are lacking. Support for this hypothesis can be made by extrapolation of the data of Fayez and Schneider (1987). The author sequentially operated on patients either with laparotomy or later by laparoscopy. Subsequently among those patients undergoing second-look laparoscopy, the incidence of adhesion development was less following laparoscopic adhesiolysis. This issue was not a goal of this chapter, and thus many faults can be attributed to attempting to make such an observation. It is mentioned here simply as a suggestion and in the hope that it will entice readers to perform the appropriate controlled clinical evaluations.

3.6 Alternatives of assisted reproduction technology

The rapid advances in assisted conception technology (*in-vitro* fertilization, gamete intrafallopian transfer, and tubal embryo transfer) has necessitated that efficacy of operative procedures, whether they be at laparotomy or at laparoscopy, also be compared with non-surgical therapy for infertility. While actual pregnancy rates following procedures vary between centres, with patient populations, and with indications for their performance, there clearly must exist a point at which patients would be more likely to conceive following assisted conception procedures compared to surgical intervention. It is not the purpose of this chapter to define what that point is. Clearly the point will continue to change in association with advances in both the conception technology and with operative procedures. What must be realized, however, is that conception technology can be performed with minimal risk to the patients from ovulation induction or from oocyte recovery and embryo transfer. The risk of clinically significant ovarian hyperstimulation in women participating in an IVF programme has been exceedingly low (Diamond, Bryan and Wentz, 1986). Furthermore, the rapid advances with transvaginal ultrasound guided oocyte recovery have essentially obviated the need for laparoscopy for oocyte recovery (Lavy *et al.*, 1988).

3.7 Concerns in endoscopic surgery

An overriding concern in the advancement of any new surgical field must be the risk of potential complications. While injuries at the time of operative laparoscopy have included damage to the bowel, the bladder, ureter and blood vessels, reports of their occurrence have been limited. In a review of over 671 patients by the Intraabdominal CO_2 Laser Adhesion Study Group, few (9 of 23 observed complications) were attributable to the operative endoscopic portion of the procedure (Diamond *et al.*, 1987). Nevertheless, as the technology continues to advance and a greater number of individuals begin to employ its use, emphasis must be placed on continued concern for safety.

Another area of concern has been the treatment of ovarian cysts at the time of laparoscopy. The concern is two-fold: firstly, whether an ovarian malignancy would be recognized and, secondly the consequences of spilling the contents of that cyst into the abdominal cavity. To date, the authors are unaware of reports in the literature in which a malignancy was treated laparoscopically; however, anecdotal reports have been described and thus this potential must be recognized. At present, there is no evidence in the literature that spill of an ovarian malignancy at the time of surgery worsens the outcome than if spill had not occurred. Nevertheless, it does change the surgical staging and also, in view of worse outcome in association with malignant ascites, does raise the concern for worsening of outcome.

Evaluation of ovarian cysts to determine whether malignancy is present is currently limited. The traditional characteristics of ovarian excrescences observed at the time of surgery is not entirely reliable. Other evaluated methods would include pre-operative ultrasound, CT or MRI evaluation, serum levels of CA-125, and potentially other serum markers such as urinary gonadotrophin fragments. However, at this time, overlap in these characteristics exists between malignant neoplasms, benign neoplasms, and non-neoplastic ovarian masses. Thus, this remains an area in need of future investigation. This need is amplified because of the increased frequency with which post-menopausal women are being identified as having small ovarian masses at the time of vaginal sonography, and the question of whether or not such ovarian cysts should be surgically treated.

3.8 The future

The future for operative laparoscopic surgery is bright. While we should continue to strive for well-controlled clinical trials, the clinical experiences emerging have clearly demonstrated a potential role for this surgical modality. There exist several areas for advancement which are awaiting improvements in technology. First is the development of a non-reactive clip which could be delivered laparoscopically. This could be utilized in lysis of vascular adhesions, to control bleeding, and to facilitate such procedures as oophorectomy and salpingectomy.

The sole remaining pelvic reproductive surgical procedure still performed at the time of laparotomy by almost all surgeons is tubal anastomosis. Several groups have experimented both in animals and in humans with the possibility of performing such a procedure at the time of laparoscopy. Potential advances which would make such a technique more of a reality include the availability of clips for anastomosis as well as such agents as a fibrin glue. What remains is a reliable way to establish precise approximation of the tubal lumen.

Salpingoscopy has emerged as a procedure which is plausible. Current salpingoscopes allow evaluation from the fimbria into the tubes down to approximately the ampullary-isthmic junction. Such examination allows identification of intraluminal tubal pathology not predicted by laparoscopic examination of the pelvis (Shapiro, 1987). Furthermore, Henry-Suchet *et al.* (1985) have shown that the observations from salpingoscopies cannot always correlate with hysterosalpingographic findings, and suggest tuboscopic findings may be of some value for future pregnancy outcome. Finally, De Bruyne *et al.* (1989) have used salpingoscopy to identify a subgroup of patients with bilateral hydrosalpinges (with mild mucosal lesions and no intratubal adhesions) in whom the pregnancy rate after neosalpingoscopy was 59%. Of even greater potential interest is the thought of treating abnormalities identified within the tubal lumen. With a multiple channel tuboscope, this could potentially be performed by passing a fibre laser with the capability of vaporizing intratubal synechiae without damaging the surrounding tubal mucosa. With the continuing advances in optics and reduction in the size of tuboscopes, the true efficacy of tuboscopy can be assessed, and therapeutic procedures initiated.

References

Acosta, A. A. Buttram, V. C. and Besch, P. K. (1973), A proposed classification of pelvic endometriosis. *Fertil. Steril.*, **42**, 19.

Betz, G., Engel, T. and Penney, L. L. (1980), Tuboplasty: Comparison of the methodology. *Fertil. Steril.*, **34**, 534.

Bruhat, M. A., Wattiez, A., Mage, G. *et al.* (1989), CO_2 laser laparoscopy. In *Baillières Clinical Obstetrics and Gynaecology*, Vol. 3 (ed. C. J. G. Sutton), pp. 499–523.

Buttram, V. C. (1979) Surgical treatment of endometriosis in the infertile female: A modified approach. *Fertil. Steril.*, **32**, 635.

Cartwright, P. S., Herbert, C. M. and Maxson, W. S. (1986), Operative laparoscopy for the management of tubal pregnancy. *J. Reprod. Med.*, **31**, 589.

Caspi, E., Halperin, Y. and Bukovsky, I. (1979), The importance of periadnexal adhesions in tubal reconstructive surgery for infertility. *Fertil. Steril.*, **31**, 296.

Daniell, J. F. (1981), Combined laparoscopic surgery and danazol therapy for pelvic endometriosis. *Fertil. Steril.*, **35**, 521.

Daniell, J. F. and Miller, W. (1989), Polycystic ovaries treated by laparoscopic laser vaporization. *Fertil. Steril.*, **51**, 232.

Davis, G. D. (1986), Instruments and methods: Management of endometriosis and its associated adhesions with the CO_2 laser laparoscope. *Obstet. Gynecol.*, **68**, 422.

DeBruyne, F., Puttemans, P., Boeckx, W. and Brosens, I. (1989), The clinical value of salpingoscopy in tubal surgery. *Fertil. Steril.*, **51**, 339.

DeCherney, A. H. and Diamond, M. P. (1987), Laparoscopic salpingostomy for ectopic pregnancy. *Obstet. Gynecol.*, **70**, 948–50.

DeCherney, A. and Kase, N. (1979), The conservative surgical management of unruptured ectopic pregnancy. *Obstet. Gynecol.* **54**, 451.

Diamond, E. (1979), Lysis of postoperative pelvic adhesions in infertility. *Fertil. Steril.*, **31**, 287.

Diamond, M. P. (1988), Surgical aspects of infertility. In *Gynecology and Obstetrics* (ed. J. J. Sciarra), Harper and Row, Philadelphia, pp. 1–23.

Diamond, M. P., Bryan, S. and Wentz, A. C. (1986), Failure of development of ovarian hyperstimulation syndrome (OHSS) in *in-vitro* fertilization attempts following human chorionic gonadotropin (hCG) administration, but without follicular aspiration. *J. In Vitro Fert. Embryo Transfer.*

Diamond, M. P., Daniell, J. F., Feste, J., Surrey, M. W., McLaughlin, D. S., Friedman, S., Vaughn, W. K. and Martin, D. C. (1987), Adhesion reformation and *de novo* adhesion formation following reproductive pelvic surgery. *Fertil. Steril.*, **47**, 864.

Diamond, M. P., Daniell, J. F., Martin, D. G., Nezhat, G., Stone R. E., Davis, G., Shirk, G., Everett, R., McLaughlin, D. S., Brand, D. A. and Feste, J. (1987), Safety of CO_2 laser laparoscopy: Report of the carbon dioxide (CO_2) laser laparoscopy study group (LLSG). 16th Annual Meeting, American Association of Gynecologic Laparoscopists, San Francisco, California, November.

Donnez, J. and Casanas-Roux, F. (1986), Prognostic factors of fimbrial microsurgery. *Fertil. Steril.*, **46**, 200.

Doyle, J. B. (1954), Paracervical uterine denervation for dysmenorrhoea *Trans. New Eng. Obstet. Gynecol. Soc.*, **8**, 143.

Fayez, J. A. (1983), An assessment of the role of operative laparoscopy in tuboplasty. *Fertil. Steril.*, **39**, 476.

Fayez, J. A. and Schneider, P. J. (1987), Prevention of pelvic adhesion formation by different modalities of treatment. *Am. J. Obstet. Gynecol.*, **157**, 1184.

Feste, J. R. (1985a), Endoscopic laser surgery in gynecology, in reproductive surgery. Postgraduate course syllabus, American Fertility Society, Chicago.

Feste, J. R. (1985b), Laser laparoscopy, a new modality. *J. Reprod. Med.*, **30**, 413.

Feste, J. R. (1989), CO_2 laser surgery treatment for endometriosis for stages I through IV. Paper presented at the International Symposium on Endometriosis, Houston, Texas, April 1989.

Frantzen, C. and Schlosser, H. W. (1982), Microsurgery and postinfectious tubal infertility. *Fertil. Steril.*, **38**, 397.

Garcia, C. R. and David, S. S. (1977), Pelvic endometriosis; infertility and pelvic pain. *Am. J. Obstet. Gynecol.*, **129**, 740.

Gjonnaess, H. (1984), Polycystic ovarian syndrome treated by ovarian electrocautery through the laparoscope. *Fertil. Steril.*, **41**, 20.

Gjonnaess, H. and Norman, N. (1987), Endocrine effects of ovarian electrocautery in patients with polycystic ovarian disease. *Br. J. Obstet. Gynaecol.*, **94**, 779.

Gomel, V. (1983), Salpingo-ovariolysis by laparoscopy in infertility. *Fertil. Steril.*, **40**, 607.

Gordts, S., Boeckx, W. and Brosens, I. (1984), Microsurgery of endometriosis in infertile patients. *Fertil. Steril.*, **42**, 520.

Grant, A. (1971), Infertility surgery of the oviduct. *Fertil. Steril.*, **22**, 496.

Greenblatt, E. and Casper, R. F. (1987), Endocrine changes after laparoscopic ovarian cautery in polycystic ovarian syndrome. *Am. J. Obstet. Gynecol.*, **156**, 279–85.

Henry-Suchet, J., Loffredo, V., Tesnier, L. and Pez, J. (1985), Endoscopy of the tube (=tuboscopy): Its prognostic value for tuboplasties. *Acta Eur. Fertil.*, **16**, 139.

Jansen, R. P. (1980), Abortion incidence following fallopian tube repair. *Obstet. Gynecol.*, **56**, 499.

Katz, M. and Cohen, B. M. (1984), Polycystic ovarian disease. *Curr. Prob. Obstet. Gynecol.*, **7**, 1.

Keckstein, J. (1989), Laparoscopic treatment of polycystic ovarian syndrome. In *Baillières Clinical Obstetrics* and *Gynaecology*, Vol. 3 (ed. C. J. G. Sutton), pp. 563–81. Baillière Tindall, London.

Kelly, R. W. and Roberts, D. K. (1983), CO_2 laser laparoscopy: A potential alternative to danazol in the treatment of stage I and II endometriosis. *J. Reprod. Med.*, **28**, 638.

Lavy, G., Restrepo-Candelo, H., Diamond, M. P., Shapiro, B. S., Grunfeld, L. and DeCherney, A. H. (1988), Laparoscopic and transvaginal ova recovery: The effect on ova quality. *Fertil. Steril.*, **49**, 1002.

Lichten, E. M. and Bombard, J. (1987), Surgical treatment of primary dysmenorrhoea with laparoscopic uterine nerve ablation. *J. Reprod. Med.*, **32**, 37.

Luciano, A. A. (1988), A comparative study of postoperative adhesions following laser surgery by laparoscopy versus laparotomy in the rabbit model (Abstract). American Association of Gynecologic Laparoscopists, Dallas, Texas, November.

Luciano, A. A., Whitman, G., Maier, D. B., Randolph, J. and Maenza, R. (1987), A comparison of thermal injury, healing patterns, and postoperative adhesion formation following CO_2 laser and electromicrosurgery. *Fertil. Steril.*, **48**, 1025–9.

Martin, D. C. (1986), CO_2 laser laparoscopy for endometriosis associated with infertility. *J. Reprod. Med.*, **31**, 1089.

Nagamani, M., London, S. and St Amand, P. (1984), Factors influencing fertility after ectopic pregnancy. *Am. J. Obstet. Gynecol.*, **149**, 533.

Nezhat, C., Crowgey, S. R. and Garrison, C. P. (1986), Surgical treatment of endometriosis via laser laparoscopy. *Fertil. Steril.*, **45**, 778.

O'Brien, J. R., Arronet, G. H. and Eduljee, S. Y. (1969), Operative treatment of fallopian tube pathology in human fertility. *Am. J. Obstet. Gynecol.*, **103**, 520.

Pouly, J. L., Mahnes, H., Mage, G., Canis, M. and Bruhat, M. A. (1986), Conservative laparoscopic treatment of 321 ectopic pregnancies. *Fertil. Steril.*, **46**, 1093.

Reich, H. and McGlynn, F. (1986), Treatment of ovarian endometriomas using laparoscopic surgical techniques. *J. Reprod. Med.*, **31**, 577.

Rock, J. A., Guzick, D. S. and Sengos, C. (1981), The conservative surgical treatment of endometriosis: Evaluation of pregnancy success with respect to the extent of disease as categorized using contemporary classification systems. *Fertil. Steril.*, **35**, 131.

Shapiro, B. S. (1987), The nonsurgical management of ectopic pregnancy. *Clin. Obstet. Gynecol.*, **30**, 230.

Sutton, C. J. G. (1989), Laser laparoscopic uterine nerve ablation. In *Operative Laser Laparoscopy and Hysteroscopy* (ed. J. Donnez), Nauwelaerts Publishers, Belgium, pp. 43–52.

Sutton, C. J. G. and Hill, D. (1990), Laser laparoscopy in the treatment of endometriosis. A 5-year study. *Br. J. Obstet. Gynaecol.*, **97**, 181–5.

Timonen, S. and Nieminen, U. (1967), Tubal pregnancy, choice of operative method of treatment. *Acta Obstet. Gynecol., Scand.*, **46**, 327.

Toaff, R., Toaff, M. E. and Peyser, M. R. (1976), Infertility following wedge resection of the ovaries. *Am. J. Obstet. Gynecol.*, **124**, 92.

Tulandi, T. (1986), Salpingo-ovariolysis: A comparison between laser surgery and electrosurgery. *Fertil. Steril.*, **45**, 489.

Wallach, E. E., Manara, L. R. and Eisenberg, E. (1983), Experience with 143 cases of tubal surgery. *Fertil. Steril.*, **39**, 609.

4 CO_2 laser laparoscopy in endometriosis

J. DONNEZ

4.1 Introduction

The endoscopic use of the laser is not new in medicine, since laser endoscopy already has been used in many disciplines. Advanced operative laparoscopy techniques for laser adhesiolysis and vaporization of endometriotic implants have been developed and laser surgeons have precisely removed endometriosis from the reproductive structure (Bruhat, Mage and Manes, 1979; Daniell and Brown, 1982; Daniell and Pittavay, 1982; Kelly and Roberts 1983; Jadir *et al.*, 1984). There are at least three advantages of laser laparoscopy over conventional operative laparoscopy: precise destruction of diseased tissue, minimal bleeding, and minimal damage to the adjacent normal tissue. Tissue reaction and post-operative adhesion formation have been shown to be no greater than with conventional methods (Donnez *et al.*, 1987a). In our department, the indications for laser laparoscopy are mainly for: endometriosis, adhesions and pelvic pain (dysmenorrhoea and dyspareunia) not relieved by hormonal therapy.

The aim of this chapter is to evaluate CO_2 laser laparoscopy in cases of endometriosis and associated pelvic adhesions.

4.2 Advantages

Used endoscopically the CO_2 laser offers some advantages over other operative techniques for endometriosis and adhesions. In order to demonstrate the safety and efficacy of such treatment, a comparison of post-operative pregnancy rates or pain relief in a prospective study with other forms of therapy (microsurgery, combined hormonal and surgical therapy) must be carried out.

In spite of the continuing development of new instrumentation to facilitate the use of the CO_2 laser via laparoscopy, there are still problems with the equipment. The system requires specialized equipment that needs good ongoing biomedical maintenance plus expert technical care in the operating room. The main problems are intraperitoneal smoke accumulation, gas leakage, and maintenance of proper beam alignment and further development and research by the manufacturers is essential.

In spite of these problems associated with the application of the CO_2 laser the advantages are numerous. The system allows precise bloodless destruction of diseased tissue and eliminates the risk of cautery. In the hands of an experienced laparoscopist, it appears safe and effective in vaporization of endometriotic lesions, uterosacral neurectomy, adhesiolysis and salpingostomy. The judicious use of these techniques, combined with carefully planned further investigations by adequately trained and experienced laparoscopists and continuing improvements in the delivery systems, will soon answer the question of the true efficacy of the CO_2 laser laparoscope. If studies continue to show pregnancy rates and pain relief to be equivalent to those patients treated by laparotomy, CO_2 laser laparoscopy will become the preferred procedure for the management of pelvic endometriosis and its associated adhesions.

4.3 Equipment

Prototype instruments for CO_2 laser laparoscopy began independently on three continents. The initial prototype proved to be unsatisfactory because of loss of carbon dioxide, accumulation of intraperitoneal smoke, and inability to keep the beam focused in the centre of the channel. Instruments were subsequently developed and tested in order to ensure safe, easy, accurate and effective procedures. Fortunately, with the development of new laparoscopic instrumentation for CO_2 laser use, the majority of technical problems have been overcome. For using the CO_2 laser with the laparoscope, two systems are now available: an operative laparoscope for single-puncture laparoscopy and two second-puncture probes.

4.3.1 SINGLE-PUNCTURE OPERATIVE LASER LAPAROSCOPY (Figure 4.1)

The operative laparoscope for laser laparoscopy is an instrument 12 mm in diameter with a 6-mm operative channel (Storz, Germany; Wolf, Germany). To use the CO_2 laser through the laparoscope, the operator simply swings the articulated arm of the laser over the operative field and attaches the black coupler containing the alignment mirror and focusing lens to the operative channel of the laparoscope. To allow free flow of fresh CO_2 down the beam channel, the CO_2 insufflation tubing

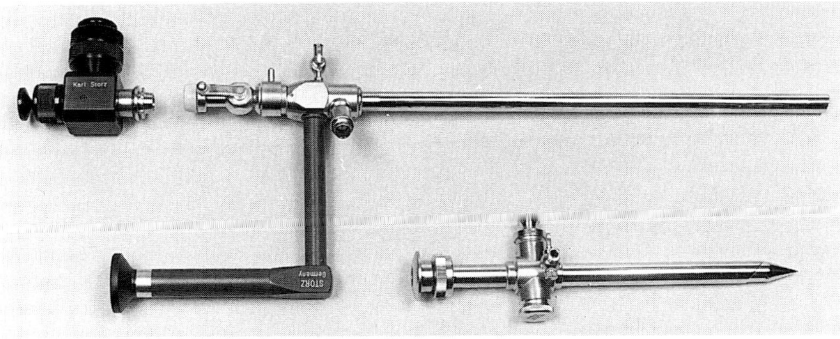

Figure 4.1 The single-puncture operative laparoscope for laser laparoscopy. The coupler contains the alignment mirror and focusing lens.

is attached to this operative channel, the flow of CO_2 from the insufflator displaces smoke which can reduce the power of the beam from the laser channel and avoids fogging the mirror and lens in the black coupler.

4.3.2 DOUBLE-PUNCTURE LASER LAPAROSCOPE (Figure 4.2)

The present second-puncture probe for using the CO_2 laser with the laparoscope is a double-ring probe that is 8 mm in external diameter. The probe attaches to the same lens and mirror that are used with the operative laparoscope. A separate second-puncture probe that has a specially designed backstop is also available for use in vaporizing adhesions. This accessory instrument, with its backstop, eliminates the risk of inadvertent injury to intraperitoneal structures and blood vessels.

The focusing lens for the standard laser laparoscope is 300 mm, with its focal point 2 cm from the end of either the operative laparoscope or the second-puncture probe. This long focal length produces a spot diameter of approximately 0.5 mm. In our series, either a Sharplan 733 apparatus or a Sharplan 1040 apparatus was used for experimental studies and clinical use. Shorter second-puncture probes are also available (Rocket, London; GV Manufacturing, London) with a 200 mm fixed focus lens (Sharplan, Tel Aviv, Israel) which are less cumbersome and easier to use (Sutton, 1989b).

(*a*) *Accessories (second- and third-puncture probes)*

The following operating instruments were developed in our department (Figure 4.3): atraumatic probe, hook for fimbrial adhesions, probe

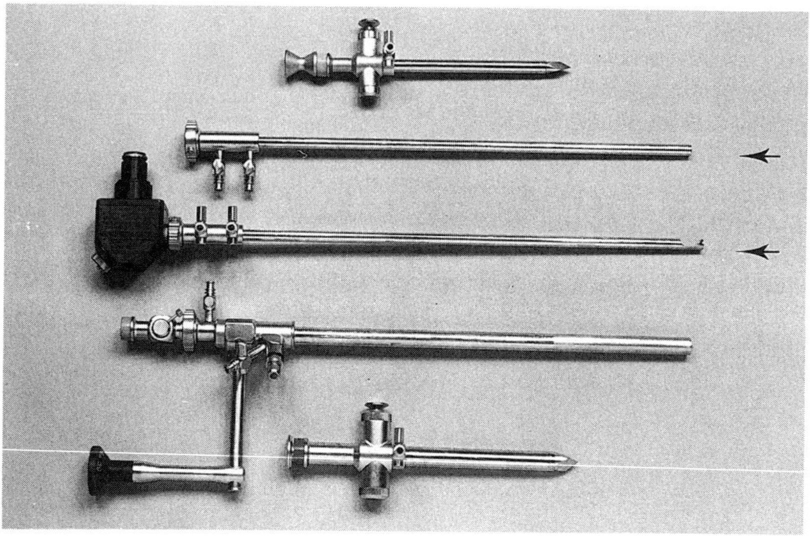

Figure 4.2 The two second-puncture probes (arrows): one with and one without the distal backstop.

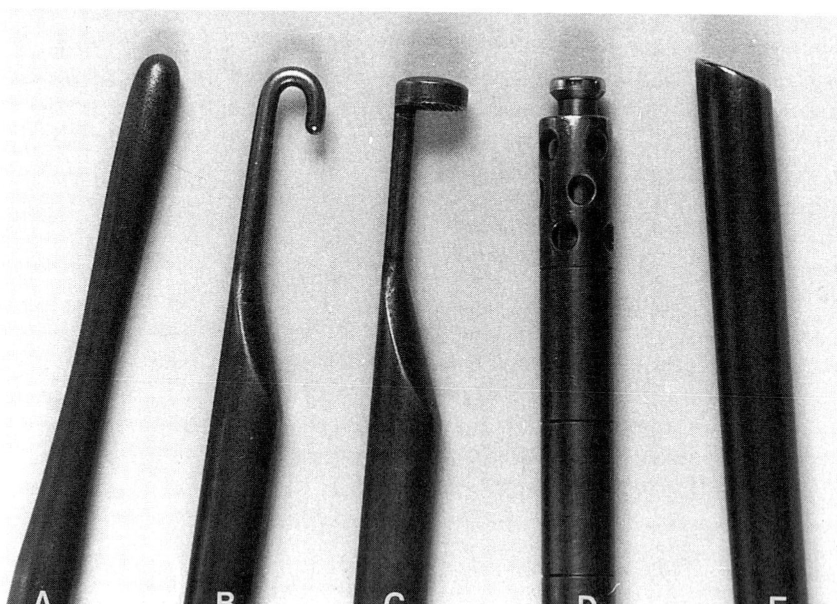

Figure 4.3 Operating instruments for second and third puncture: (A) atraumatic probe; (B) hook; (C) probe with backstop; (D) smoke suction and rising tube; (E) double channel probe for rinsing and suction.

with backstop for use in vaporizing adhesions near large blood vessels, smoke suction and irrigating tube, and double-channel probe for lavage of the pelvis and suction.

4.4 Methods

Mild and moderate endometriosis (Acosta, Buttram and Besch, 1973) can be treated with the CO_2 laser at laparoscopy. The CO_2 laser laparoscope offers several advantages over cautery of endometriotic implants. With cauterization, the laparoscopist is unable to control the 'star burst' effect of the unipolar or bipolar cautery and to evaluate the depth of cauterization. With the CO_2 laser, the laparoscopist is able to control the process of vaporization by seeing the three-dimensional boundaries of the lesion and by alternately irrigating to remove charcoal and then vaporizing with the laser. It is possible to remove all the endometriotic tissue completely.

In general, power densities between 2500 and 5000 W/cm^2 are used. Debulking endometriotic implants is best performed by using a continuous firing mode. However, if a lesion is overlying a vital structure, such as the ureter, urinary bladder, colon, or larger blood vessels, single or repeat pulse modes of 0.05–0.1 s in duration provide safer vaporization of the lesions. This duration allows a 100–200 μm depth of vaporization, thus substantially limiting the depth of penetration and allowing a degree of precision that could not be achieved with electrodiathermy (Wilson, 1988).

4.4.1 PERITONEAL ENDOMETRIOTIC IMPLANT

The impact of the laser on endometriotic implant provokes the explosive vaporization of old blood, followed by the appearance of a curdy white material representing vaporization of the stromal layer. After the entire endometriotic lesion has been vaporized, retroperitoneal fat is encountered, and the appearance of the 'bubbling of water' confirms the complete vaporization of the lesion. The absorption of the CO_2 laser by water prevents deeper penetration of the laser beam for a few seconds after the complete destruction of the implant. Firing the laser at the surface of the implant allows the chocolate-coloured material to drain from the lesion. In the peritoneal and utero-sacral sites, the endpoint of vaporization is the absence of any further visible pigment or the appearance of normal fibrous tissue. Bladder lesions and lesions overlying the colon or ureter should be treated in a similar fashion. It is important to eradicate deep nodular implants in the utero-sacral ligaments and to continue to vaporize until an assistant with fingers in the

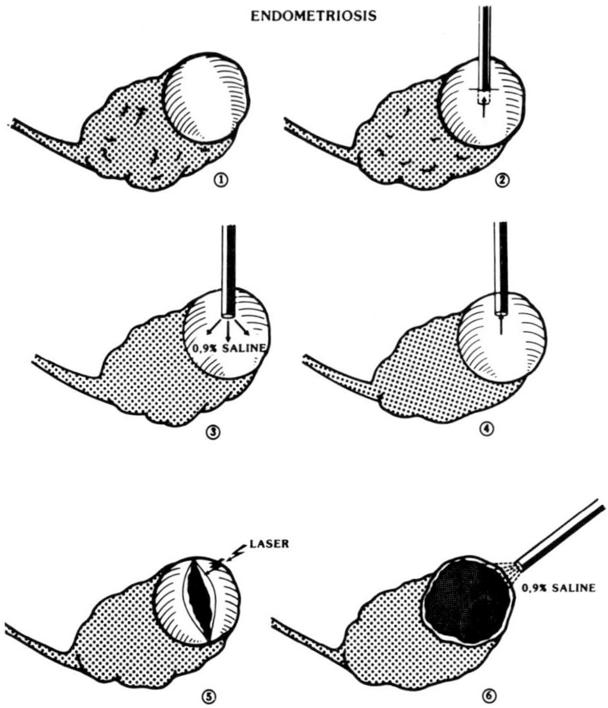

Figure 4.4 Ovarian endometriosis (1) treated by the CO_2 laser laparoscope. Any chocolate material is aspirated with the help of an aspirating canula (2) and the cyst is washed with irrigation fluid (3,4). The vaporization of the interior wall of the endometrioma is then carried out until follicles are encountered (5). At the end of the laser procedure, copious irrigation (6) is carried out to remove deposits of carbonized particles.

posterior cul-de-sac signifies complete disappearance of palpable deposits (Sutton, 1989a). Intermittent irrigation with a jet of 0.9% saline or Ringer lactate is helpful throughout the procedure to wash off debris and provide a backstop for the laser beam.

4.4.2 OVARIAN ENDOMETRIOSIS (Figure 4.4)

Ovarian endometriosis is treated if no greater than 3 cm of penetration into the ovary and no larger than 3 cm of diameter cyst are present. Pulses of laser energy are fired into the endometriomas. Small endometriotic implants on the surface of the ovary are vaporized until follicles containing fluid are encountered or no further pigmented tissue is seen. Large endometriomas are destroyed as follows: a 3- to 4-mm portion of the top of the cyst is excised, the chocolate-coloured material aspirated, and the cyst washed out with irrigation fluid. After washing, the interior wall of the cyst is carefully examined to confirm the absence of any suspected intracystic lesion (ovarian cystoscopy). With a power setting of 25–30 W and continuous mode application, the interior wall of the cyst is then vaporized to destroy the mucosal lining of the cyst. The vaporization continues until no further pigment is seen. The ovarian incision is left open to heal by secondary intention or if the endometrioma is large the incision edges are sealed with a fibrin glue (Tissucol).

As a safety measure, irrigation fluid (0.9% saline or Ringer lactate) can be introduced into the pelvis to protect the bowel and pelvic sidewalls from the inadvertent scatter of the laser beam. At the end of the laser procedure, copious irrigation of the pelvic cavity is carried out to prevent deposits of carbon-containing plume which may be irritating to the peritoneum. At the end of the procedure and following the removal of blood from the cul-de-sac, 100–200 ml of 32% Dextran 70 can be instilled into the peritoneal cavity.

4.4.3 'ENDOMETRIOTIC' ADHESIONS (Figure 4.5)

In many patients, post-operative or post-infectious adhesions are amenable to vaporization by laser laparoscopy. When compared with the standard technique of cautery and the use of the laparoscopic scissors or blunt dissection, there is probably no difference in the outcome when the adhesions are small and avascular. With more vascular adhesions or particularly thick tubo-ovarian adhesions, however, the CO_2 laser allows more precise destruction of the adhesions with minimal injury to the adjacent normal tissue. Filmy peritubal and periovarian adhesions are easily vaporized with the operative laser laparoscope or the laser probe with its backstop (Figure 4.5). When this probe is used, the adhesion is placed across the 'firing' platform and the laser is fired to vaporize the band.

Salpingolysis is usually performed by applying traction to adhesions by suprapubic grasping forceps or by the smooth manipulating probe. Frequently, adhesions are incised without the need of a separate backstop. Manipulating the Fallopian tube is avoided as much as possible.

Ovariolysis is performed by applying traction to the utero-ovarian ligaments with the smooth manipulating probe. Elevation and rotation of the ovary are made while continuing traction and torsion. Adhesions can be easily dissected from the ovarian surface and vaporized. Care is taken to apply traction only to adhesions and not to the ovary

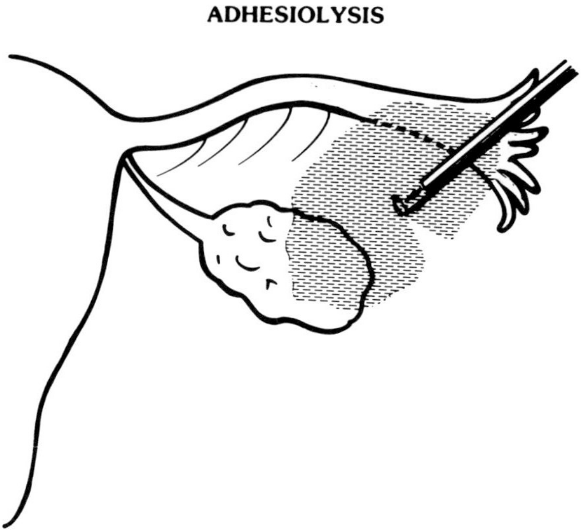

Figure 4.5 Filmy peritubal and periovarian adhesions. When the probe with its backstop is used, the adhesion is placed across the 'firing' platform and the laser is fired to vaporize the band.

or the Fallopian tube. Care is also taken not to apply too much traction, for fear of tearing the adhesion at its attachment. This results in bleeding which, in this very vascular area, can be difficult to stop. In a first series, a pregnancy rate of 60 and 50% was obtained, respectively, after adhesiolysis for adhesions of degree I (filmy and avascular) and II (dense and vascular but not very thick) (Donnez, 1987a).

4.4.4 SAFETY MEASURES

During adhesiolysis, the use of the probe with a backstop eliminates the risk of inadvertent injury to intraperitoneal structures. Irrigation fluid can be introduced into the pelvis to protect the bowel from inadvertent scatter of the laser beam.

4.4.5 PRECAUTIONS

At the end of the procedure, the peritoneal cavity is irrigated with Ringer's solution to remove carbonized particles and to avoid their implantation and 'phagocytosis' by macrophages (Figure 4.6). Thereafter, following the removal of fluid from the cul-de-sac, 100–200 ml of 32% Dextran 70 is instilled into the peritoneum.

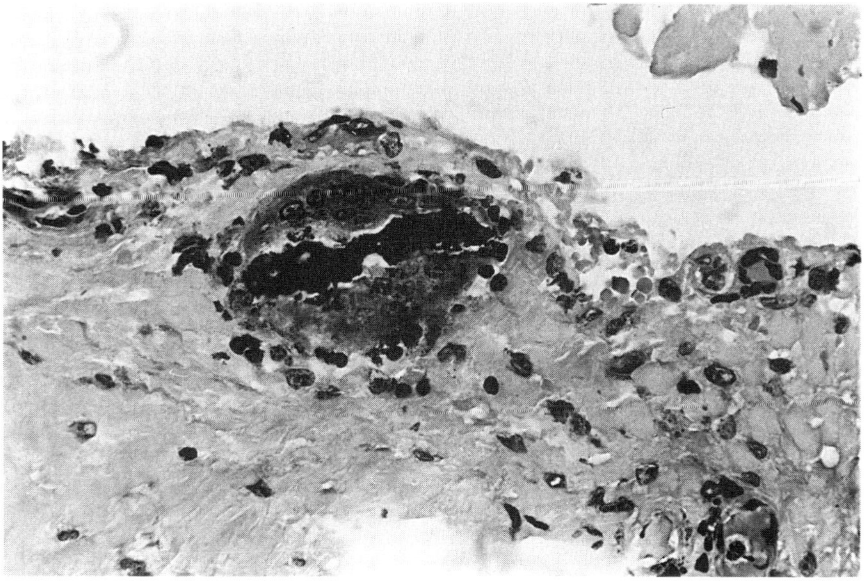

Figure 4.6 Peritoneal biopsy taken after 2 months implant vaporization. Presence of carbonized particules and macrophages. (Gomori's Trichrome, × 260.)

4.5 Results

In a first series of 1000 laser laparoscopies (Table 4.1), 487 patients underwent laser laparoscopy for endometriosis. In this series, no complication such as bladder injury, bowel injury or ureteral injury occurred.

Results of a first study (Donnez *et al.*, 1987a,b) with a follow-up of more than 18 months are shown in Table 4.2. Considering pregnancies resulting in full-term infants, the pregnancy rate in patients with endometriosis (group I) was 57% for a follow-up period of 18 months. A viable pregnancy rate of 62% was attained in mild endometriosis. The viable pregnancy rates in moderate and severe endometriosis were 52 and 42%, respectively. No ectopic pregnancy occurred. There were three spontaneous abortions. In group II (pelvic adhesions without endometriosis), a viable pregnancy rate of 57% was achieved. The pregnancy rates were 62 and 50%, respectively, after adhesiolysis for adhesions of degrees I and II. The operating time varied from 30 to 60 min. All patients were released in good condition the following day. Typical post-laparoscopy pain, such as pelvic discomfort and signs of

Table 4.1 Indications for laser laparoscopy in 1000 consecutive patients

Indication	*n*
Luna	101
Tuboplasty	139
Fimbrioplasty	112
Salpingoneostomy	27
Endometriosis	488
Mild (peritoneal only)	271
Moderate (ovarian cyst)	—
Severe (ovarian cyst)	217
Pelvic adhesions	266
Salpingolysis	112
Salpingo-ovariolysis	154
Tubal pregnancy	6

Table 4.2 Viable pregnancy rate in 124 patients for a follow-up period of 18 months

	No. of patients	*No. of pregnancies (%)*
Endometriosis		
Mild	42	26 (62)
Moderate	21	11 (52)
Severe	7	3 (42)
Total	70	40 (57)
Adhesions		
Degree I	32	20 (62)
Degree II	22	11 (50)
Total	54	31 (57)
Total	124	71 (57)

diaphragmatic irritation, was the most common post-operative complaint and was relatively short-term.

In the first series of 70 patients with endometriosis, eight of them underwent a second-look laparoscopy 3 months after the laser procedure. Absence of both endometriosis and adhesions was confirmed. In some sites where vaporization of endometriotic implants or cysts had been carried out, black pigments were visualized. Biopsy of such

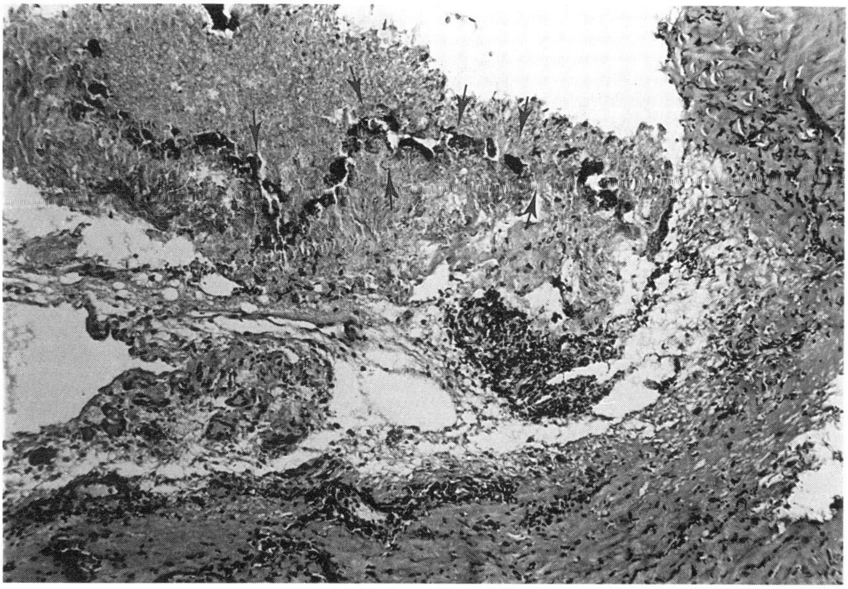

Figure 4.7 Ovarian biopsy in a site where vaporization of an endometriotic cyst (3 cm in diameter) has been carried out. The line (arrows) with black pigments represents the walls of the cyst after healing. (Gomori's Trichrome, × 110.)

implants was performed for histologic study. Presence of carbonized particles (Figure 4.7) was proved without plasma cell infiltration. Absence of endometriosis was confirmed by serial sections.

Table 4.3 shows studies in which women were treated with laser therapy only, resulting in a 54% overall pregnancy rate. Our results confirm other studies and suggest that laser laparoscopy can be as efficacious as laparotomy in experienced hands. However, no data exist regarding its value when compared with expectant management and particularly in cases of mild endometriosis where a number of reports indicate that a relatively high rate of pregnancy may be expected in patients with mild endometriosis, although their monthly fecundity rate is considerably less than that of the general population. As suggested by Olive and Haney (1986), the institution of future randomized trials should help to clarify these issues.

In our study, efficient removal of endometriosis and absence of adhesions were confirmed in patients by a second-look laparoscopy. The finding of black pigment at the site of laser vaporization probably results from insufficient irrigation of the pelvic cavity to prevent deposits of carbonized particles. Nevertheless, no adhesions were found

Table 4.3 Surgical treatment of endometriosis via laser laparoscopy

Reference	*No. of patients*	*No. of pregnancies (%)*
Kelly and Roberts (1983)	10	6 (60)
Feste (1985)	58	30 (52)
Davis (1986)	65	37 (57)
Martin and Olive (unpublished data)	80	33 (41)
Nezhat *et al.* (1986)	102	62 (60)
Donnez (1987a)	70	40 (57)
Sutton and Hill (1990)	56	45 (80)
Total	441	253 (58)

around the deposits which were covered by a new peritoneal layer. The absence of lymphocyte and plasma cells established that complete healing had occurred without an inflammatory reaction (Figure 4.7). In an experimental study the same histologic data were found in the mouse ovary after CO_2 laser treatment (Donnez *et al.*, 1987a). Other advantages were found in this study. The precision achieved by the CO_2 laser allows the experienced operator to remove superficial endometriosis near the ureter or on the bowel. The magnification attained with the laparoscope and the precision of the CO_2 laser beam allows precise removal of diseased tissue in many sites which could not be treated by electrocautery.

4.5.1 HORMONAL AND MICROSURGICAL THERAPY

Although the definition of conservative surgery is still 'the destruction of as much endometriosis as possible while preserving childbearing function', the technical advances of *in-vitro* fertilization, embryo transfer and embryo donation allow the maintenance of the uterus as the sole prerequisite for the implantation and delivery of a viable infant. This means that the surgical removal of endometriosis in women who wish to have children will change dramatically. The tools of surgery are also expanding from the scalpel to include the laser, for both laparoscopy and laparotomy. Critical studies on the use of lasers in endometriosis are still limited, so that a review of the more traditional surgical interventions has to serve as a basis for comparison.

(a) Conservative surgery

Without taking into account the stage of endometriosis, pregnancy rates after conservative surgery range from 33.3 to 87.5% (Olive and

Haney, 1986). However, the figures for the different stages of the disease show the chances of conception to be 66–75% for mild, 37–74% for moderate, and 0–40% for severe endometriosis. Improved pregnancy rates have been reported with atraumatic microsurgery. This was used in 176 women whose cumulative pregnancy rates, using life table methods, were 28.8% after 1 year and 40.5% after 2 years (Gordts, Boeckx and Brogens, 1984) Gordts *et al.* (1984) suggested that careful reconstruction of the tubo-ovarian interface and the surrounding peritoneum, without incidental appendicectomy or presacral neurectomy, may make the chances of conception in the different stages (American Fertility Society, 1979, 1985) of endometriosis more equal.

(b) *Combined (hormonal and microsurgical) therapy*

The concept of combining pre-operative hormonal therapy with microsurgery was suggested by us in 1978. Combined therapy probably improves the post-operative pregnancy rate because it facilitates surgery and possibly lowers the risk of post-operative adhesions by decreasing pelvic vascularity.

The hormonal management of endometriosis has undergone significant evolution in the two past decades (Sutton and Hill, 1990). In the 1960s, the introduction of 'progestogen only' regimens resulted in a marked improvement in the medical management of endometriosis. In the last decade, three new agents: Danazol, Gestrinone and gonadotrophin releasing hormone (GnRH) agonist, have created further options in the hormonal treatment of endometriosis. In a recent study (Donnez *et al.*, 1987b; Donnez, Nisolle and Casanas-Roux, 1990), the use of different hormonal agents was evaluated in order to compare the resolution of disease after 6 months of therapy and the pregnancy rates after combined (hormonal and microsurgical) therapy.

Resolution of ovarian disease was based upon the decrease in size of ovarian endometriomas. Although the effect of Danazol in decreasing active endometriotic tissue has been well documented in other studies (Dmowski and Cohen, 1975; Barbieri, Canick and Makris, 1977; Buttram and Reiter, 1981; Seibel, Berber and Weinstein, 1982), the efficacy of Danazol was not proven in our study (Donnez, Nisolle and Casanas-Roux, 1990). Indeed, ovarian endometriosis regressed in only 30% of cases. Moreover, the lesions were more severe after Danazol in 27% of cases. Buttram and Reiter (1981) found also that ovarian disease >1 cm (typically invasive endometrioma) responded less well to Danazol than peritoneal and superficial ovarian endometriosis. The results obtained with Gestrinone were similar to those obtained with Danazol. When compared, Buserelin (GnRH analogue) emerged superior to Danazol or Gestrinone treatment. Indeed, ovarian endometriotic

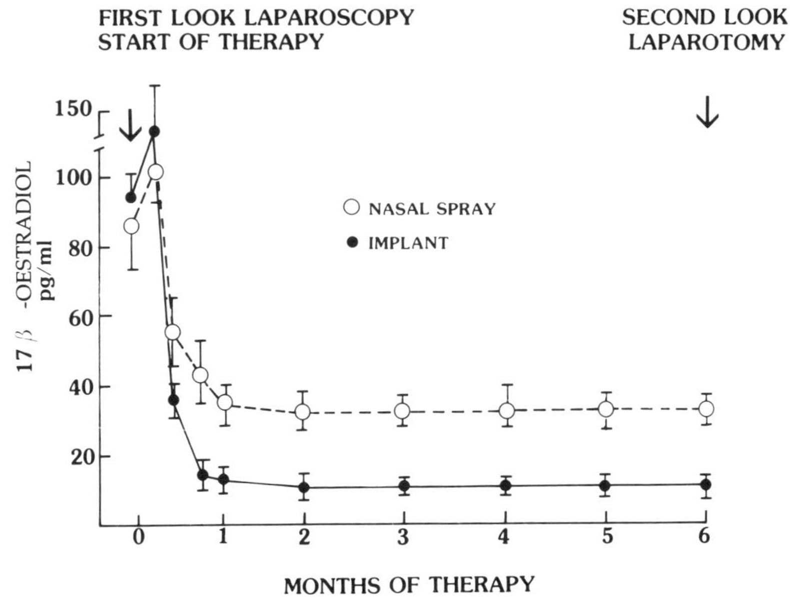

Figure 4.8 E_2 serum concentrations during GnRH agonist therapy.

lesions regressed in more than 70% of cases in moderate endometriosis and 66% of cases in severe endometriosis.

The classification schemes [Acosta (Acostra, Buttram and Besch, 1973), AFS (American Fertility Society, 1979) and RAFS (American Fertility Society, 1985)] were not helpful in documenting resolution of ovarian endometriosis following hormonal therapy. They are based upon the total area of endometriosis involving the peritoneum and/or ovaries; frequently the implants and cysts appeared less active surrounded by reduced pelvic vascularity and inflammation, although the total amount of disease and the size did not decrease.

In moderate endometriosis, when the scores found before and after hormonal therapy were compared, the most important difference between the scores before and after therapy was found among women treated with Buserelin. The data were in agreement with a previous study (Nisolle, Casanas-Roux and Donnez, 1988) in which a lower mitotic index was found in ectopic glandular epithelium after Buserelin therapy than that observed after either Lynestrenol or Gestrinone therapy. The 'medical oophorectomy' caused by GnRH agonist allows temporary suppression of ovarian function. Two weeks after first administration, the production of gonadal steroids reaches post-oophorectomy levels, lower than <30 pg/ml (Figure 4.8).

In our series of 180 infertile women with moderate and severe

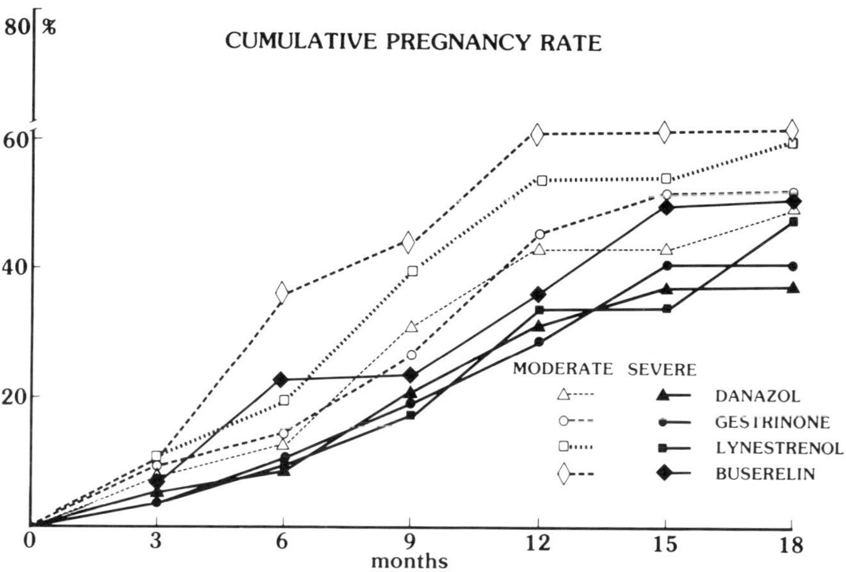

Figure 4.9 Cumulative pregnancy rates obtained after combined (hormonal and microsurgical) therapy.

endometriosis (AFS, 1979), hormonal therapy was given for 6 months prior to microsurgery for endometriosis resection (Lynestrenol, Gestrinone, Danazol, or Buserelin, a potent GnRH agonist). They were followed for a period of 18 months (Donnez, Nisolle and Casanas-Roux, 1989).

4.5.2 PREGNANCY RATES (Figure 4.9)

Considering pregnancies resulting in viable infants, the pregnancy rate was 50% for a follow-up period of 18 months. The pregnancy rate in moderate endometriosis (53%) differed significantly ($P < 0.05$) from the rate obtained in severe endometriosis (45%). Spontaneous abortion rate was less than 5%. No ectopic pregnancy occurred. The pregnancy rate (58%) obtained after Buserelin is significantly higher ($P < 0.05$) than those obtained after Danazol (45%) or Gestrinone (47%). Among women with moderate endometriosis, the following pregnancy rates were found: group Danazol 48%; group Gestrinone 48%; group Lynestrenol 53% and group Buserelin 61%. Among women with severe endometriosis, the following pregnancy rates were found: group Danazol 38%; group Gestrinone 42%; group Lynestrenol 49% and group Buserelin 53%.

In terms of pregnancy rates, significant differences were noted, depending on the type of drug used. In moderate endometriosis, the pregnancy rate varies from 48% (Danazol) to 61% (Buserelin). In cases of severe endometriosis, the rate varies from 38% (Danazol) to 53% (Buserelin).

When the data of the present study are compared with data reported by Olive and Haney (1986) (moderate endometriosis, pregnancy rate 50%; severe endometriosis, pregnancy rate 39%), it seems clear that pre-operative hormonal treatment (when effective as in the Buserelin group) improves the conception rate after surgery. As suggested in a previous study, the advantage of an efficacious hormonal treatment consists of a reduction of pelvic vascularity and inflammation, often present around endometriosis foci. Unfortunately, these parameters are not evaluated in any staging system. The improved pelvic environment facilitates the technical aspects of surgery and we believe it reduces the risk of post-operative adhesion formation.

In conclusion, the high percentage of 'responders' and the decreased severity scores observed in the Buserelin group suggest that LHRH analogues are the most effective agents in the resolution of disease. But menopausal symptoms (hot flushes, vaginal thinning and bone loss) are also induced. Bone loss was reversible and complete recovery was obtained 4 months after the cessation of therapy (De Vogelaer *et al.*, 1987).

Despite its relative better efficacy, when compared to other drugs, Buserelin was unable to completely suppress endometriotic cells because ectopic foci are not governed by the normal control mechanisms governing the uterine endometrial glands and stroma. This fact provides the scientific basis for the surgical removal of invasive ovarian endometriosis which is performed most effectively and precisely by the CO_2 laser.

4.6 Conclusion: the future

New delivery systems are now under clinical investigation (Donnez *et al.*, submitted). Indeed, sustained release systems for LHRH analogues can be administered by injection with implants or microcapsules. Sustained Buserelin release from implants of polyhydroxybutyric acid or polylactic-glycolic acid has been effective in suppressing oestrogen or androgen secretion.

Resolution of ovarian disease is based upon the decrease in size of endometriomas. Increments of 25% are considered sufficient to discriminate between and evaluate the two delivery systems. When compared, the Buserelin implant emerged superior to the Buserelin spray.

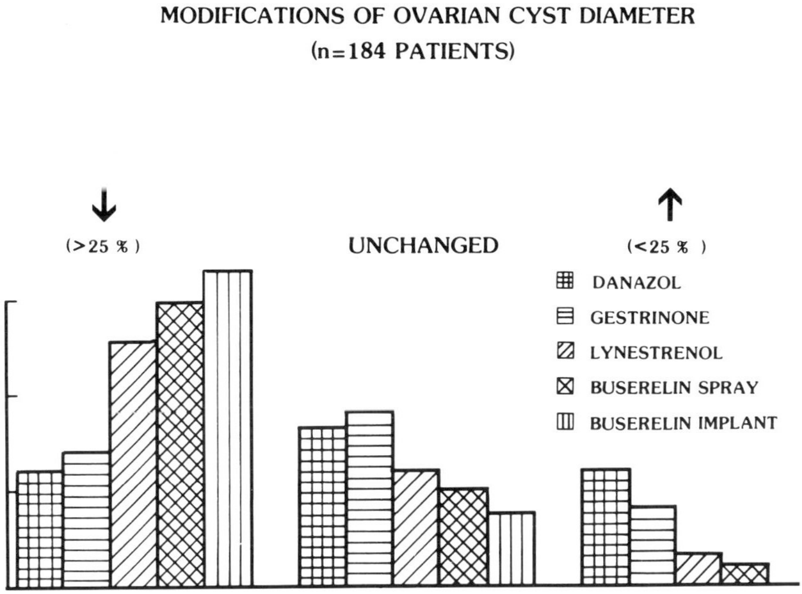

Figure 4.10 Modifications of ovarian cyst diameter (n = 184 patients) by 6 months of hormonal therapy: Danazol, Gestrinone, Lynestrenol, Buserelin spray and Buserelin implant.

Indeed, ovarian endometriosis regressed more often in the Buserelin implant group than in the Buserelin spray group (Figure 4.10).

A significant lower incidence of active endometriosis and lower mitotic index was observed in the Buserelin implant group when compared to data from the nasal spray group (Donnez *et al.*, 1988). The differences observed in this study between the intranasal group and the subcutaneous group demonstrate that lower circulating levels of E_2 during therapy are correlated with a greater resolution of the disease. Although intranasal Buserelin (900 μg/daily) was effective in producing low serum oestrogen levels (<30 pg/ml), anovulation and amenorrhoea, the E_2 levels obtained by the sustained release delivery system are significantly lower than those obtained with the intranasal therapy (Figure 4.8). The difference between the intranasal and subcutaneous group can be explained by variation in patient compliance, by decreased bioavailability of medication delivered by nasal spray or by more constant Buserelin serum levels obtained by the subcutaneous implant.

LHRH agonist therapy is effective in reducing endometriotic size to a greater extent than is possible with other drugs. The subcutaneous implant method of administration achieved a more consistent inhibition

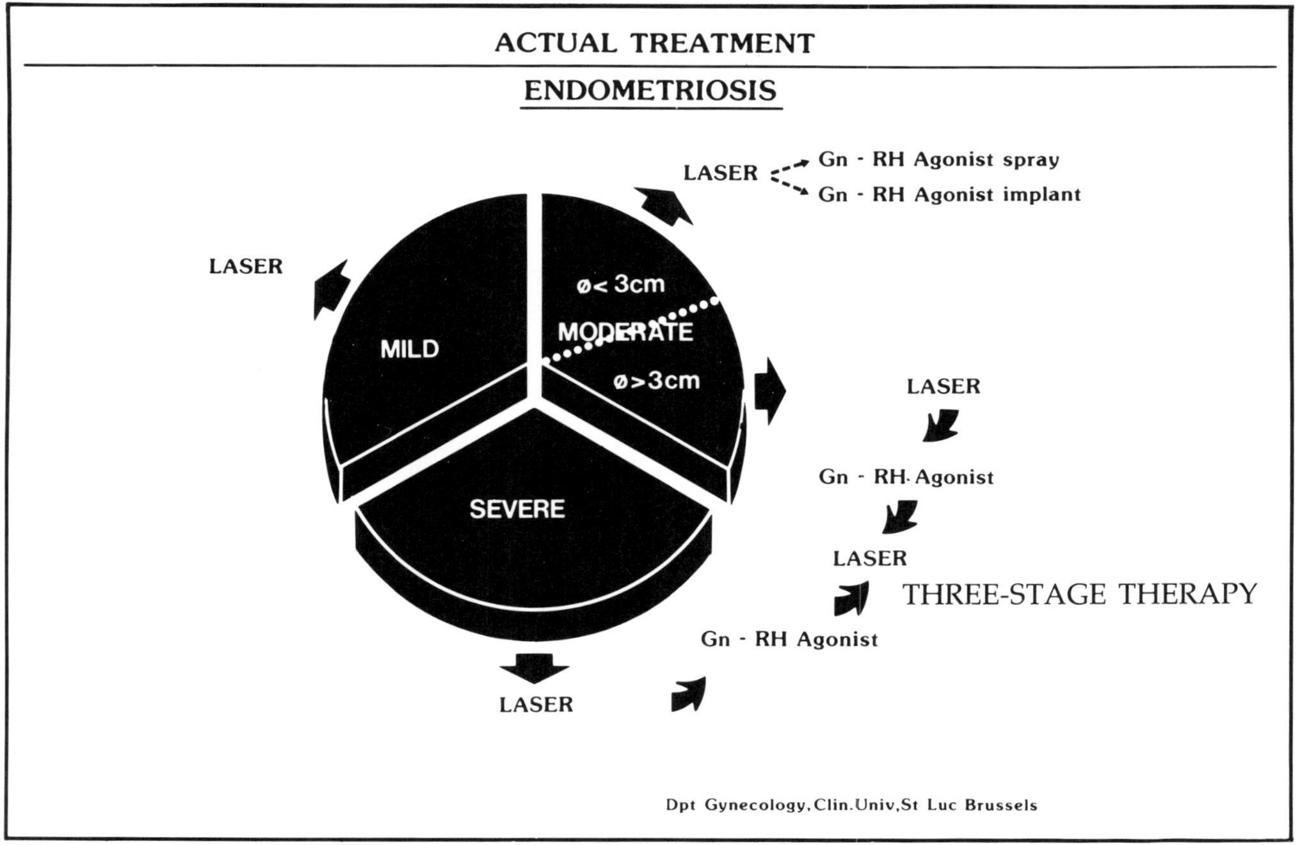

Figure 4.11 Treatment in infertile women with endometriosis according to the severity of the disease (AFS classification). *Mild* endometriosis: laser laparoscopy. *Moderate* endometriosis (ovarian endometrial cyst <3 cm in diameter): laser laparoscopy following by hormonal (GnRH agonist) therapy. *Moderate* endometriosis (ovarian cyst >3 cm in diameter) and *severe* endometriosis: three-stage therapy (see text).

of the pituitary ovarian axis than nasal administration. We feel that treatment by sustained release preparations is an effective, and probably superior, alternative to existing steroid hormones prior to laser laparoscopy (De Vogelaer *et al.*, 1987; Donnez *et al.*, 1988). Indeed, the effectiveness of the Buserelin subcutaneous implant is such that it permits an important reduction of large ovarian cyst diameter so that a second-look laparoscopy can be carried out for laser vaporization or residual endometriosis without a high risk of subsequent periovarian adhesion formation.

After several modes of treatment have been evaluated, the therapeutic regimen according to the schema of Figure 4.11 has been employed in our department. Combining hormonal and surgical treatment seems to be the best approach to infertility associated with moderate and severe endometriosis. In cases of mild/AFS endometriosis, CO_2 laser laparoscopy permits vaporization of peritoneal implants. In cases of moderate/AFS endometriosis (with ovarian cyst diameter <3 cm), lysis of adhesions and vaporization of the interior wall of the endometrial cyst are carried out by CO_2 laser laparoscopy. In cases of more severe endometriosis (moderate/AFS with ovarian cyst <3 cm or severe/AFS), three-stage therapy is proposed as the optimal approach to treatment.

1. Adhesiolysis, vaporization of peritoneal implants and small ovarian (<3 cm) endometriomas as much as possible. Fenestration, irrigation and removal of chocolale fluid from ovarian cysts <3 cm in diameter.
2. Hormonal therapy for 3 months (GnRH agonist implant).
3. Second-look laparoscopy and laser vaporization of residual ovarian cyst.

So far, this *three-stage therapy* has been performed in more than 200 cases of ovarian endometriomas. If our study continues to show pregnancy rates to be equivalent to those treated by laparotomy, CO_2 laser laparoscopy will become the preferred procedure for the management of pelvic endometriosis-associated infertility.

Endometriosis continues to baffle both scientists and clinicians. It is hoped that further insight into many areas of research will resolve both the pathogenesis and the relationship between endometriosis and infertility.

References

Acosta, A. A., Buttram, C. J. Jr and Besch, P. K. (1973), A proposed classification of pelvic endometriosis. *Obstet. Gynecol.*, **42**, 19.

American Fertility Society (1979), Classification of endometriosis. *Fertil. Steril.*, **32**, 633.

American Fertility Society (1985), Revised American Fertility Society classification of endometriosis. *Fertil. Steril.*, **43**, 351.

Barbieri, R. L., Canick, J. A. and Makris, A. (1977), Danazol inhibits steroidogenesis. *Fertil. Steril.*, **28**, 809.

Bruhat, M., Mage, G. and Manes, M. (1979), Use of the CO_2 laser via laparoscopy. In *Laser Surgery III*. Proceedings from the Third International Society for Laser Surgery (ed. I. Kaplan), International Society for Laser Surgery, Tel Aviv, p. 275.

Buttram, V. C. Jr and Reiter, R. C. (1981), Uterine leiomyomata: etiology, symptomatology and management. *Fertil. Steril.*, **36**, 433.

Daniell, J. F. and Brown, D. H. (1982), Carbon dioxide laser laparoscopy: initial experience in experimental animals and humans. *Obstet. Gynecol.*, **159**, 761.

Daniell, J. F. and Pittaway, D. E. (1982), Use of the CO_2 laser in laparoscopy surgery: initial experience with the second puncture technique. *Infertility*, **5**, 15.

Davis, G. D. (1986), Management of endometriosis and its associated adhesions with the CO_2 laser laparoscope. *Obstet. Gynecol.*, **68**, 422.

De Vogelaer, J. P., Nagant de Deuxchaisnes, C., Donnez, J. and Thomas, K. (1987), LH-RH analogues and bone loss. *Lancet*, I, 1498.

Dmowski, W. P. and Cohen, M. R. (1975), Treatment of endometriosis with an antigonadotropin, danazol: A laparoscopic and histologic evaluation. *Obstet. Gynecol.*, **46**, 147.

Donnez, J. (1987a), CO_2 laser laparoscopy in infertile women with adhesions or endometriosis. *Fertil. Steril.*, **48**, 390.

Donnez, J. (1987b), *CO_2 Laser in Intraepithelial Neoplasia and in Infertility* (ed. J. Donnez), Nauwelaerts Printing, Leuven, Belgium.

Donnez, J., Fernandez, C., Willems, T. and Casanas-Roux, F. (1987a), Experimental ovarian CO_2 laser surgery. In *CO_2 Laser in Intraepithelial Neoplasia and in Infertility* (ed. J. Donnez), Nauwelaerts Printing, Leuven, Belgium, p. 25.

Donnez, J., Lemaire, M., Karaman, Y., Nisolle-Pochet, M. and Casanas-Roux, F. (1987b), Combined (hormonal and microsurgical) therapy in infertile women with endometriosis. *Fertil. Steril.*, **48**, 239.

Donnez, J., Nisolle-Pochet, M., Clerckx-Braun, F. and Casanas-Roux, F. (1988), Combined (hormonal and microsurgical) therapy in endometriosis. *Gynecol. Endocrinol.*, **2**, 81.

Donnez, J., Nisolle, M. and Casanas-Roux, F. (1990), Endometriosis associated infertility. Evaluation of preoperative use of Danazol, Gestrinone and Buserelin. *Int. J. Fert.*, **35**, 297–301.

Donnez, J., Schrurs, B., Gillerot, S., Sandow, J. and Clerckx, F. (1989), Treatment of uterine fibroids with implants of gonadotropin releasing hormone agonist: assessment hysterography. *Fertil. Steril.*, **51**, 947–50.

Feste, J.R. (1985), Laser laparoscopy: a new modality. *J. Reprod. Med.*, **30**, 413.

Gordts, S., Boeckx, W. and Brosens, I. (1984), Microsurgery of endometriosis in infertile patients. *Fertil. Steril.*, **42**, 520.

Kelly, R. W. and Roberts, D. K. (1983), CO_2 laser laparoscopy; a potential alternative to danazol in the treatment of stage I and II endometriosis. *J. Reprod. Med.*, **28**, 638.

Nezhat, C., Crowgey, S. R. and Garrison, C. P. (1986), Surgical treatment of endometriosis via laser laparoscopy. *Fertil. Steril.*, **45**, 778.

Nisolle, M., Casanas-Roux, F. and Donnez, J. (1988), Histologic study of ovarian endometriosis after hormonal therapy. *Fertil. Steril.*, **49**, 423.

Olive, D. L. and Haney, A. F. (1986), Endometriosis-associated infertility: a critical review of therapeutic approaches. *Obstet. Gynecol. Surv.*, **41**, 538.

Seibel, M. M., Berber, M. J. and Weinstein, F. G. (1982), The effectiveness of Danazol on subsequent fertility in minimal endometriosis. *Fertil. Steril.*, **38**, 534.

Sutton, C. J. G. (1989a), Laser uterine nerve ablation. In *Laser Operative Laparoscopy and Hysteroscopy*. (ed. J. Donnez), Nauwelaerts, Leuven, Belgium, pp. 43–52.

Sutton, C. J. G. (1989b), Carbon dioxide laser laparoscopy in the treatment of endometriosis. In *Baillière's Clinical Obstetrics and Gynaecology*, Vol. 3. (ed. C. J. G. Sutton), Baillière Tindall, London, pp. 449–523.

Sutton, C. J. G. and Hill, D. (1990), Laser laparoscopy in the treatment of endometriosis. A 5-year study. *Br. J. Obstet. Gynaecol.*, **97**, 181–5.

Tadir, Y., Kaplan, I., Zuckerman, Z., Edelstein, T. and Ovadia, J. (1984), New instrumentation and technique for laparoscopic carbon dioxide laser operations: a preliminary report. *Obstet. Gynecol.*, **63**, 582.

Wilson, E. A. (1988), Surgical therapy for endometriosis. *Clin. Obstet. Gynaecol.* **31**, No. 4.

5 *Adhesions and laser laparoscopic adhesiolysis*

RUSSELL MACDONALD and CHRIS SUTTON

5.1 Introduction

The clinical and pathological effects of intra-abdominal adhesions have not been elucidated. There are a number of reasons for this. Adhesions within the abdominal cavity are common and it is likely that in the majority of locations they are incidental. Adhesions are also the inevitable consequence of any laparotomy, regardless of how meticulous and painstaking the surgeon's technique. Even following microsurgical adhesiolysis, significant adhesions remain in 75% of cases (Decherney and Mezer, 1984) and *de novo* adhesions, i.e. new adhesions, form in over 50% of cases (Diamond *et al.*, 1987). An inability to perform effective adhesiolysis, coupled with the likelihood that the situation may actually be made worse has, not surprisingly, led to the virtual extinction of adhesiolysis as a general surgical procedure.

Gynaecologists, however, have not been so dismissive. Pelvic adhesiolysis is still commonly practised and is indicated both for the treatment of pelvic pain and infertility. But how effective are these gynaecological procedures? Are they justified by post-operative results, and, if so, can patient care be improved by altering technique?

5.2 What is the mechanism of adhesion formation?

The incidence of intra-abdominal adhesions has been established in a large post-mortem study involving 252 cadaver examinations (Weibel and Majno, 1973). Adhesions were categorized as either spontaneous or post-operative. Spontaneous adhesions were found in 28% of cases not previously having undergone surgery. Significantly more spontaneous adhesions were identified in patients over 60 years old. Post-operative adhesions were much more common – an incidence of 67% and in cases having undergone multiple procedures this rose to 93%.

These figures have recently been corroborated by a prospective clinical study carried out at the time of laparotomy (Menzies and Ellis, 1989a), which estimated the incidence of spontaneous and post-operative adhesions to be 10.4 and 93%, respectively. An aetiological link with age and a strong association with intra-abdominal surgery can therefore be concluded.

A number of more specific factors predisposing to adhesion formation have also been identified. Peritoneal inflammation regardless of how it is caused, whether due to tissue injury, infection or reaction to chemical agents or a foreign body, will cause adhesions (Ellis, 1971). Tissue ischaemia, due to ligatures or peritoneal grafts, is particularly likely to cause adhesions (Ellis, 1962). Superficial peritoneal injury, either due to drying or abrasion (Ryan, Grobety and Majno, 1971), will also lead to adhesion formation, but only in the presence of fresh clotted blood or plasma. Peritoneal damage due to drying and superficial abrasion is not easily prevented during laparotomy. Keeping the peritoneum moist with normal saline or Ringer's solution will not prevent adhesions forming (Ryan *et al.*, 1971). Possibly other factors, simply associated with opening the abdominal cavity, are implicated.

It has long been recognized that fresh blood alone, even in large quantities, without adjacent peritoneal damage, will not produce adhesions (Adams, 1913). Defibrinated blood, plasma or serum, washed erythrocytes and heparinized blood products are also insufficient (Ryan *et al.*, 1971), even in the presence of peritoneal damage. Fresh blood or plasma plus peritoneal damage is required. Therefore, an intact coagulation system is also fundamental to adhesion formation.

What is the effect of peritoneal damage? Traditional theory dictates that this promotes coagulation and fibrin deposition. However, there is substantial evidence that the critical defect associated with peritoneal damage is diminished fibrinolysis rather than enhanced fibrin deposition. Normal peritoneum produces fibrinolysins and will lyse fibrinous adhesions. Fibrinolysin production in damaged peritoneum is defective and is insufficient to stop transformation to permanent fibrous adhesions.

The hypothesis that adhesions are a manifestion of defective healing and repair rather than directly due to tissue damage is not new. However, the mechanisms which support this theory, have only recently been established and are outlined in Figure 5.1.

What is the evidence for this pathway? Following peritoneal insult a fibrin-rich serosanguinous exudate is produced (Trompke and Siegner, 1956). This exudate coagulates, usually within 3 hours, forming a fibrinous mesh which tethers adjacent peritoneal surfaces. The fibrinous attachments to normal peritoneum are lysed within a few days (Jackson, 1958). If lysis does not occur, the fibrinous adhesions become organ-

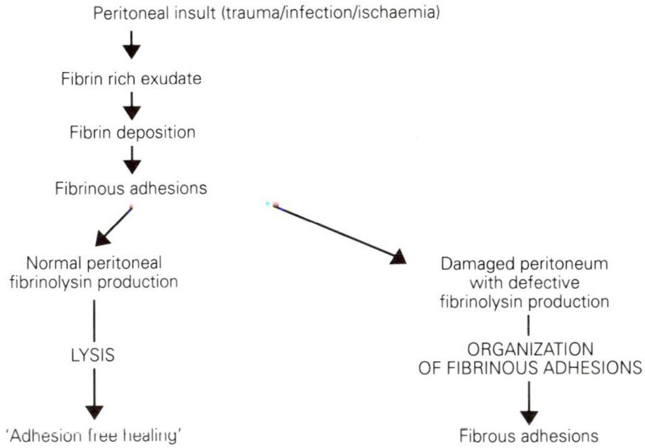

Figure 5.1 The pathogenesis of intra-abdominal adhesions. (From Menzies and Ellis, 1989b.)

ized – fibroblast proliferation takes place and collagen is laid down (Milligan and Raferty, 1974). The adhesions become fibrous, are insensitive to fibrinolysins and are therefore permanent.

The ability of the peritoneum to absorb fibrinous agglutinations has been recognized for some time (Hertzler, 1919). How fibrinolysis occurred was unknown until plasminogen activator activity (PAA) was demonstrated within the peritoneal mesothelium (Myhre-Jensen, Larsen and Astrup, 1969; Porter *et al.*, 1969). This activator converts an enzyme precursor, plasminogen, which is found freely circulating in blood and in interstitial fluid, to a fibrin splitting protease, plasmin (Dano *et al.*, 1985). The concentration of plasminogen activator varies greatly in different tissues, reflecting quite different fibrinolytic potential. For example, particularly high levels are found in vascular connective tissue (Astrup, 1966). Activity is also present in blood vessels (Todd, 1959) and in various serosal and synovial membranes (Myhre-Jensen *et al.*, 1969). Although the activity exhibited by serosal surfaces is less than that of vascular endothelium, it is still thought to be sufficient to clear these surfaces of any fibrin laid down following peritoneal insult. Without this fibrinolytic capability effective healing and repair would be impossible and fibrous adhesions would be the inevitable consequence of any serosal damage.

To substantiate the above theory it must be possible to demonstrate that any peritoneal insult, likely to produce adhesions, is associated with a reduction in plasminogen activator activity and that artificial replacement of this deficit is associated with less adhesion formation.

Significantly reduced levels of peritoneal fibrinolytic activity have been demonstrated following peritoneal trauma due to abrasions, excisional defects, peritoneal grafting, crushing, diathermy and ischaemia (Gervin, Puckett and Silver, 1973; Buckman *et al.*, 1976; Rafferty, 1981). Reduced peritoneal fibrinolytic activity has also been demonstrated in the presence of inflammation (Thomspon *et al.*, 1989). Recently, recombinant plasminogen activator (rt-PA) has become available and animal studies have shown that when this agent is applied to areas of peritoneal injury likely to produce adhesions or following adhesiolysis, subsequent adhesion formation is greatly reduced (Doody, Dann and Buttram, 1989; Menzies and Ellis, 1989c). A key role for PAA in the prevention of adhesions is therefore apparent. The lack of side effects interfering with healing led these authors to conclude that their findings should initiate clinical trials involving the use of rt-PA for adhesion prophylaxis.

5.3 What are the clinical implications of adhesions?

Though the vast majority of intra-abdominal adhesions are clinically insignificant, in certain locations they may have pathological effects. There is little doubt that adhesions can precipitate bowel obstruction. They are therefore an accepted cause of acute abdominal pain. However, their association with chronic abdominal pain is a different matter and is controversial. Chronic abdominal pain is a common complaint and often a satisfactory explanation is not found. Intra-abdominal adhesions are also common and may be simply an incidental finding in a patient with chronic pain. However, adhesions which tether previously mobile viscera will produce pain and discomfort when put under tension. For instance, pelvic adhesions which tether the female reproductive organs are a recognized cause of dyspareunia. Is it reasonable to extend this argument to include adhesions which tether and restrict the mobility of the bowel? A case has been put forward to suggest this, particularly concerning intra-abdominal adhesions as a cause of chronic post-operative abdominal pain. At present this association is hypothetical: definite evidence is lacking. Properly controlled and randomized clinical trials are therefore needed.

Adhesions which tether viscera may also restrict function. For instance, tubo-ovarian adhesions impair fertility due to anatomical distortion causing interference with ovum pick-up and this constitutes the main indication for pelvic adhesiolysis in women.

5.4 Adhesions and abdominal pain

Although bowel obstruction secondary to adhesions is not common, it accounts for an appreciable proportion of the general surgical workload. Due to an overall increase in the incidence of abdominal surgery, there is evidence that the magnitude of this problem is increasing (Bevan, 1984). About 0.9% of all general surgical adult admissions are for adhesive obstruction. Surgery is indicated in half of these cases and they account for 3.3% of all laparotomies (Menzies and Ellis, 1989a). The procedure simply involves the release of offending adhesions and resection of any bowel which may have undergone irreversible ischaemic injury. Even if surgery is kept to a minimum, further adhesion formation is inevitable and the recurrence of intestinal obstruction may be as high as 32% (Brightwell, McFie and Aust, 1977). There would therefore seem to be a need for improvement in the treatment of this problem.

At present it is impossible to predict which type of adhesions are likely to cause obstruction. Even if this was possible, the risk of producing more adhesions outrules the possibility of prophylactic adhesiolysis employing standard surgical techniques. Surgery is only indicated in the presence of persistent obstruction and is essentially an emergency procedure.

The association between chronic abdominal pain and adhesions is less certain. A common view is that the association is nothing more than a poorly substantiated myth (Alexander-Williams, 1987). Supporting this myth is a retrospective study which examined a series of 100 consecutive laparoscopies for pelvic pain and compared these with 85 laparoscopies for infertility (Rapkin, 1986). There was no difference, with respect to location and adhesion density, between the groups. The report concluded that these findings questioned the role of pelvic adhesions as a cause of chronic abdominal pain. There were, however, some problems with the design of the study which made an acceptable conclusion difficult. The study was retrospective and patients with infertility were used as a control. Infertility patients will inevitably have a high incidence of adhesions and because of selection bias the majority will be asymptomatic. In the study 39% of the infertility patients exhibited pelvic adhesions as the only abnormal finding, compared with only 26% in the pain group. Only four of the 34 patients with infertility and adhesions complained of any pain. Perhaps it would have been more appropriate to have used a group of women undergoing laparoscopic sterilization as a control. Another report following a series of laparotomies for pelvic pain concluded that adhesions were likely to cause pain if the pelvic viscera were in some way immobilized or tethered (Chan and Wood, 1985), a conclusion more in line with current thinking, but the evidence presented in the paper scarcely justified such a conclusion. Unaccountable variables such as the removal of diseased viscera may have been the reason for symptomatic improvement.

5.5 Laparoscopic adhesiolysis for abdominal pain

The ineffectiveness of adhesiolysis by laparotomy means there is little place for this type of surgery in the treatment of chronic abdominal pain. Laparoscopic adhesiolysis is a different technique and seems to be worthwhile (Kleinhaus, 1984; Mecke, Semm and Lehman-Willenbrock, 1988; Daniell, 1989). Mecke *et al.* (1988) reported on 200 diagnostic laparoscopies for pelvic pain and identified adhesions without other pathology in 33% of cases. This is the expected proportion when laparoscoping women with pelvic pain (Kresch *et al.*, 1984; Rapkin, 1986). Eighty-four per cent of these women underwent complete adhesiolysis and of the 75% who were available for follow-up at 6 months, 58% were pain free or improved. Kleinhaus (1984) and Daniell (1989) only referred to post-operative adhesions associated with chronic pain. These adhesions usually involved bowel and the abdominal wall. Kleinhaus reported immediate and lasting relief of symptoms in two patients following lysis of post-appendicectomy adhesions and Daniell, in a much larger study involving 42 patients, reported either no symptoms or improved symptoms in 67% of cases.

In Guildford we have used laparoscopic adhesiolysis for the past 8 years employing the CO_2 laser and latterly the KTP-532 visible light laser which can be passed down flexible fibres to improve access in difficult situations. In 1986 we reported our initial experience with laser laparoscopic adhesiolysis (Sutton, 1986) and were impressed by the fact that 71% of the women treated claimed to be pain free following this relatively simple procedure and we were encouraged to find that none were actually made worse by the operation, there were no serious complications and, most importantly, there were no bowel injuries.

We have recently reviewed our results and, although latterly we have had an increase in secondary and even tertiary referrals who almost invariably have multiple adhesions, we have found that the overall success rate has remained virtually the same (Table 5.1). We have followed up a group of 118 patients between 1 and 5 years following laser laparoscopic adhesiolysis. All these patients presented with abdominal pain and at laparoscopy the site of the adhesions appeared to correlate with the patient's symptoms. Of the 118 patients treated eight were lost to follow-up but 84 (76%) claimed that they were better and the pain had gone, seven reported improvement in symptoms and the remaining 19 were not helped at all. No patients were made worse and all were treated as day cases or stayed in hospital for the first post-operative night and were discharged the following morning. One patient had to have a mini-laparotomy because the backstop of the adhesiolysis probe fractured in the valve

Table 5.1 Laser laparoscopic adhesiolysis for abdominal pain

Number of patients treated	118
Adhesions involving bowel	41
Associated endometriosis	36
Patients lost to follow up	8
Results of treatment	
Better	84 (76%)
Improved	7
No improvement	19
Total followed up (1–5 years)	n = 110

mechanism of the trochar and could not be retrieved laparoscopically. Another patient had a severe surgical emphysema which took 10 days to absorb, suggesting that it was due to a relatively insoluble gas such as air, nitrous oxide or nitrogen. Although we were never exactly certain from where this gas emanated it was probably due to the fact that the early lasers used nitrogen to cool the expensive laser lens to prevent thermal damage. We have never been able to explain why the gas leaked into the patient nor why it only happened to this one woman and has never been seen, even to a minor degree, in over 900 cases of laser laparoscopy performed before and since. Apart from these two patients who had a slightly prolonged recovery, the remainder returned to work or domestic activity within 48 h, although a few reported discomfort lasting about a week.

It must be stressed that the adhesions we were treating were not mere omental adhesions but thick adhesive bands that were tethering the viscera and impeding function, either bowel motility of the small or large bowel or ovum pick-up if they involved the Fallopian tube and ovary. In 36 patients the adhesions were associated with endometriosis and in 41 they involved the bowel, most of these being associated with a previous surgical operation. Although there is considerable scepticism over the significance adhesions have in the causation of abdominal pain it would require a prospective randomized trial to determine the answer. This would have to be performed in both men and women and would be difficult to organize due to the large number of variables involved. One would have to consider the type of laser used, the skill of the operator, the extent of the adhesions and the difficulty in assessing whether or not the procedure has been satisfactorily completed. This is easy when dividing a thick adhesive band but is difficult when adhesions are completely enveloping the ascending colon and binding it down to the peritoneal surface of the para-colic gutter. It would also be difficult to ethically justify a 'no-treatment' arm when three-quarters of our patients appear to have been helped by a simple procedure performed at the same time as the diagnostic laparoscopy.

5.6 Adhesions and infertility

There is little doubt that the gross anatomical distortion caused by extensive pelvic adhesions causes infertility. However, the effect less extensive tubo-ovarian adhesions have on fertility is not so clear. The common risk factors associated with this problem are previous surgery and salpingitis occurring in 59 and 42% of patients, respectively (Lacos, 1988). It has been estimated that after one pelvic infection the chance of infertility is 12.9%, after two infections 35% and following the third infection a huge 75% (Westrom, 1985). Ovulation is less likely to take place in patients with tubo-ovarian adhesions (Devroey *et al.*, 1985). In addition, tubo-ovarian adhesions may restrict movement of the tube and ovary and it is likely that this further impairs function. The mesotubarium ovarica (MTO), the structure which connects the ovary to the fimbrial end of the Fallopian tube, contains bundles of smooth muscle cells (Okamura, Morkawa and Oshima, 1977). Contraction of these fibres will bring the fimbriae closer to the ovary, facilitating ovum pick-up. Contractile activity varies throughout the menstrual cycle, but is significantly higher ($P < 0.01$) (Morikawa *et al.*, 1980) in the ovulatory phase. Contractile strength also peaks during this phase. Tonic contraction of these muscle bundles can be produced *in vitro* by PGF2α, acetylcholine and noradrenaline (norepinephrine). *In vivo*, culdoscopic observation in women has demonstrated that the transvaginal adminstration of PGF2α initiates movement of the fimbria towards the ovary to cover the pre-ovulatory follicle (Iwahashi, 1978). It is not known how essential tubal movement is for successful conception, but it is logical to assume that adhesions which restrict tubo-ovarian mobility will impair fertility.

To complicate matters tubo-ovarian adhesions may only be one manifestation of more extensive pelvic pathology. The initial peritoneal insult which caused the adhesions, particularly if due to salpingitis, is likely to have damaged the tubal mucosa. This may have induced intra-tubal adhesions or caused the formation of hydrosalpinges. Regardless of how well adhesiolysis is performed, function will not be restored unless attempts are also made to treat these additional problems. Even then, if damage has been extensive the probability of a viable intra-uterine pregnancy is reduced considerably.

5.7 How should adhesiolysis be performed?

The multifactorial nature of pathology associated with adhesions causes problems when assessing the effectiveness of treatment. We can only do this by looking at the results of reported case series. Grouping these reports for the purposes of comparing different techniques is commonly done, but the influence of uncontrollable variables within and between the patient series severely questions the validity of such an exercise. For example, it is difficult to classify adhesions, therefore this is either not done or is unsatisfactorily done. Also, other factors impairing fertility are often inadequately excluded. Quite apart from these problems is the more fundamental question of comparing treatment with no treatment. Adhesions, unless associated with complete tubal blockage, are only a relative and not an absolute cause of infertility. Although a history of infertility pre-operatively can safely be assumed, a proportion of patients with adhesions will always conceive without surgery. It is important to establish this proportion in any study. This should then be compared with pregnancy rates following surgery in a matched group of patients. Only by doing this will it be possible to calculate the true value of adhesiolysis in the treatment of infertility.

5.7.1 ADHESIOLYSIS BY LAPAROTOMY

The results of traditional surgery, employing laparotomy without using microsurgical techniques, are outlined in Table 5.2. Seven case series have been grouped to accumulate a total of 601 patients. The combined term pregnancy rate is 33% with an ectopic rate of 4%. Corticosteroids and antihistamines were prescribed in two of the studies (marked *).

Microsurgical techniques seem to offer some improvement, but is this enough to justify a major operation, particularly when simpler laparoscopic techniques are available (Table 5.3)?

5.7.2 ADHESIOLYSIS BY LAPAROSCOPY

Laparoscopic adhesiolysis offers a useful alternative to laparotomy techniques. This type of surgery can be performed at the time of diagnostic laparoscopy; it is a simpler technique and seems to be as effective as microsurgery. From the point of view of patient inconvenience and post-operative morbidity, laparoscopic surgery must be more acceptable than techniques requiring laparotomy. However, as with microsurgery, its real clinical value has yet to be demonstrated in a randomized trial. Such a study would be required to firmly establish

Table 5.2 Results of salpingolysis by conventional surgery

Reference	*Year*	*No. of patients*	*Term pregnancy (%)*	*Ectopic (%)*
Martius	(1959)	138	57 (41)	7 (5)
Ozaras	(1968)	34	7 (20)	1 (3)
Arronet *et al.*	(1969)	46	20 (43)	1 (2)
Young	(1970)	47	15 (32)	2 (4)
Horne *et al.**	(1973)	81	28 (35)	3 (4)
Bronson and Wallach*	(1977)	35	20 (57)	1 (3)
Diamond	(1979)	220	N/A (25)	8
Total		601	202 (33)	23 (4)

N/A = absolute figures not available, to calculate totals, estimation has been made from percentage.
* Corticosteroids and promethazine given.

Table 5.3 Results of salpingolysis by microsurgery

Reference	*Year*	*No. of patients*	*Term pregnancy (%)*	*Ectopic (%)*
Diamond	(1979)	140	80 (57.1)	1
Frantzen and Schlosser	(1982)	49	19 (38.8)	2 (4.1)
Donnez and Casanas-Roux	(1986)	42	27 (64)	1 (2)
Total		231	126 (54)	4 (1)

the clinical significance of adhesions. Ethical restrictions have so far prevented such a trial employing microsurgical techniques, but these restrictions would not necessarily apply to laparoscopic techniques. Various techniques can be employed to perform laparoscopic adhesiolysis and each seems equally effective (Table 5.4).

(a) Scissors

The simplest technique is to use scissors, but this method is not without problems. Scissors have no haemostatic function and bleeding can occur making visualization and continuation of the procedure difficult. Of course, bleeding into the abdominal cavity during laparoscopy may not present the same risk of inducing adhesions as bleeding at the time of laparotomy. This may explain the apparent effectiveness of using scissors to perform adhesiolysis. If diathermy is used to stop

Table 5.4 Results of laparoscopic salpingo-ovariolysis

Reference		*No. of patients*	*Term pregnancy (%)*	*Ectopic (%)*
Scissors				
Gomel	(1983)	92	54 (58.7)	5 (5.4)
Bruhat *et al.*	(1983)	93	*48 (51.6)	7 (5.2)
Scissors and electro-dissection				
Reich	(1987)	12	9 (75)	1 (8)
CO_2 laser				
Donnez	(1989)	186	†108 (58)	N/A
Total		383	219 (57)	13 (3)

* Intra-uterine pregnancy rate.
† Total pregnancy rate.
N/A = Data not available.

bleeding, particularly if monopolar diathermy is used, tissue necrosis will occur and this will inevitably increase the risk of further adhesion formation. Bipolar laparoscopy diathermy forceps are available and theoretically will induce haemostasis with much less tissue necrosis. Other problems with laparoscopy scissors concern design. A scissors action involving movement of both blades is not available. Only scissors with one fixed and one moving blade exist, and these will not self-sharpen. These instruments need repeated maintenance which, for practical purposes, means that the laparoscopic surgeon often has to work with blunt scissors.

(b) The CO_2 laser

An alternative and easier means of performing adhesiolysis is to use the CO_2 laser. Although the equipment is expensive, adhesiolysis can be performed rapidly and safely with minimal tissue necrosis. Unless the adhesions are very vascular, bleeding is rarely troublesome. Plates 1, 2 and 3 show a sequence from a salpingolysis procedure. This patient had a perforated appendix with extensive peritonitis when she was a young girl, resulting in extensive omental adhesions covering the surface of the tubes and preventing any possibility of tubal motility and ovum pick-up. The tubes were patent on hystero-salpingography and once the adhesions had been precisely vaporized with the CO_2 laser, salpingoscopy revealed normal intra-luminal folds. This patient became pregnant 6 weeks after this procedure although she had been trying for a pregnancy for 4 years prior to the operation.

In order to avoid causing damage to tissue distal to the adhesion a backstop is inserted on the end of the adhesiolysis probe. In certain situations this can be difficult to place and an alternative is to position a flexible blackened probe through a third or fourth portal trochar or to stretch the adhesion over a pool of fluid which will absorb laser energy. During salpingolysis the operator should use relatively high power densities, preferably on a superpulse mode, to achieve precise cutting. Care must be taken between the tube and ovary where the mesosalpinx is extremely vascular and troublesome bleeding is encountered if the thin-walled veins are accidentally punctured. In this situation the bleeding is difficult to stop with electrodiathermy without causing damage to the tube. The blunt-tipped endocoagulator probe is more effective here but has to be cooled by running irrigant fluid to prevent it from sticking to the tissues and forming a coagulum which starts to bleed again when the probe is pulled off.

In most patients the damaged tubes are a result of salpingitis and the damage to the endothelium and cilia lining the tube ensures uniformly poor results. Similarly, adhesions due to endometriosis are associated with other, poorly understood, infertility aspects of endometriosis itself. There are, however, a small group of patients who have tubal adhesions due to extrinsic infection, usually peritonitis secondary to appendicitis, which are associated with a relatively high pregnancy rate following laparoscopic adhesiolysis. In Guildford we have treated 26 such patients and although one was lost to follow-up, 18 (72%) became pregnant mostly within the following 3 months. Donnez (1989) reported similar success rates when the peri-tubal or peri-ovarian adhesions were thin but he felt that if the adhesions were thick and vascular microsurgical adhesiolysis performed by laparotomy was more effective. These latter adhesions, however, are often associated with extensive tubal damage which will severely diminish the chance of successful conception and thus brings into question the value of performing any surgery at all and the patient may best be advised to opt for assisted conception techniques.

One disadvantage of the CO_2 laser is that it cannot for practical purposes be transmitted through a flexible fibre. The beam can only be transmitted in a straight line and reflection is needed to alter its direction. Access to many locations is therefore difficult. Wave guides have been developed to direct the laser beam, but they again are straight instruments and therefore do not significantly improve access.

(c) Visible light lasers

Other wavelengths of laser energy, for example the potassium titanyl phosphate (KTP-532) laser, may be transmitted through a flexible fibre

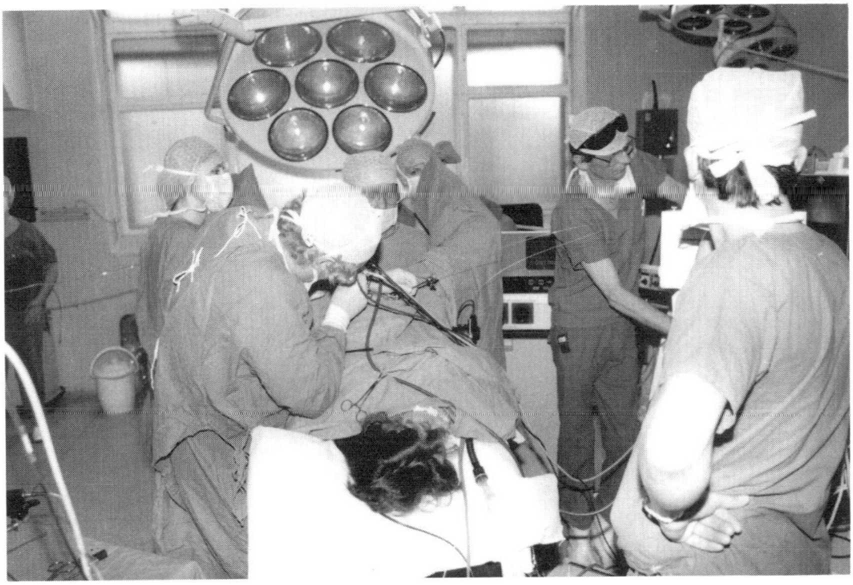

Figure 5.2 Flexible fibre laser laparoscopy. At a flick of a mirror the fibre will transmit Nd-YAG or KTP-532 laser wavelengths.

(Figures 5.2 and 5.3). The KTP laser will also divide vascular adhesions in a relatively bloodless manner. This laser has both tissue-cutting and coagulation effects unlike the CO_2 laser which is principally a vaporizing or cutting instrument. However, the price of haemostasis is greater coagulative and thermal damage with increased tissue necrosis. Tissue necrosis will predispose to further adhesion formation and it remains to be seen if this laser is as effective a means of performing adhesiolysis as the CO_2 laser, particularly in so far as recurrence is concerned.

(d) Electrodiathermy

Consider the use of diathermy through the laparoscope. After all, this is the established cutting instrument of choice for microsurgical adhesiolysis. Monopolar diathermy was used extensively in the 1970s in the USA and Europe for laparoscopic sterilization. It was associated with many reports of unforeseen injury to the bowel and urinary tract (Cheng, 1976; Chamberlain and Carron-Brown, 1982). These complications may have been due to aberrant electrical conductivity or simply poor technique. Despite inadequate explanation, monopolar diathermy has been deemed unsuitable for laparoscopic use and the

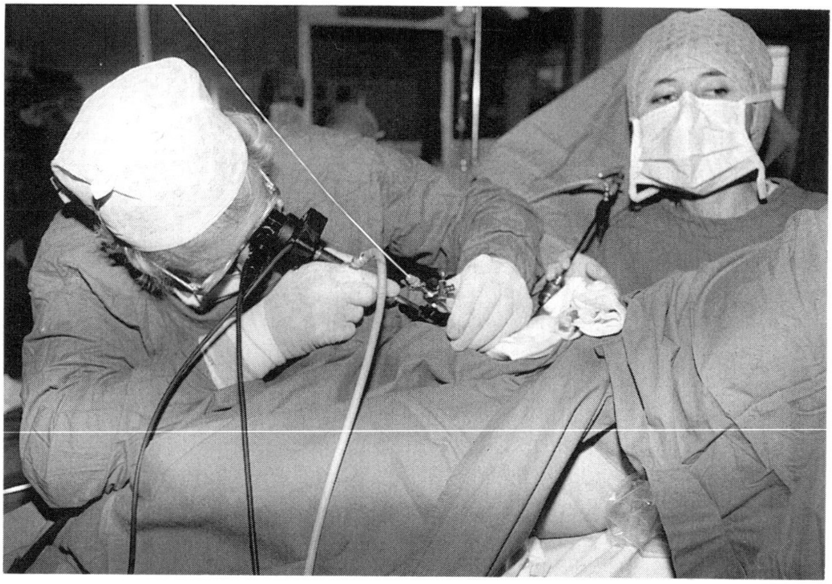

Figure 5.3 The KTP-532 laser being used in a hazardous situation near the ureter requires the surgeon to 'eyeball' the target for maximum safety. The assistant retracts tissues guided by the TV monitor.

alternative technique of endocoagulation is the recommended means of securing haemostasis (Semm and O'Neill-Freys, 1989). However, high-frequency monopolar diathermy is a good cutting instrument. It is simple to use and inexpensive. There are also reports that laparoscopic electrocautery is a safe and effective way of treating endometriosis (Seiler, 1986) and high-frequency laparoscopic electrodissection using a pure cutting current has also been successfully employed to perform tubo-ovariolysis and neosalpingostomy (Reich, 1987). Further technical developments with particular regard to safety may see the return of this instrument as a means of performing laparoscopic adhesiolysis. Bipolar diathermy is an alternative and theoretically should give a precise cut. However, suitably refined bipolar laparoscopy forceps have not yet been developed and until they are available, the CO_2 laser will remain the optimum method of performing laparoscopic adhesiolysis.

5.7.3 CONTROVERSIAL ASPECTS

(a) CO_2 laser vs diathermy

Are there theoretical as well as practical reasons why the CO_2 laser should be used for adhesiolysis? Initial animal studies on the tissue effects of this laser were carried out during laparotomy (Bellina *et al.*, 1984). Compared to microsurgical diathermy, which produced significant tissue damage and adhesions, the CO_2 laser produced less tissue injury and no adhesions. Other similar studies have failed to produce such convincing evidence. No significant difference between the laser and microdiathermy has been reported with respect to post-operative adhesion formation (Pittaway, Mayson and Daniell, 1983), the effectiveness of adhesiolysis (Filmar, Gomel and McComb, 1986) and total tissue damage in the acute and healing phases (Luciano *et al.*, 1987). To complicate matters, the American intra-abdominal laser study group (Diamond *et al.*, 1984), reporting on a group of 106 women undergoing laparotomy infertility surgery, concluded that although adhesions were reduced at second-look laparoscopy in both groups, non-laser microsurgery may have been a more efficient means of treating adhesions. Other laparotomy studies (Barbot *et al.*, 1987; Tulandi, 1987) comparing these techniques found significant and comparable reduction in post-operative adhesion scores.

(b) Laparoscopy vs laparotomy

Is there evidence that tissue effects are different when the procedure is carried out laparoscopically? Standard tissue injury with scissors, whether inflicted during laparotomy or laparoscopically, produces similar adhesions (Filmar, Gomel and McComb, 1987). On the other hand, an excellent controlled study on rabbits (Luciano *et al.*, 1989) comparing CO_2 laser adhesiolysis during laparoscopy and laparotomy demonstrated that post-operative adhesion scores were significantly greater in the laparotomy group. This study also showed that laparotomy, but not laparoscopy adhesiolysis was associated with *de novo* adhesions, that is adhesion formation in sites not directly associated with the surgical procedure. Pre-operative adhesion scores were different in each group (Table 5.5). Although the adhesions were worse and the relative improvement in score was better in the laparoscopy group, it was not possible to conclude that laparoscopic adhesiolysis was better. The evidence only allowed the authors to say that these methods were equally effective.

5.8 Does adjuvant therapy improve the effectiveness of adhesiolysis?

There is vast and often conflicting information on the value of adjuvant therapy. All publications to date refer to laparotomy adhesiolysis, mainly involve animal studies and may not be applicable to laparoscopic

Table 5.5 Adhesion scores pre- and post-CO_2 laser adhesiolysis by laparoscopy and by laparotomy (from Luciano *et al.*, 1989)

	Adhesion scores		
	pre-op	*post-op*	*P*
Laparoscopy	2.7	0.9	0.001
Laparotomy	1.13	1.0	0.465

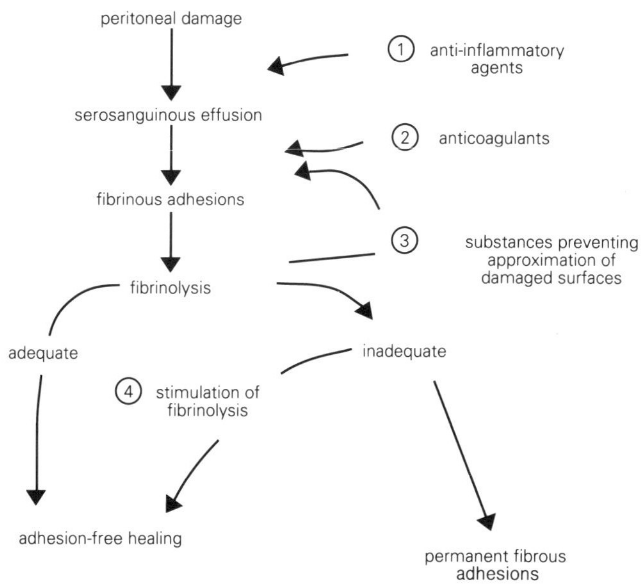

Figure 5.4 How adjuvant therapy affects adhesion formation.

techniques. Agents presently available act at various stages of the adhesion formation pathway. The majority of publications also concern ways in which the early phases of the pathway, the formation of a serosanguinous effusion and formation of fibrinous adhesions, can be prevented (Figure 5.4). In effect, an attempt is made to attenuate the physiological response to tissue injury. The magnitude of this response is, of course, an important indicator of the severity of eventual adhesion formation; however, it is also part of the normal process of tissue healing and repair. Attempts to manipulate this response may therefore be harmful. Adverse effects were not reported when dexamethazone and promethazine were initially recommended (Replogle, Johnson and Gross, 1966), but since then there have been reports of excessive morbidity from infection (Grossfeld *et al.*, 1973). The possibility that these agents will worsen or increase the likelihood of an infection must be considered whenever they are used as adjuvant therapy.

The natural fate of fibrinous adhesions within the abdominal cavity is lysis and complete resolution. Treatments acting on the latter stages of adhesion formation augment rather than attenuate this physiological process. Agents which delay the apposition of damaged peritoneal surfaces will allow more time for peritoneal regeneration to take place and peritoneal fibrinolysin will have more time to take effect. In addition, the use of exogenous fibrinolysins or rt-PA will also assist lysis of fibrinous adhesions prior to irreversible fibrosis occurring.

Corticosteroids and other anti-inflammatory agents principally act by reducing the body's response to tissue damage. Release of the mediators of inflammation is diminished, lysosome membranes are stabilized and vascular permeability is decreased. There is therefore a smaller serosanguinous effusion and less likelihood of a fibrinous meshwork of adhesions forming. Corticosteroids may also affect fibroblast function and will have a delayed effect on the formation of fibrous adhesions.

The value of corticosteroids has clearly been shown in animal studies (Luciano, 1983), but a beneficial effect has not been shown in human infertility surgery (Jansen, 1985). Inconclusive evidence of benefit plus the risk of potential side effects must surely question the routine use of these agents, particularly when other forms of prophylaxis are available. Similar comments also apply to the use of anticoagulants. Heparin has been used systemically in high doses and will effectively reduce adhesions, but this form of therapy is associated with haemorrhagic complications (Holtz, 1980). Heparin is also empirically added to irrigant solutions to reduce fibrin deposition, but how effective this practice is has yet to be determined.

Substances which prevent the apposition of damaged peritoneal surfaces either work through a hydroflotation principle or by forming a protective film and exerting a temporary 'siliconization' effect. A number of agents are available. All are hydrophilic polymers of high molecular weight. The commonest of these agents is Hyskon 32% Dextran 70), but there is evidence that this may not be the most efficacious. A prospective and randomized study involving a large group of women undergoing infertility surgery has demonstrated the effectiveness of instilling into the abdominal cavity 250 ml of this solution compared with a similar volume of normal saline (Adhesions Study Group, 1983). Excellent pregnancy rates have been achieved using 500 ml of this solution in a large microsurgery series (Donnez and Casanas-Roux, 1986). Normal saline itself seems to have hydroflotation properties and will improve the effectiveness of adhesiolysis. In certain prospective clinical trials when this has occurred, no additional benefit was found following the instillation of Hyskon (Larsson *et al.*, 1985). This finding is worthy of consideration, particularly when anaphylactic shock has been associated with Hyskon (Trimbos-Kemper and Verring, 1989).

Carboxymethyl cellulose (CMC) and chondroitin sulphate (CDS) are both high molecular weight solutes which are used to prevent corneal adhesions following eye surgery. Animal studies have shown both these agents to be useful adjuncts to laparotomy adhesiolysis. CMC seems to be better than Hyskon, particularly when larger volumes and more concentrated solutions are used (Diamond *et al.*, 1988). CDS seems to be a particularly potent adjunct and has been shown to be significantly more effective than Hyskon, CMC and normal saline. When used in high concentration (25% solution) adhesiolysis is highly effective even without microsurgical techniques (Delsner *et al.*, 1987).

Another approach is to insert an absorbable adhesion barrier made of oxidized regenerated cellulose (Interceed, TC7, Johnson & Johnson, New Brunswick, USA). A randomized prospective study with 134 patients in each arm of the trial has shown that 51% of pelvic sidewalls (n = 68) treated with Interceed after 'state-of-the-art' surgery were completely free of adhesions whereas only 24% (n = 32) were free of adhesions when treated with surgery alone (Interceed (TC7) Adhesion Barrier Study Group, 1989). The main problem is that the fabric has to be applied dry and flat to the surface following adhesiolysis and meticulous haemostasis. This is difficult enough to achieve at a microsurgical laparotomy and requires a surgeon who is a technical virtuoso to perform the same procedure at laparoscopy. For this reason some of the second-look laparoscopies that we have witnessed have been far from impressive.

The rationale behind using fibrinolysins has already been explained. To date efficacy has only been demonstrated in animal studies. The high cost of the presently available rt-PA is likely to prevent immediate clinical evaluation, but the theoretical reasons for employing this agent are attractive and pose a strong case for its use.

5.9 Conclusions

Although it has not been shown that laparoscopic surgery is any better than laparotomy and microsurgery, clinical results following intra-abdominal adhesiolysis are comparable. Regardless of which modality is employed to perform laparoscopic adhesiolysis – the CO_2 laser, KTP-532 laser, diathermy or scissors – subsequent clinical results are also similar. Patient morbidity and hospital stay are both greatly re-

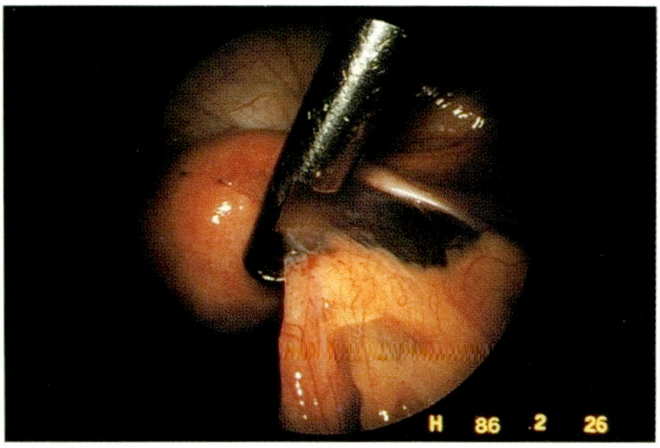

Plate 1: CO_2 laser adhesiolysis with back stop.

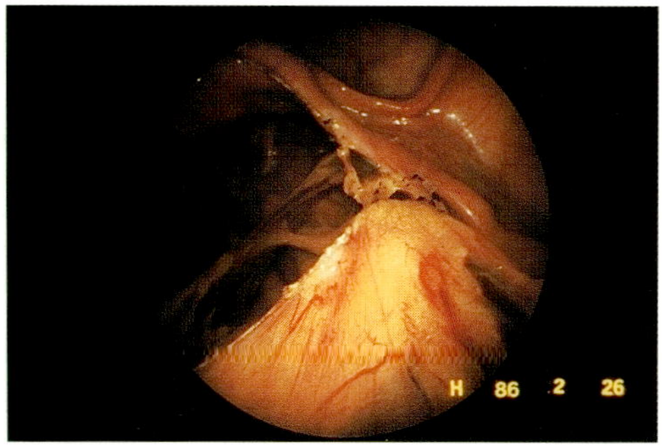

Plate 2: Adhesiolysis partially completed. Note absence of bleeding and minimal tissue damage.

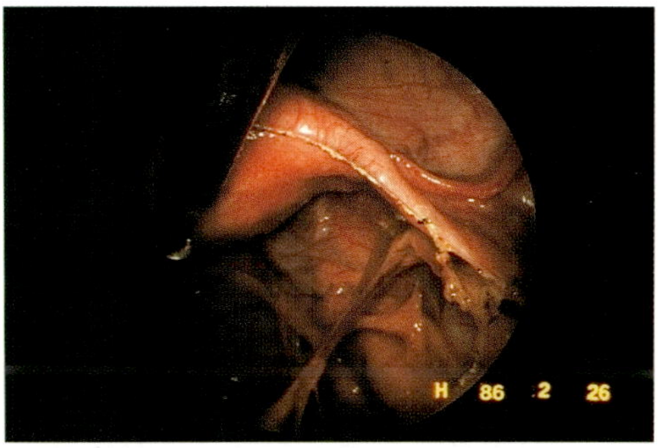

Plate 3: Laser adhesiolysis completed.

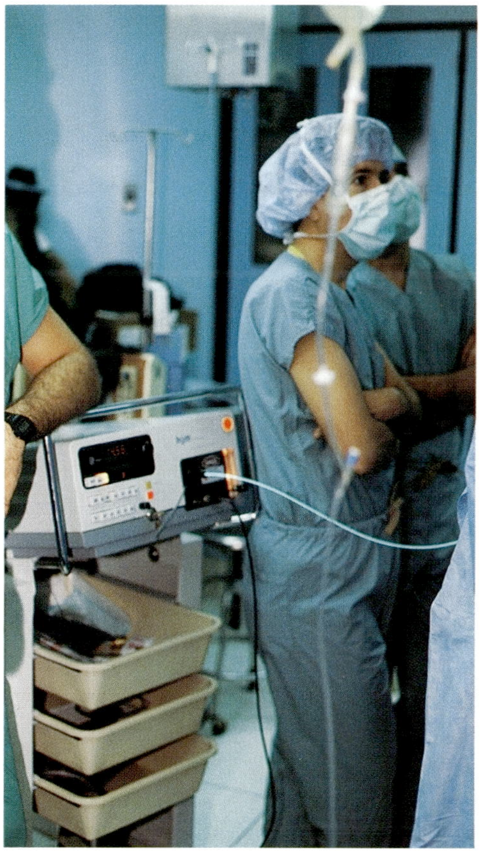

Plate. 4. Argon laser

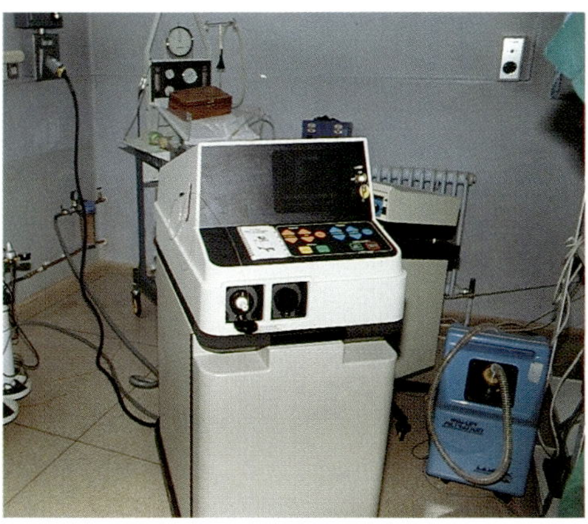

Plate. 5. KTP/532 laser

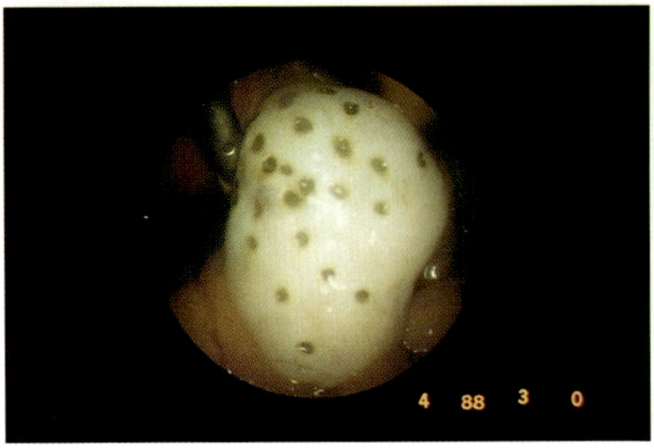

Plate. 6. Polycystic ovary with KTP laser drill.

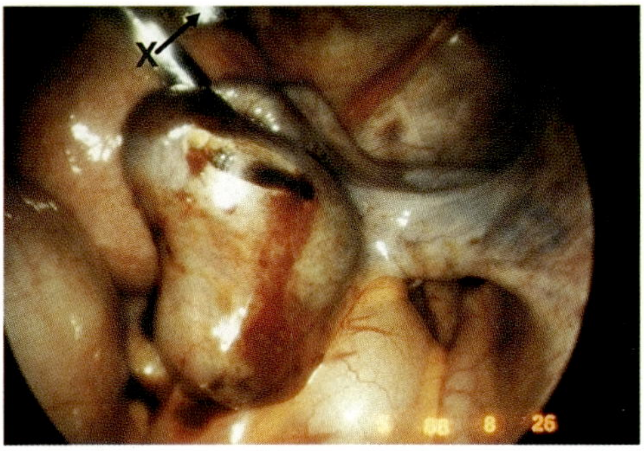

Plate. 7(a) Laparoscopic view of the distended distal part of the tube. Salpingotomy has been done with the CO_2 laser (×) resulting in a precise incision of the tubal wall with minimal coagulation effect. Trophoblastic tissue in view already.

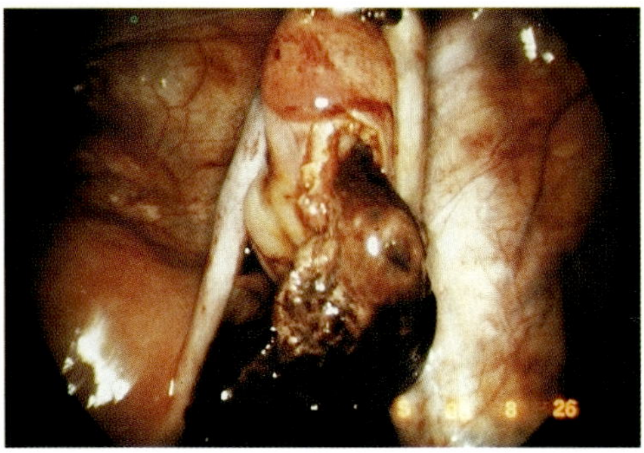

Plate. 7(b) Trophoblastic tissue is almost entirely expelled by saline irrigation.

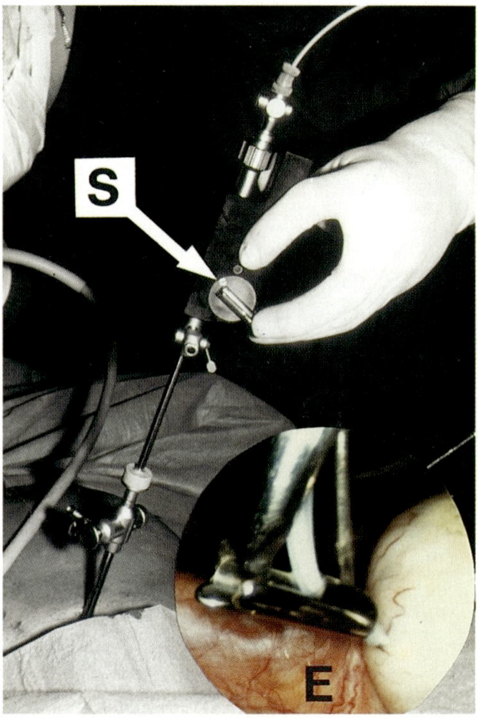

Plate. 8. Laser fibre steering probe for fibre optic lasers. Tip deflection (E) can be achieved by special mechanism (S).

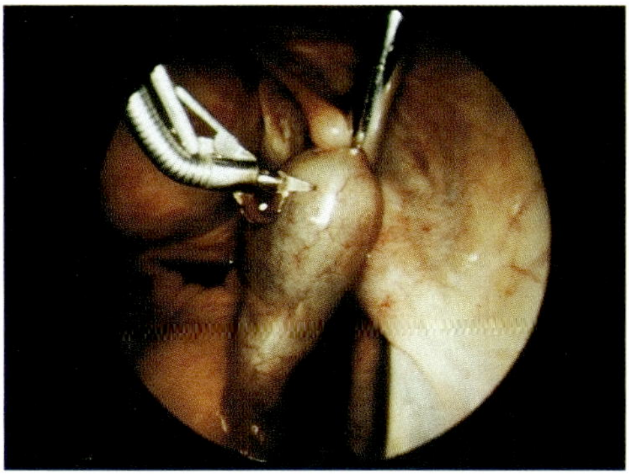

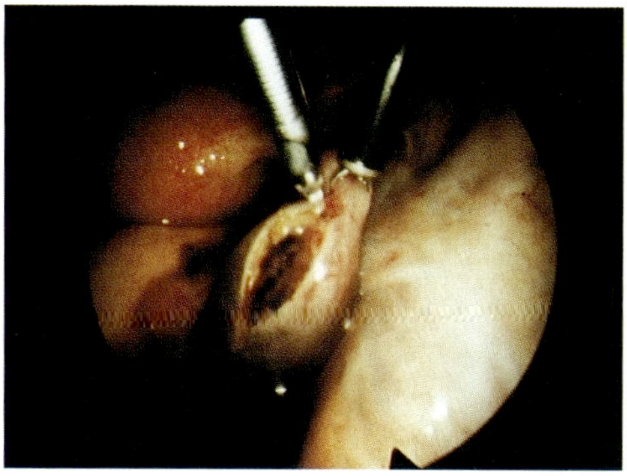

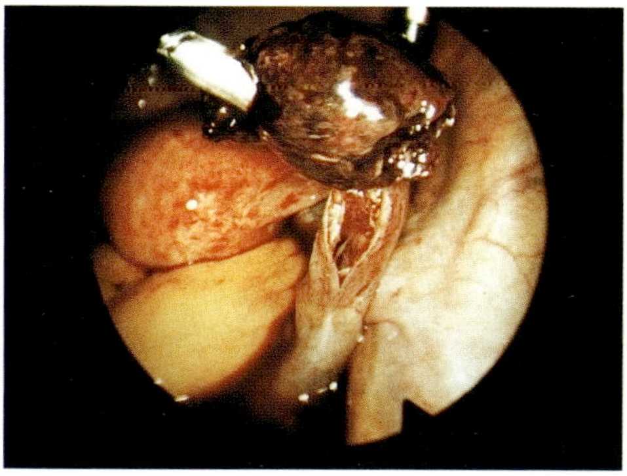

Plate. 9. View of the tube before (a) and after (b) salpingotomy with the contact Nd-YAG laser. The wound margins (c) are precise and damage to adjacent tissue is minimal.

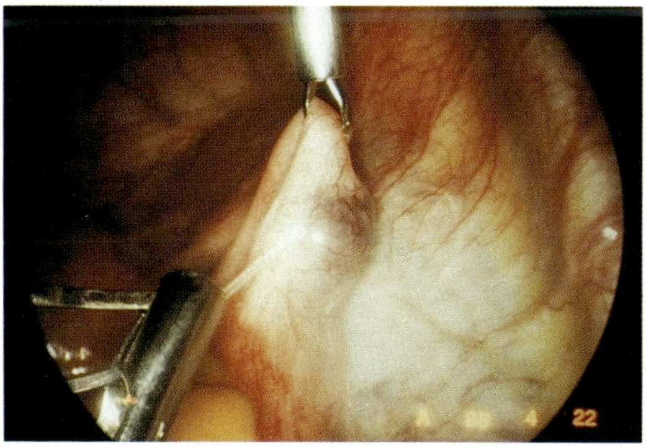

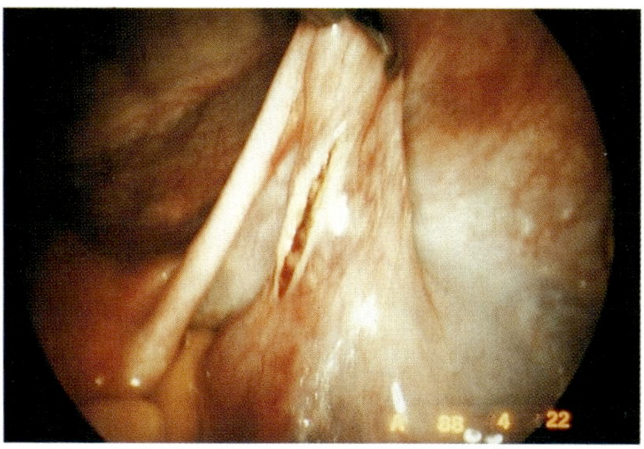

Plate. 10. a and b. Incision of unruptured ectopic pregnancy in the right tube with the argon laser. A minimal coagulation zone can be seen.

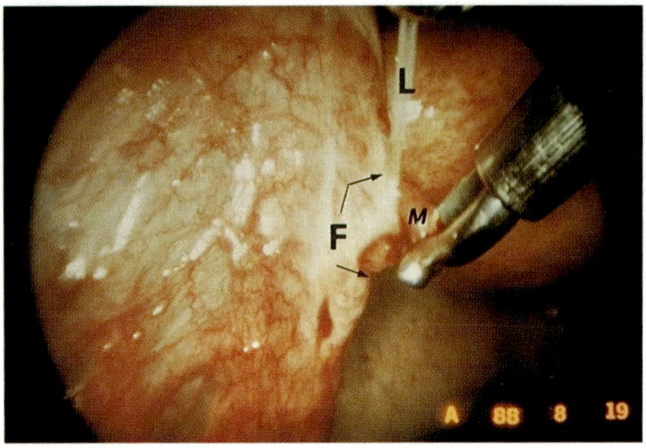

Plate. 11. View of the ampullary portion of the left tube. Extension of a fistula (F) is marked (arrows). Extruding mucosa (M), held by the grasping forceps, is resected with the 300 μm laser fibre (L) with contact technique.

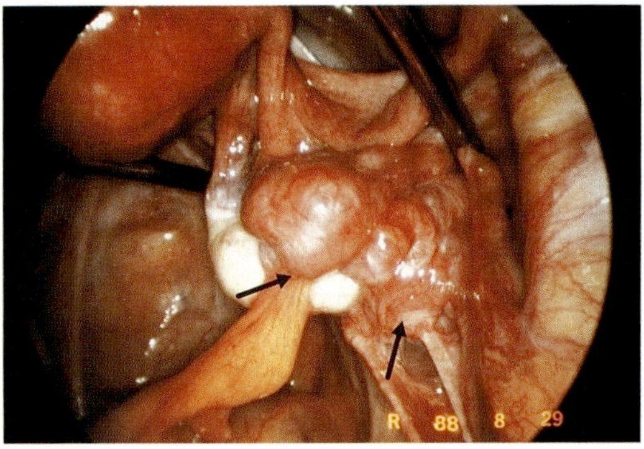

Plate. 12. View of the right tube after treatment of tubal pregnancy with 'classic' instruments (thermocoagulation). Note adhesions (arrow) covering the distal part of the tube and incision site of salpingotomy.

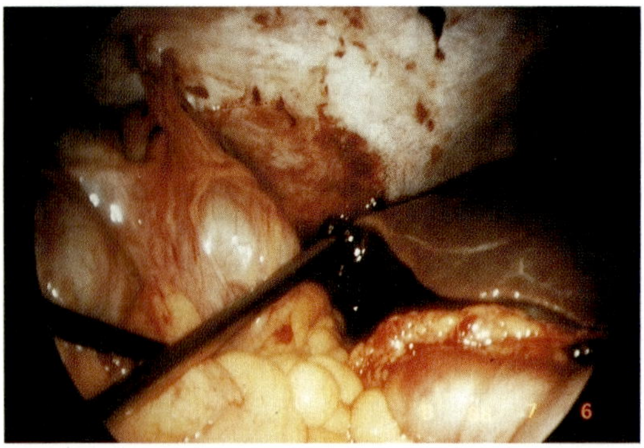

Plate. 13. View of the right upper abdominal cavity. Secondary implantation of trophoblast tissue has occurred in the omentum. Blood clots can be seen between the right hepatic lobe and omentum.

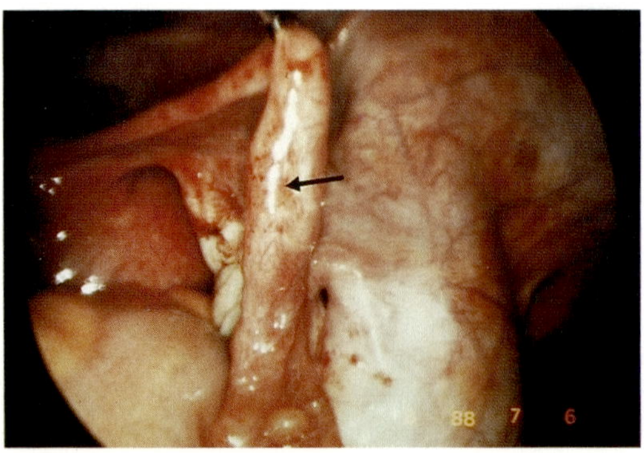

Plate. 14. View of the right tube in second-look laparoscopy after laser salpingotomy. Minimal scarring on the antimesenterial side of the tube (arrow) without any adhesions.

duced following laparoscopy. From the patient's point of view laparoscopy is therefore a much more acceptable technique. This means that any procedure which can be performed laparoscopically should not be done by laparotomy. Adhesiolysis, when required for the treatment of infertility or chronic abdominal pain should therefore be performed laparoscopically.

At present the CO_2 or KTP-532 laser seems to be the optimal way of performing laparoscopic adhesiolysis, but in the future improved instrumentation, better laparoscopy scissors, laparoscopy staple ligatures and more precise diathermy instruments may mean that these alternative methods will be as suitable.

References

Adams, J. (1913), Peritoneal adhesions. *Lancet*, **i**, 663–8.

Adhesions Study Group (1983), Reduction of post-operative pelvic adhesions with intraperitoneal 32% dextran 70: a prospective, randomised chemical trial. *Fertil. Steril.*, **40**, 612–19.

Alexander-Williams, J. (1987), Do adhesions cause pain? *Br. Med. J.*, **294**, 659–60.

Arronet, G., Eduljee, S. and O'Brien, J. (1969), A nine-year survey of fallopian tube dysfunction in human infertility. *Fertil. Steril.*, **20**, 901–17.

Astrup, T. (1966), Tissue activators of plasminogen. *Fed. Proc.*, **25**, 42–51.

Barbot, J., Parent, B., Dubuisson, J. and Aubriot, F. (1987), A clinical study of the CO_2 laser and electrodiathermy for adhesiolysis in 172 cases followed by early second-look laparoscopy. *Fertil. Steril.*, **48**, 140–2.

Bellina, J., Hemmings, R., Voros, J. and Ross, L. (1984), Carbon dioxide laser and electrosurgical wound study with an animal model: A comparison of tissue damage and healing pattern in peritoneal tissue. *Am. J. Obstet. Gynecol.*, **148**, 327–34.

Bevan, P. G. (1984), Adhesive obstruction. *Annals Royal Coll. Surg*. Eng., **66**, 164–9.

Brightwell, N., McFie, A. and Aust, J. B. (1977), Bowel obstruction and the long tube stent. *Arch. Sang.*, **112**, 105–11.

Bronson, R. and Wallach, E. (1977), Lysis of periadnexal adhesions for correction of infertility. *Fertil. Steril.*, **28**, 613–19.

Bruhat, M., Mage, G., Manhes, H., Soualhat, C., Ropert, J. and Pouly, J. (1983), Laparoscopy procedures to promote fertility. Ovariolysis and salpingolysis. Results of 93 selected cases. *Acta Euro. Fert.*, **14**, 113–15.

Buckman, R., Woods, M., Sargent, L. and Gervin, A. (1976), A unifying pathogenic mechanism in the etiology of intra-peritoneal adhesions. *J. Surg. Res.*, **20**, 1–5.

Chan, C. and Wood, C. (1983), Pelvic adhesiolysis – the assessment of symptom relief by 100 patients. *Aust. N.Z.J. Obstet. Gynecol.*, **25**, 295.

Daniell, J. (1989), Laparoscopic enterolysis for chronic abdominal pain. *J. Gynecol. Surg.*, **5**, 61–6.

Dano, K., Andreason, P. Grondahl-Hansen, J., Fristensen, P., Neilsen, L. and Skriver, L. (1985), Plasminogen activators: tissue degradation and cancer. *ADU Cancer Res.*, **44**, 139–266.

DeCherney, A. and Mezer, H. (1984), The nature of post-tuboplasty pelvic adhesions as determined by early and late laparoscopy. *Fertil. Steril.*, **41**, 643–6.

Devroey, P., Zimmerman, M., Naaktgeboren, N. and Van Steirteghem, A. (1985), Ovarian adhesions impair ovulation. *Acta Euro. Fert.*, **16**, 183–6.

Diamond E. (1979) Lysis of postoperative adhesions in infertility. *Fertil. Steril.*, **31**(3), 287–95.

Diamond, M., Daniell, J., Feste, J., Surrey, M., McLaughlin, D., Friedman, S., Vaughn, W. and Martin, D. (1987), Adhesion reformation and *de novo* adhesion formulation after reproduction surgery. *Fertil. Steril.*, **47**, 864–6.

Diamond, M., Daniell, J., Martin, D., Feste, J., Vaughn, W. and McLaughlin, D. (1984), Tubal patency and pelvic adhesions at early second look laparoscopy following intra-abdominal use of the CO_2 laser: initial report of the intra-abdominal laser study group. *Fertil. Steril.*, **42**, 717–23.

Diamond, M., Decherney, A., Linsky, C., Cunningham, T. and Constantine, B. (1988), Assessment of carboxymethyl cellulose and 32% dextran 70 for prevention of adhesions in a rabbit uterine horn model. *Int. J. Fertil.*, **33**, 278–82.

Donnez, J. (1989), CO_2 laser laparoscopy in infertile women with adnexal adhesions and women with tubal occlusion. *J. Gynecol. Surg.*, **5**, 47–53.

Donnez, J. and Casanas-Roux, F. (1986), Prognostic factors of fimbrial microsurgery. *Fertil. Steril.*, **46**, 200–4.

Doody, K., Dann, R. and Buttram, V. (1989), Recombinant tissue plasminogen activator reduces adhesion formation in a rabbit uterine horn model. *Fertil. Steril.*, **51**, 509–12.

Ellis, H. (1962), The aetiology of post-operative abdominal adhesions. *Br. J. Surg.*, **50**, 10–6.

Ellis, H. (1971), The cause and prevention of post-operative intraperitoneal adhesions. *Surg. Gynecol. Obstet.*, **133**, 497–511.

Filmar, S., Gomel, V. and McComb, P. (1986), The effectiveness of CO_2 laser and electromicrosurgery in adhesiolysis: a comparative study. *Fertil. Steril.*, **45**, 407–11.

Filmar, S., Gomel, V. and McComb, P. (1987), Operative laparoscopy versus open abdominal surgery: a comparative study on post-operative adhesion formation in the rat model. *Fertil. Steril.*, **48**, 486–9.

Frantzen, C. and Schlosser, H. (1982), Microsurgery and post-infectious tubal infertility. *Fertil. Steril.*, **38**, 397–402.

Gervin, A., Puckett, C. and Silver, D. (1973), Serosal hypofibrinolysis. *Am. J. Surg.*, **125**, 80–8.

Gomel, V. (1983), Salpingo-ovariolysis by laparoscopy in infertility. *Fertil. Steril.*, **40**, 607–11.

Grosfeld, J., Berman, I., Schiller, M. and Morse, T. (1973), Excessive morbidity resulting from the prevention of intestinal adhesions with steroids and antihistamines. *J. Paed. Surg.*, **8**, 221–6.

Hertzler, A. (1919), Nature and genesis of peritoneal adhesions. In *The Peritoneum*, Vol. 1, C. V. Mosby, St. Louis, p. 278.

Holtz, G. (1980), Prevention of post-operative adhesions. *J. Reprod. Med.*, **24**, 141.

Horne, H., Clyman, M., Debrouner, C., Griggs, G., Kistner, R., Kosasa, T., Stevenson, C. and Taymor, M. (1973), The prevention of post-operative pelvic adhesions following conservative operative treatment for human infertility. *Fertil. Steril.*, **28**, 613–14.

Interceed (TC7) Adhesion Barrier Study Group (1989), Prevention of post-surgical adhesions by Interceed (TC7), an absorbable adhesion barrier: a prospective randomized multicenter clinical study. *Fertil. Steril.*, **51**, 933–8.

Iwahashi, G. (1978), Culdoscopic observation of fimbrial movement induced by transvaginal prostaglandin F2 in the human. *Sanfu-jinka-sekai*, **30**, 175.

Jackson, B. (1958), Observations on intraperitoneal adhesions. *Surgery*, **44**, 507–14.

Jansen, R. P. S. (1985), Failure of intraperitoneal adjuvants to improve the outcome of pelvic operations in young women. *Am. J. Obstet. Gynecol.*, **153**, 363.

Kleinhaus, S. (1984), Laparoscopic lysis of adhesions for post-appendicectomy pain. *Gastro-Endosc.*, **5**, 304.

Kresch, A., Seifer, D., Sachs, L. and Barrese, I. (1984), Laparoscopy in 100 women with chronic pelvic pain. *Obstet. Gynaecol.*, **64**, 672–4.

Lacos, O. (1988), Risk factors for tubal infertility among fertile and infertile women. *Eur. J. Obstet. Gynecol.*, **29**, 129–36.

Larsson, B., Lalos, O., Marsk, L., Tronstad, S.-E., Bygdeman, M., Pearson, S. and Joelsson, I. (1985), Effect of intraperitoneal instillations of 32% dextran 70 on post-operative adhesion formulation after tubal surgery. *Acta Obstet. Gynecol. Scand.*, **64**, 437–47.

Luciano, A., Hauser, K. and Benda, J. (1983) Evaluation of commonly used adjuvants in the prevention of post operative adhesions. *Am. J. Obstet. Gynecol.*, **146**(1), 88–92.

Luciano, A., Maier, D., Koch, E., Nillsen, J. and Whitman, F. (1989), A comparative study of post-operative adhesions following laser surgery by laparoscopy versus laparotomy in the rabbit model. *Obstet. Gynecol.*, **74**, 220–4.

Luciano, A., Witman, G., Mater, D., Randolph, J. and Maenza, R. (1987), A comparison of thermal injury, healing patterns and post-operative adhesive formation following CO_2 laser and electromicrosurgery. *Fertil. Steril.*, **48**, 1025–9.

Martius, H. (1959), Surgical technique in the treatment of sterility in women. *Int. J. Surg.*, **4**, 70.

Mecke, H., Semm, K. and Lehman-Willenbrock, E. (1980), Die pelviskopische adhesiolyse. *Geburtsk. u. Frauenheitk.*, **48**, 155–9.

Menzies, D. and Ellis, H. (1989a), Intestinal obstruction from adhesions – how big is the problem? *Ann. R. Coll. Surg. Engl.*, **72**, 60–3.

Menzies, D. and Ellis, H. (1989b), Intra-abdominal adhesions and their prevention by topical tissue plasminogen activator. *J. R. Soc. Med.*, **82**, 534–5.

Menzies, D. and Ellis, H. Adhesion prevention: The risk of plasminogen activator (in preparation).

Milligan, D. and Rafferty, A. (1979), Observations on the pathogenesis of peritoneal adhesions: a light and electron microscopical study. *Br. J. Surg.*, **61**, 274–80.

Morikawa, H., Okamura, H., Takenaka, A., Morimoto, K. and Nishimura, T. (1980), Physiological study of the human mesotubarium ovarica. *Obstet. Gynecol.*, **55**, 493–6.

Myhre-Jensen, O., Larsen, S. B. and Astrup, T. (1969), Fibrinolytic activity in serosal and synovial membranes. *Arch. Path.*, **88**, 623–30.

Oelsner, G., Graebe, R. Pan, S.-B., Haseltine, F., Barnea, E., Fakih, H. and DeCherney, A. (1987), Chondroitin sulphate. A new intraperitoneal treatment for post-operative adhesion prevention in the rabbit. *J. Reprod. Med.*, **32**, 812–4.

Okamura, H., Morikawa, H. and Oshima, M. (1977), A morphological study of the mesotubarium ovarica in the human. *Obstet. Gynecol.*, **49**, 197.

Ozaras, H. (1968), The value of plastic operations on the fallopian tubes in the treatment of female infertility. *Acta Obstet. Gynecol. Scand.*, **47**, 484–500.

Pittaway, D., Mayson, W. and Daniell, J. (1983), A comparison of the CO_2 laser and electrocautery on post-operative intra-peritoneal adhesions formation in rabbits. *Fertil. Steril.*, **40**, 366–8.

Porter, J., McGregor, F., Mullen, D. and Silver, D. (1989), Fibrinolytic activity of mesothelial surfaces. *Surgical Forum*, **20**, 80–2.

Rafferty, A. (1981), The effect of peritoneal trauma on peritoneal fibrinolytic activity and intra-peritoneal adhesion formation. *Eur. Surg. Res.*, **13**, 397–401.

Rapkin, A. (1986), Adhesions and pelvic pain. A retrospective study. *Obstet. Gynecol.*, **68**, 13–15.

Reich, H. (1987), Laparoscopic treatment of extensive pelvic adhesions, including hydrosalpinx. *J. Reprod. Med.*, **32**, 736–42.

Replogle, R., Johnson, R. and Gross, R. (1966), Prevention of post-operative intestinal adhesions with combined promethazine and dexamethasone therapy. *Annals Surg.*, **163**, 580–8.

Ryan, G., Grobety, J. and Majno, G. (1971), Post-operative peritoneal adhesions. *Am. J. Path.*, **65**, 117–37.

Semm, K. and O'Neill-Freys (1989), Conventional operative laparoscopy. In *Laparoscopic Surgery* (ed. C. J. G. Sutton), *Baillière's Clinical Obstetrics and Gynaecology, Vol. 3*, Baillière Tindall, London, pp. 663–9.

Sutton, C. J. G. (1986), Initial experience with carbon dioxide laser laparoscopy. *Lasers Med. Sci.*, **1**, 25–31.

Thompson, J., Paterson-Brown, S., Harbourne, T., Whawell, S., Kalodike, E. and Dudley, H. (1989), Reduced human peritoneal plasminogen activator activity: possible mechanism of adhesion formation. *Br. J. Surg.*, **76**, 382–5.

Todd, A.S. (1959), The histological localisation of fibrinolytic activator. *J. Path. Bact.*, **78**, 281–3.

Trimbos-Kemper, T. and Veering, B. (1989), Anaphylactic shock from intracavitary 32% dextran 70 during hysteroscopy. *Fertil. Steril.*, **51**, 1053–4.

Trompke, R. and Siegner, R. (1954), Ein Betrag zu den Verhutungsmabnahmen postoperativer interabodmineller Verwachsungen. *Langenbeck's Arch. Dtsch. Chir.*, **281**, 323–32.

Tulandi, T. (1987), Adhesion formation after reproductive surgery with and without the CO_2 laser. *Fertil. Steril.*, **47**, 704–6.

Weibel, M. A. and Majno, G. (1973), Peritoneal adhesions and their relation to abdominal surgery. *Am. J. Surg.* **126**, 345–53.

Westrom, L. (1985), Effect of acute pelvic inflammatory disease in infertility. *Am. J. Obstet. Gynecol.*, **121**, 707–13.

Young, P. E., Egan, J. E., Barlow, J. J. and Mulligan, W. S. (1970) Reconstructive surgery for infertility in the Boston Hospital for Women. *Am. J. Obstet. Gynecol.*, **108**, 1092.

6 *Advanced operative laser laparoscopy*

JAMES F. DANIELL

6.1 Introduction

Lasers have now been used laparoscopically for a decade. Initial use of the CO_2 laser beam through the laparoscope began independently in France (Bruhat, Mage and Manhes, 1979), Israel (Tadir *et al.*, 1982) and North America (Daniell and Brown, 1982). The first commercial laser laparoscope was marketed by Eder Instrument Co. in North America in early 1983. Since that time, almost all endoscopic manufacturers have introduced their own systems for aiming and firing the CO_2 laser beam through the laparoscope or through second-puncture probes. Following the introduction of the CO_2 laser, investigators have subsequently reported use of the argon (Keye, Matson and Dixon, 1983; Diamond, DeCherney and Polan, 1986), neodymium-yttrium aluminium garnet (Nd-YAG) (Lomano, 1983) and the potassium titanyl phosphate (KTP) (Daniell, 1986; Daniell *et al.*, 1986) lasers for laparoscopic laser surgery. All four of these lasers are now widely available and are used clinically for various laparoscopic procedures.

This chapter will review the advanced operative procedures that are possible using flexible visible laser light energy from the argon and the KTP lasers.

6.2 History of the development of visible light lasers for laparoscopy

Keye *et al.* (1983) at the University of Utah were the first to begin clinical evaluations of the argon laser at laparoscopy (Plate 4). Working with a local manufacturer of the argon laser (HGM, Salt Lake City, Utah), Keye began to evaluate an argon laser that could be aimed and fired through flexible optical fibres at laparoscopy. After initial animal investigations, he reported the use of this new visible light laser beam for the vaporization of endometriosis. Soon after, other authors reported other uses for the argon laser at laparoscopy (Diamond *et al.*, 1986). In the autumn of 1985, the KTP laser (Laserscope, Santa Clara, California) became available for clinical investigations in gynaecology in North America (Plate 5). This laser initially had been evaluated in ophthalmology and ENT, but because of its specific characteristics of vaporization, it was felt that it might be of benefit in gynaecological surgery. Initial evaluations were carried out in rabbits (Daniell, 1986), and laparoscopically for treatment of endometriosis as well as other pelvic conditions (Daniell *et al.*, 1986). These two visible light lasers, the argon and the KTP, are now commercially available and used for several operative laparoscopic procedures.

6.3 Physics and tissue interaction of the argon and KTP lasers

Both the KTP and the argon lasers are in the visible light spectrum. The KTP wavelength is 532 nm and the argon is 515 and 500 nm. These lasers do not require a helium–neon laser for aiming purposes since the laser light generated is in the visible spectrum. The argon is bluish–green while the KTP is more of a lime-green colour. Both of these lasers can pass through flexible fibreoptic fibres for delivery to the tissue through endoscopes. They pass through clear fluids and their primary tissue effect is coagulation. The tissue depth of penetration is less than with the Nd-YAG laser but more than with the CO_2 laser.

The argon laser beam is generated from a resonator chamber filled with argon gas, whereas the KTP laser beam is produced by pumping a Nd-YAG laser at 50 W through a crystal of KTP. From this crystal a green beam is generated, which at 532 nm is double the wavelength of the Nd-YAG. Thus, the KTP laser has also been called the frequency-doubled YAG laser.

For clinical use in laparoscopy, the energy of these two lasers can be delivered through flexible fibres. The argon can be delivered through a 600 or a 300 μm fibre, and the KTP laser is delivered through either a 400 or 600 μm fibre. Fibres of both these lasers are reusable. They can be cleaved for repeated use until the entire fibre is used. Both of these lasers generate bright visible light with significant backscatter from tissue impact. Thus, it is necessary to work with safety lenses to protect the operator's eyes and to allow adequate visual observation of the effects of the laser when fired. Tissue penetration does not exceed 2 mm and the primary effects are coagulation or vaporization when direct tissue contact with the fibre tip occurs.

6.4 Advantages and disadvantages of visible light laser energy for laparoscopy

From working initially with the CO_2 and then more recently the KTP and the argon lasers, we have found distinct advantages of the visible

Table 6.1 Advantages of fibre lasers for laparoscopy

1. Laser delivery via flexible fibres
2. No backstop necessary
3. Effective under fluids
4. Minimal smoke formation
5. Excellent haemostasis
6. Both vaporization and coagulation possible
7. Shortened operating time

light lasers for laparoscopy. These are listed in Table 6.1. The main advantage we have found of the visible light lasers is the tremendous ease with which the energy of these lasers can be delivered to tissue compared to the more cumbersome coupling devices needed with the CO_2 laser. The fibre is simply delivered either through the operating channel of the laparoscope or through an alternative probe into the pelvis and placed on or close to the impact site (Figure 6.1). There are no cumbersome alignment steps needed for the application of laser energy. Since visible light laser energy passes through clear fluids in the pelvis, the amount of smoke generated is reduced when performing operative procedures at laparoscopy compared to the CO_2 laser. This simpler delivery system combined with less smoke generation means that operative procedures can usually be performed in a much shorter period of time than with the CO_2 laser. Another advantage of visible light lasers is the ability to either incise, vaporize or photocoagulate very rapidly by merely pulling the fibre tip back away from the tissue slightly. We also feel that there is less potential for bleeding, since both these lasers have greater haemostatic effects than the CO_2 laser.

As with all technology, there are certain disadvantages of the visible light lasers for laparoscopy. These include the necessity for running water to cool the lasers and the need for special electrical wiring. In addition, an eye safety filter must be placed over the laparoscope before firing. This eye filter reduces the diameter of the field of view for the operator and adds an extra encumberment to the eyepiece of the laparoscope as well as an extra cord running out from the operating field. The initial filters developed by these manufacturers somewhat obscured the view, but the filters that are now commercially available do not impede the view of the operator or video monitors when used. Another disadvantage of these two lasers is that their cost is more than CO_2 lasers that can be used for laparoscopic surgery. Both the KTP and the argon laser at time of writing cost more than US$70 000.

In spite of the above disadvantages of visible light laser energy, we

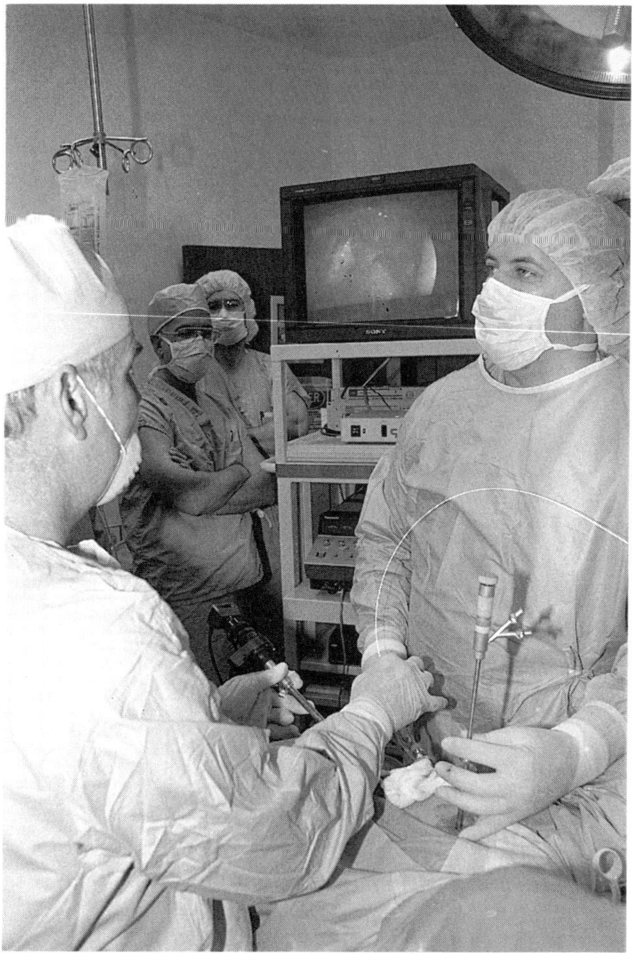

Figure 6.1 Laser laparoscopy using a visible light laser.

feel that the ease and simplicity of certain procedures combined with the reduced operative time far outweighs the disadvantages. This has led us to discard use of the CO_2 laser for laparoscopic surgery except in some certain specific instances or when training physicians in use of the CO_2 laser.

6.5 Delivery techniques

Since the laser energy from visible light lasers can be delivered through flexible fibres, it is simple to get the fibre into the peritoneal cavity for laparoscopic surgery. The method used by most surgeons when only a minimum amount of laser firing is necessary, is to deliver the fibre down the operating channel of a standard laparoscope. The advantages of this system are that it only requires one extra puncture, usually in the lower abdomen, and it allows the operator to have a good angle of attack into the pelvis by passing the fibre down the coaxial channel of the laparoscope. The disadvantage of this method is that it reduces the visible light available through the optics of the scope, since an operating scope is being used. In addition, the depth perception of the operator is reduced because the fibre is passing down the axis of his line of sight.

The alternative method of using these fibres is to deliver them through another puncture site while using a standard diagnostic laparoscope. The manufacturers themselves have designed specific small probes or trocars for bringing in their fibres. As an alternative, the fibres can be passed through the central channel of a 5 mm probe marketed for suction and irrigation at CO_2 laser laparoscopy. These double-channelled suction probes are available from most endoscopic manufacturers. Recently, a 5 mm steerable probe (Marlow Medical, Willoughby, Ohio) has been designed that allows passage of the fibre as well as suction and irrigation of smoke. The probe tip can be moved to any degree from 180° to 90° with the fibre thus being directed at whatever angle is necessary. This probe is especially helpful for treating posterior ovarian surfaces. Alternatively, the probe can be used as a backstop for the fibre or to accomplish traction on tissues in the pelvis. We have found this probe to be particularly helpful in advanced laparoscopic procedures such as salpingostomy, extensive adhesiolysis, or treatment of advanced stages of endometriosis.

Since most advanced operative laparoscopy demands the placement of extra probes, it is important to select and arrange the location of probe entry carefully. We normally will place our first extra probe in the midline suprapubically and use this with 5 mm instruments for retraction and dissection as necessary. If inspection of the pelvis reveals a need for a third probe, we will usually place it 2–3 in. lateral to the umbilicus and at that same level on the side opposite to the major portion of disease. If a fourth probe is needed, we will place it on the opposite side. Occassionally, three probes can be placed in the midline, but this often leads to problems with clashing of the instruments during pelvic manipulations. Care should be taken to avoid inferior epigastric arteries when placing the lateral probes. This potential problem can be reduced by trans-illuminating the abdominal wall and identifying the vessels in a briefly darkened operating room. Multiple ancillary instruments have been developed for laparoscopy, and many have specific uses. We feel that the minimum necessary instruments

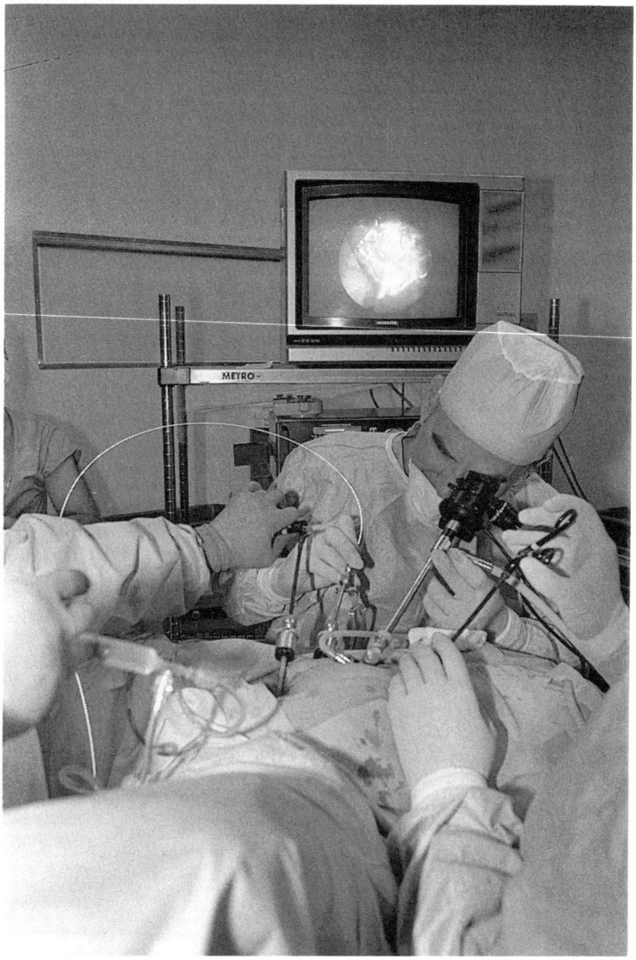

Figure 6.2 Laser laparoscopy with the use of video.

are at least three 5 mm trochars with scissors, atraumatic grasping forceps, and the ability to pass cautery forceps for both unipolar and bipolar use. Certainly, any gynaecologist who plans to undertake extensive operative laser laparoscopy should be experienced with multiple punctures and with the use of both unipolar and bipolar cautery at laparoscopy.

The use of video can be very helpful when doing operative laparoscopy with lasers (Figure 6.2). There are many advantages of video, some of which are listed in Table 6.2. Since multiple punctures and

Table 6.2 Advantages of video use for endoscopy

1. Allows assistant to really 'help'
2. Resident able to do more
3. Greater involvement of operating room personnel
4. Teaching potential improved
5. Educational tapes can be produced
6. Patient enlightenment
7. Increases referrals for surgery

extensive operative procedures require more than two hands, it is mandatory to have a co-ordinated, knowledgeable assistant. The only way that the assistant can reasonably assist is to visualize what is actually occurring and anticipate the actions necessary to optimize the results with a minimum of complications. The use of video can either be with a direct coupler which requires the operator to work while looking directly at the T.V. monitor, or with a beam splitter which allows the option of either looking directly through the laparoscope or at the monitor. We prefer the beam splitter, since it gives the operator the chance to look into the pelvis directly when necessary. A 90–10 beam splitter which directs 90% of light to the video monitor and 10% through to the eye of the operator has been adequate for us, giving good diameter of view as well as enough light for good visibility on the monitor and for recording purposes (Wolf Instrument Company, Chicago, Illinois). If the operator prefers to work directly off the video monitor, it is best to place the monitor between the patient's legs so that the orientation is the same as the operator would have if looking directly into the pelvis. Although the term 'video laser laparoscopy' has been coined in North America, we feel that this is a silly term which has no real bearing on what is being performed. A more accurate term would be 'laparoscopic surgery performed under video control'. The idea that a flat video monitor being viewed by two eyes would give better depth of perception and finer colour discrimination than that of the human eye looking directly through the laparoscope seems impossible to believe. In my opinion, no monitor or camera system will ever approach the visual acuity of the human eye. Because of this, we like to always retain the ability to look directly into the pelvis when we feel we are in a tight spot or a particularly difficult dissecting area. Having the beam splitter attached makes this very simple and saves the need to remove the camera and replace it intermittently.

6.6 Specific procedures performed laparoscopically

Almost every procedure that has been done laparoscopically with scissors, cautery and CO_2 lasers has now been reported using the visible light lasers. This list includes the treatment of polycystic ovaries, correction of hydrosalpinx, conservative treatment of ectopic pregnancy, extensive adhesiolysis, and treatment of all stages of endometriosis.

6.6.1 TREATMENT OF POLYCYSTIC OVARIES

Following reports of successful use of laparoscopic ovarian cautery (Gjönnaess, 1984), and ovarian biopsy to treat polycystic ovaries (Campo *et al.*, 1983), we began investigating the use of laser energy to treat polycystic ovaries in 1984. Initially, we used the CO_2 laser for this technique and had satisfactory results. However, the volume of tissue vaporized produced a tremendous amount of smoke and, in addition, any bleeding induced was difficult to stop. Thus this procedure required a fairly long operating time. With the availability of KTP and argon lasers, we began to use lasers of this wave length for laparoscopic treatment of polycystic ovaries. We have been able to reduce operating time while still selectively destroying portions of the ovarian stroma satisfactorily. In a series of 85 patients, we have been able to produce spontaneous ovulation post-operatively in 71% and successful pregnancy in 56% of these patients. These data, summarized in Table 6.3, have recently been reported (Daniell and Miller, 1989).

Our present technique for treating polycystic ovaries involves laparoscopy with a three-puncture technique. A 5 mm grasping forceps is used to fix the ovary and the flexible fibre from either the argon or KTP laser is introduced through a 5 mm probe and used to vaporize multiple sites symmetrically over each ovary. Some of the subcapsular cysts are opened and the follicular fluid removed and aspirated. Likewise, the ovarian stroma itself is vaporized. Small craters in the range of 3–5 mm are thus drilled on the ovarian surface with the laser energy (Plate 6). The procedure can usually be accomplished in less than an hour and the majority of the patients are discharged within 8 h. We feel that this is an excellent procedure in those patients who desire immediate pregnancy and who have failed to respond to Clomiphene in adequate doses, or who have responded to Clomiphene but need a laparoscopy to complete their infertility evaluation. It gives these patients a 'window of opportunity' during which they might conceive without the need for expensive ovulation induction therapy or wedge resection. The effect is transient, as almost all patients have reverted back to anovulatory status within 6 months to 1 year after the laparoscopic treatment (Keckstein, 1989). We have had no complications in this

Table 6.3 Pregnancy after laparoscopic laser vaporization of polycystic ovaries

	Patients	*Post-operative results*			
		No CC		*CC given*	
		(ovulated)	*(conceived)*	*(ovulated)*	*(conceived)*
Patients ovulating on CC prior to laparoscopy	47	40	20	7	2
Patients not ovulating prior to laparoscopy	38	20	15	17*	10
Total	85	60 (71%)	35	24	12

CC, clomiphene citrate; HMG, human menopausal gonadotrophin; HCG, human chorionic gonadotrophin.
Total conception = 48 (56%) – spontaneous, CC, HMG, HCG.
* One patient was anovulatory with CC and required HMG for ovulation and conception.

procedure in over 120 cases and now recommend it for all of our patients with polycystic ovarian syndrome who meet the criteria of failure to respond to Clomiphene, with or without human chorionic gonadotrophin or otherwise need a laparoscopy while desiring immediate post-operative pregnancy.

Switching from the CO_2 laser to the use of visible light lasers has made this an easier, safer and quicker procedure at laparoscopy. This is of particular advantage because many of these patients are extremely obese and thus somewhat difficult subjects on whom to perform operative laparoscopy with a reasonable degree of safety. The advantages to these patients are obvious compared to the risks and discomfort that they would undergo from a formal wedge resection performed at laparotomy. In addition, it avoids the expense involved with Pergonal therapy as well as the risks of hyperstimulation and multiple pregnancies.

6.6.2 TREATMENT OF HYDROSALPINX

In the past, surgical treatment of hydrosalpinx had uniformly poor results with even the best microsurgeons reporting no more than 30% pregnancy rates with long-term follow-up in controlled series (Bateman, Nunley and Kitchin, 1987). Laparoscopic treatment of hydrosalpinges has been attempted since the late 1970s with the first reports by Gomel (1977) and others (Mettler, Giesel and Semm, 1979; Fayez, 1983). Following the reports of Mage and Bruhat (1983) on using the CO_2 laser for repair of hydrosalpinx at laparotomy, we began investigating the use of laser energy through the laparoscope for treatment of hydrosalpinges. Our initial results with the CO_2 laser were reported in 1984 (Daniell and Herbert, 1984). More recently we have switched to using the visible light laser fibres for this technique and have obtained better results by being more selective in our attempts at salpingostomy and by refining our techniques using the fibreoptic laser delivery systems. The problems that we encountered with the CO_2 laser were bleeding that required cautery to the opened edges of the tubes and the inability in some tubes to evert the edges out successfully. Using the small diameter visible light laser fibres with four puncture techniques, we find it easier and quicker to do salpingostomy. A small haemostatic incision is made in the distal end of the tube and either one or two radial cuts performed using the fibre. After the tube is opened, the 5 mm steerable probe is placed into the tube and used as a backstop and for traction so that the thinner portions of the tube can be identified and the proper site for the next incisions selected. After the tube is opened, the fibre is then held 2 cm from the lateral edges of the peritoneum of the open fimbria and the defocused laser energy used to constrict the peritoneum. This causes the tubes to evert outwards like the petals of a flower. This 'Bruhat technique' is much easier in our opinion to accomplish laparoscopically using a fibre than with the CO_2 laser. Our recent results in patients in which the primary treatment of their tubal blockage was carried out laparoscopically using the KTP laser with a minimum of 18 months follow-up are given in Table 6.4. As can be seen, a reasonable pregnancy rate has been obtained with an acceptable level of ectopic pregnancies in these patients. Most pregnancies in these patients do not occur until 9 months to a year and a half after surgery, so a relatively long-term follow-up is necessary before any meaningful data can be presented.

It is our opinion that in this age of increasing availability of office-based ultrasound IVF with acceptable pregnancy rates, that laparotomy for hydrosalpinges should only be offered to those patients who cannot afford or do not desire IVF and in situations where the Fallopian tubes cannot be repaired by a laparoscopic approach. Certainly the advantages to the patients in reduced discomfort, minimum recuperation time, and reduction of cost and time off work are tremendous. Although further work and evaluation by other authors is needed, it appears that laparoscopic treatment of hydrosalpinges using laser energy is a reasonable alternative to laparotomy in the hands of experienced operative laparoscopists.

6.6.3 LAPAROSCOPIC TREATMENT OF TUBAL PREGNANCY USING LASER ENERGY

Although this subject is covered in depth in another chapter of this book, we do feel that the techniques that we have used with visible light laser energy have some advantages for treatment of ectopic pregnancies. Certainly there have been many reports of successful treatment of tubal pregnancy using laparoscopic cautery (Reich *et al.*, 1987) and the CO_2 laser (Pouly *et al.*, 1986; Loffer, 1987). In our experience, the risk of bleeding from the tube is reduced when using visible light laser energy delivered through the small diameter fibre compared with that of the CO_2 laser. In addition, the trauma to the tube appears to be less with the visible light laser fibres than when using the needle electrodes presently available for laparoscopic use. Table 6.5 lists our results at West Side Hospital in Nashville, Tennessee using laser energy for ectopics treated by laparoscopy. All cases after 1985 were performed with visible light laser energy. We certainly agree with others that laparoscopic treatment of ectopic pregnancy is well tolerated by patients and very cost-effective (Brumsted *et al.*, 1988).

Table 6.4 Results of laparoscopic neosalpingostomy with lasers. West Side Hospital, Nashville, Tennessee (18 month minimum follow-up)

Laser type	*Year*	*No. of patients*	*Open tubes at 6 weeks HSG*	*Attempting pregnancy*	*Pregnancy results*		
					IUP	*Abortions*	*Ectopics*
CO_2	1982–85	104*	58/71 (82%)	88	22 (25%)	11 (13%)	11 (13%)
KTP	1985–86	36†	24/28 (86%)	32	10 (31%)	3 (9%)	5 (16%)
Totals		140	82/99 (83%)	120	32 (28%)	14 (12%)	16 (13%)

* Sixty procedures were in recurrent hydrosalpinges with at least 2 year follow-up.
† Only three procedures were recurrent hydrosalpinges.
HSG, hysterosalpingogram; IUP, intra-uterine pregnancy.

Table 6.5 Laparoscopic treatment of ectopics. Hospital Corporation of America, West Side Hospital, Nashville, Tennessee. January 1984 to January 1988

Total patients	36
Ruptured tubes	2
Salpingectomy	6
Salpingostomy	30
Laparotomies done	0

Tubal patency on hysterosalpingogram: 18 of 20 tested, 90% post operatively. Repeat ectopics: 2 of 20 attempting pregnancy (10%). Intra-uterine pregnancy: 8 of 20 (40%).

6.6.4 OPERATIVE LAPAROSCOPY AT THE TIME OF ASSISTED CONCEPTION

Many patients who are infertile also have other symptoms related to either endometriosis or adhesions. These patients often come to laparoscopy either because of persistence of their infertility or recurrence or persistence of pain or a combination of both. The ability to offer patients an attempt at conception (GIFT) and treatment for their primary disease (operative laparoscopy with adhesiolysis, vaporization of endometriosis or uterine nerve ablation), seems very appealing. The main problem at a laparoscopy done with GIFT is that the ovaries have been stimulated and therefore are enlarged and tend to bleed if too much manipulation is attempted. In addition, uterine manipulators should not be used and chromotubation cannot be carried out. Because of this, the operator is limited as to what can be accomplished at the time of the GIFT procedure with laparoscopic treatment. Often, however, endometriosis and adhesions can be treated. The use of visible light laser energy is particularly helpful in working around ovaries in these patients because of the increased vascularity related to the multiple follicles that have been produced by hormone stimulation before the laparoscopy. After aspirating the follicles and while the laboratory personnel are identifying and preparing the gametes for transfer into the tube, the surgeon has an opportunity to perform indicated laparoscopic procedures. The fibres can be easily brought in through one of the accessory probes and used for adhesiolysis and/or vaporization of endometriosis in a minimal period of time. This does not prolong the anaesthesia time and if the surgeon is careful, should not increase risks of bleeding from manipulation in the pelvis. It is even possible to transect the uterosacral ligaments in these patients if one is careful to reflect the ovaries laterally and lift the uterus up with accessory probes. We feel that this ability to give the chance of conception to the patient via GIFT as well as accomplish treatment of her pelvic pathology is logical and intelligent and an option that many patients will embrace and elect if given the choice.

6.6.5 TREATMENT OF ENDOMETRIOSIS WITH VISIBLE LIGHT LASERS

Pelvic endometriosis is an ideal condition to be treated with laparoscopic surgery of any type. It is usually multifocal and often associated with adhesions that cannot be successfully treated with drug therapy. The ability to perform laparoscopic surgery condenses the patient's therapy into one event. The laparoscopy can accomplish the diagnosis and staging of the disease, and then by bringing in the laser fibre, the experienced operator can treat the patient and accomplish successful adhesiolysis and destruction or reduction of diseased tissue. Endometriomas can be opened, drained and/or vaporized and other associated pathology corrected at the time of the procedure. The choice for post-operative drug suppressive therapy will then depend on the amount of disease remaining and the patient's desires and symptoms. Patients who desire pregnancy can begin attempts at conception immediately without long delays associated with drug therapy or recovery from major surgery. In addition, the likelihood of post-operative adhesions forming in the pelvis is probably less when the procedure is done laparoscopically as compared with the same techniques performed at laparotomy.

The techniques for treating endometriosis depend on the location and amount of disease present. Surface implants can usually be photocoagulated using the larger fibres held close to the tissue. If vaporization is desired, the tip can actually be touched to the tissue. An alternative method is to use accessory forceps to grasp the implants of endometriosis, put them on traction and dissect them from the area of implantation using the tip of the laser fibre. The most important fact to remember is that the areas of endometriosis often tunnel out and some active disease that is not visible may be located in the margins of visible implants. Because of this, we treat each implant in a similar fashion to viral lesions on the perineum using an 'airbrush' technique around the periphery of the visible lesions. Care must be taken when working over the bladder, close to the ureter and overlying bowel. In other areas, laser energy can be used with good margins of safety with little risk of damage to underlying tissues. Endometriomas need to be carefully dissected from their usual attachments to the lateral pelvic sidewalls. In our experience, it has usually been the sidewall that bleeds and not the ovary itself, so putting gentle traction on the ovary and using the laser energy to vaporize the ovary off the sidewall seems to be more effective than bluntly freeing up the ovary. Care must be taken to identify the ureter along its path and to avoid the major uterine vessels lateral to the ovary. Once the ovary is freed from its adherence to the sidewall, the endometrioma can be opened and the chocolate contents aspirated or irrigated. The method of handling the endometrioma depends on whether the capsule can be stripped from the ovarian stroma or not. By using grasping forceps, if it is possible to tease the capsule free, it can be grasped and usually removed from the ovary with gentle traction. This is basically a non-laser technique. If the capsule is too adherent to the ovarian stroma, we then use the fibreoptic laser fibre to vaporize the capsule by holding the fibre very close to the surface of the inside of the endometrioma and gently passing it over the entire surface. The endometrioma bed, if under 5–6 cm, will usually constrict and close and thus is left without any laparoscopic sutures. Occasionally laparoscopic sutures can be placed using the techniques described by Semm and O'Neill-Freys (1989). Endometriomas larger than 8 or 9 cm are probably still best handled by laparotomy because of the large open ovarian surface areas that result from opening the cyst.

6.6.6 ADHESIOLYSIS WITH VISIBLE LIGHT LASERS

Adhesions associated with endometriosis are handled in a similar fashion as other adhesions. The advantage of the visible light laser fibres is that the energy dissipates from the tip very rapidly so that any structures more than 2 cm beyond the tip will not be affected by impact of the laser beam. This means that it is not so important to maintain a backstop behind adhesions that are not closely overlying vital structures. However, when working close to the bowel or the fimbria, it is necessary to use a backstop because of the potential for damage close behind the beam. The best instrument for providing this extra safety is a 5 mm steerable probe with the titanium tip which can be placed through a 5 mm second puncture site and manipulated as needed to provide both a backstop and traction behind the adhesion while firing the laser. Gentle traction is usually necessary on the adhesion so that the bands can be easily vaporized. The KTP and argon lasers are particularly advantageous for this technique because of the speed with which the adhesions can be taken down, with minimal risk of bleeding and with minimal smoke production.

There has not been an organized prospective study using second-look laparoscopy to evaluate early healing after laparoscopic surgery of any type. A multicentre prospective study is now under way evaluating the early second-look laparoscopic appearance in patients undergoing extensive operative laser laparoscopy. Hopefully in the future this study will shed some light on the actual amount and location of adhesions that occur following laparoscopic adhesiolysis with various different techniques.

Perihepatic adhesions are often seen in patients who have had infectious pelvic pathology (Fitzhugh–Curtis syndrome). Some of these may be symptomatic; however in most cases they are an incidental finding. Our policy is to routinely remove these adhesions which is a very simple matter using the visible light laser fibres. In this case, since the pathology is high in the upper abdomen, it is much simpler to introduce the fibre through the operating channel of the laparoscope. The laparoscope is swung around into the upper abdomen and the fibre introduced under direct visual control. Since the energy dissipates from the tip of the fibre very rapidly, there is no need for a backstop and one does not need to be concerned about damaging the diaphragm. In addition, the haemostatic properties of the beam reduce the potential for bleeding from the liver.

6.6.7 LASER LAPAROSCOPIC ENTEROLYSIS

Laparoscopic bowel adhesiolysis following post-surgical or infectious processes can also be accomplished successfully in many cases using visible light laser energy. We have operated on a significant number of patients over the last decade who have been referred to us for attempts at laparoscopic adhesiolysis after multiple abdominal operations. Many of these patients have had previous bowel obstructions and are at extremely high risk for potential complications at attempted laparoscopy. We routinely counsel these patients concerning the risks of bowel injury and the possible need for immediate laparotomy and/or diverting colostomy. We do a bowel preparation and have them on clear liquids for 48 h before surgery. We will not perform surgery on these patients without having a consenting adult present in the waiting area to giving us immediate consent for laparotomy if indicated and without having a general surgeon standing by to repair any bowel injuries that we might encounter during attempted enterolysis through the laparoscope. We do not routinely do an open laparoscopy, but initially will try to accomplish pneumoperitoneum in a standard fashion, and then introduce a 5 mm laparoscope for initial inspection. After confirming that we are in the correct peritoneal space and noting the proper site for placement of the 10 mm laparoscopic trocar, the larger laparoscope is inserted. The laser fibre is brought in through accessory probes and placement is based on the location of any abdominal wall adhesions. Many of these patients can be helped, although some have such extensive adhesions with bowel so adherent to the internal surface of the abdominal wall that it is impossible to establish a plane of cleavage to vaporize the adhesions. However, those patients who do have significant pain from post-surgical adhesions who undergo successful laparoscopic lysis do have improvement in the majority of cases. We have not yet had any late complications and have only had one bowel perforation that required immediate laparotomy in a series of over 40 patients treated with extensive laser laparoscopic bowel adhesiolysis.

Although some authors have reported the treatment of bowel endometriosis using laser energy through the laparoscope, we have no experience with this. Since most bowel implants are somewhat indurated, we feel that the risk of later bowel perforation is greater than the potential for successful destruction of the entire lesion. For this reason, we limit laparoscopic treatment of bowel endometriosis to those lesions that are exophytic or on epiploic fat or on the tip of the appendix. We will perform an appendectomy through the laparoscope if the tip of the appendix is affected with endometriosis and if we feel we can safely get an endoloop around the proximal appendix and mobilize it enough for removal in one piece through the laparoscopic 10 mm trocar. We do not remove infected appendices or perform elective appendectomy through the laparoscope, as we feel this is better left to general surgeons at open laparotomy.

6.6.8 REMOVAL OF ADNEXAL STRUCTURES WITH LAPAROSCOPIC LASER ENERGY

We have had good experience with use of endoloop sutures for oophorectomy, salpingectomy, or removal of periadnexal structures. In these cases, the technique is mainly non-laser. However, we will occasionally use the KTP or argon laser to excise the ovary away from its pedicle, or to vaporize the pedicle after the bulk of the tissue has been removed. These lasers can be very helpful for cutting pedunculated fibroids into smaller pieces after the fibroid has been constricted with endoloop sutures.

6.6.9 UTEROSACRAL ABLATION WITH LASER ENERGY

One of the more common operations that we perform is transection of the uterosacral ligaments using laparoscopic laser energy (LUNA). We offer this procedure to all patients who have dysmenorrhoea and who are planning laparoscopy. Doyle (1955) was the first to report successful relief from dysmenorrhoea by separating the uterosacral ligaments.

Table 6.6 Laparoscopic uterosacral nerve ablation (LUNA) results with KTP laser (6 month follow-up)

	Worse	*Same*	*Improved*
Endometriosis 80 Patients	3 (4%)	17 (21%)	60 (75%)
Primary dysmenorrhoea 20 Patients	2 (10%)	6 (30%)	12 (60%)
Total 100 Patients	5 (5%)	23 (23%)	72 (72%)

Data from several authors have shown laser transection via laparoscopy to be a successful therapy for dysmenorrhoea, either with or without endometriosis (Feste, 1984; Lichten and Bombard, 1987; Sutton, 1989). We initially used the CO_2 laser for this, but encountered several cases of bleeding that required cautery. As of this writing, there have been two deaths in North America resulting from bleeding from uterosacral ligaments that occurred when these were transected with CO_2 laser energy. Neither of these reports has been published in the literature at this time. We feel that the haemostatic properties of visible light laser energy add some degree of safety when the uterosacral ligaments are being transected. Our technique is to identify the uterosacral ligaments, trace them out to the pelvic brim, trace the ureters out, and note the area of insertion of the uterine artery into the lateral cervix. We then take a 5 mm probe and push against the posterior cervix to tent up the uterosacral ligaments. The laser fibre is then used to transect the ligaments at right angles just as the ligaments insert into the posterior cervix. Sometimes the ligaments will be attenuated and difficult to identify. In these cases we may refrain from cutting if we feel it is unsafe or the landmarks cannot be identified. Occasionally, rectosigmoid obliteration of the cul-de-sac in cases of endometriosis will preclude the ability to cut the uterosacrals in this area. Our follow-up has been satisfactory in the majority of patients, with at least 70% having reduction in their menstrual pain (Table 6.6). Most patients will have a somewhat painful initial period post-operatively, which probably reflects the tissue swelling in the healing phase. We have not noted any effect on bowel or bladder function in these patients, and no patients have reported any reduction in ability to enjoy intercourse or obtain orgasm. It is important to carefully counsel these patients preoperatively and make certain that they are aware that success is not guaranteed in all cases.

6.7 Future possibilities for visible light lasers for advanced operative laparoscopic techniques

Since the KTP laser contains a 50 W Nd-YAG laser, it is possible to utilize both the Nd-YAG or the KTP energy sources independently from the one laser generator. This opens up the possibility of using the Nd-YAG component for ablation of the endometrium at hysteroscopy as well as using the Nd-YAG laparoscopically in selected indications. For example, if bleeding was occurring from an ectopic pregnancy, this might be better treated with the Nd-YAG laser fibre delivered through laparoscopic energy. The potassium titanyl phosphate crystal doubles the frequency from the 1 064 nm infra-red wavelength of a Nd-YAG laser to the 532 nm emerald-green light of the KTP laser and the interposition of a mirror in the system allows energy of either wavelength to emerge from the laser generator.

Other lasers may become available for laparoscopic use in the future. Some of these include the carbon monoxide laser which has tissue effects similar to those of the CO_2 laser, but which can be delivered through a fibre. In addition, the gold vapour laser, tuneable dye laser, the free electron laser and excimer laser all have future potential uses through the laparoscope. As of this writing, none of these has been evaluated either experimentally or in humans for laparoscopic surgery.

6.8 Safety in advanced laser laparoscopy

The safe use of these visible light lasers at laparoscopy includes the proper use of eye filters and protection for both the patient, the surgeon, and the assistants in the operating room. Since the laser energy through the argon and KTP is a visible beam, it is less likely that damage will be done to the operator's eyes. Any inadvertent firing of the laser without eye filters will be immediately recognized because of the bright green colour that is seen. This improves the safety of use of these lasers compared to the Nd-YAG laser which is infra-red and therefore not visible when fired. When working in a closed abdominal cavity, we do not require people in the operating room to wear safety glasses. The fibre itself is coated with a special coating which protects leakage of the energy except from the tip of the fibre. The operator is the only person at risk when the beam is being fired intraperitoneally through the laparoscope, and his eyes are protected by the fail-safe eye filter that is placed over the eyepiece of the laparoscope. With both the argon and the KTP laser, the laser cannot be fired if the eye filter is not working properly. If an attempt is made to

Table 6.7 Shifting trends in gynaecologic endoscopy

	Old therapy	*New therapy*
Menorrhagia	Hysterectomy	YAG ablation or hysteroscopic electrodiathermy
Severe endometriosis	Laparotomy	Laparoscopy
Ectopic gestation	Laparotomy	Laparoscopy
Uterine septum	Abdominal metroplasty	Hysteroscopic resection
Hydrosalpinx	Laparotomy	Laparoscopy
Cornual blockage	Cornual reanastomosis	Hysteroscopic probing and dilatation
Pelvic adhesions	Laparotomy	Laparoscopy
Ovarian pathology requiring removal	Laparotomy Oophorectomy	Laparoscopic Oophorectomy

override the eye filter (this can be done for instance by placing the eye filter on another laparoscope that might be on the table), the operator will immediately be aware of this problem because of the intense brightness that he sees when he attempts to fire the laser in the pelvis without the eye filter. Other considerations are the proper handling of smoke in the operating room because of the potential harmful effects on those breathing the plume. We vent off the smoke through a specially designed suction-irrigation probe that is used to aspirate fluid and pass it through a filter into the disposable plastic canisters on the floor (PumpVac, Marlow Medical, Willoughby, Ohio). By using inline filters, we protect the hospital filter system from being plugged by particulate matter that might be in the plume.

Other safety precautions are those that one would undertake with any sort of operative laparoscopy, such as gentle tissue handling, use of the proper instruments in the proper situations, and proper use of both bipolar and unipolar cautery when necessary. With proper attention to safety, the careful endoscopist can perform extensive operative laparoscopic procedures with good results in the majority of cases with minimal complications and good patient recuperation.

6.9 Conclusions

We agree with Dr Alan DeCherney, who said in his editorial in *Fertility and Sterility* entitled 'The Leader of the Band is Tired,' that the obituary for laparotomy for infertility surgery had been written but not yet

Table 6.8 Benefits of out-patient surgery

1. Reduces cost to patient, insurance company and government
2. Removes psychological stress associated with hospitalization
3. Uses physician's (and patient's) time more effectively
4. Eliminates bed congestion
5. Lessens chance for medication error or therapeutic misadventure
6. Rapid return to full activity by patient

published. Certainly, many gynaecologists now are becoming interested in doing more aggressive operative laparoscopic surgery. We are finding that procedures which in the past required open laparotomy to be successfully performed, can now be done with combinations of hysteroscopy and/or laparoscopy. Table 6.7 lists the so-called old methods of treatment for some of these disease processes compared to the new available techniques that are achieving good results in the hands of experienced operators.

In this time of concern for cost containment in medicine, it seems particularly of benefit to interested physicians to try to reduce costs without cutting corners or compromising patient care. Careful selective use of lasers as well as non-laser laparoscopic techniques in gynaecology can certainly help in cost containment by giving compatible results while avoiding major surgery with its concomitant expense, increased risks, and morbidity and discomfort for patients. The benefits of outpatient surgery are many. Some of these are listed in Table 6.8. All forward-thinking gynaecologists should investigate the potential for using advanced operative laparoscopic laser surgery in their practices.

References

Bateman, B. G., Nunley, W. C. and Kitchin, J. D. (1987), Surgical management of distal tubal obstruction – are we making progress? *Fertil. Steril.*, **48**, 523.

Bruhat, M., Mage, C. and Manhes, M. (1979), Use of the CO_2 laser via laparoscopy. In *Laser Surgery III, Proceedings of the Third International Society for Laser Surgery* (ed. I. Kaplan), International Society for Laser Surgery, Tel Aviv, p. 275.

Brumsted, J., Gibson, C., Gibson, M. *et al.* (1988), A comparison of laparoscopy and laparotomy for the treatment of ectopic pregnancy. *Obstet. Gynecol.*, **71**, 889.

Campo, S., Garcea, N., Caruso, A. and Siccardi, P. (1983), Effect of celioscopic ovarian resection in patients with polycystic ovaries. *Gynecol. Obstet. Invest.*, **15**, 213–22.

Daniell, J. F. (1986), Laparoscopic evaluation of the KTP/532 Laser for treating endometriosis – Initial report. *Fertil. Steril.*, **46**, 373.

Daniell, J. F. and Brown, D. H. (1982), Carbon dioxide laser laparoscopy: Initial experience in experimental animals and humans. *Obstet. Gynecol.*, **49**, 761.

Daniell, J. F. and Herbert, C. M. (1984), Laparoscopic salpingostomy utilizing the CO_2 laser. *Fertil. Steril.*, **4**, 558.

Daniell, J. F., Meisels, S., Miller, W. and Tosh, R. (1986), Laparoscopic use of the KTP/532 laser in nonendometriotic pelvic surgery. *Colpo. Gynecol. Laser Surg.*, **2**, 107–11.

Daniell, J. F. and Miller, W. (1989), Polycystic ovaries treated by laparoscopic laser vaporization. *Fertil. Steril.*, **51**, 232–6.

Diamond, M. P., DeCherney, A. H. and Polan, M. L. (1986), Laparoscopic use of the argon laser in nonendometriotic reproductive pelvic surgery. *J. Reprod. Med.*, **31**, 1011.

Doyle, J. B. (1955), Paracervical uterine denervation by transection of the cervical plexus for the relief of dysmenorrhea. *Am. J. Obstet. Gynecol.*, **70**, 1.

Fayez, J. A. (1983), An assessment of the role of operative laparoscopy in tuboplasty. *Fertil. Steril.*, **39**, 476.

Feste, J. R. (1984), CO_2 laser neurectomy for dysmenorrhea. *Lasers Surg. Med.*, **3**, 327.

Gjönnaess, H. (1984), Polycystic ovarian syndrome treated by ovarian electrocautery through the laparoscope. *Fertil. Steril.*, **41**, 20–5.

Gomel, V. (1977), Salpingostomy by laparoscopy. *J. Reprod. Med.*, **18**, 265.

Keye, W. R., Matson, G. A. and Dixon, J. (1983), The use of the argon laser in the treatment of experimental endometriosis. *Fertil. Steril.*, **39**, 26.

Keckstein, J. (1989), Laparoscopic treatment of polycystic ovarian syndrome. In *Baillières Clinical Obstetrics and Gynaecology*. International Practice and Research, Vol. 3 (ed. C. S. G. Sutton), Tindall, London, pp. 563–81.

Lomano, J. M. (1983), Laparoscopic ablation of endometriosis with the YAG Laser. *Lasers Surg. Med.*, **3**, 179.

Lichten, E. M. and Bombard, J. (1987), Surgical treatment of primary dysmenorrhea with laparoscopic uterine nerve ablation. *J. Reprod. Med.*, **32**, 37.

Loffer, F. D. (1987), Outpatient management of ectopic pregnancies. *Am. J. Obstet. Gynecol.*, **156**, 1467.

Mage, G. and Bruhat, M. A. (1983), Pregnancy following salpingostomy: comparison between CO_2 laser and electrosurgery procedures. *Fertil. Steril.*, **40**, 472.

Mettler, L., Giesel, H. and Semm K. (1979), Treatment of female infertility due to tubal obstruction by operative laparoscopy. *Fertil. Steril.*, **32**, 384.

Pouly, J. L., Mahnes, H., Mage, G. *et al.* (1986), Conservative laparoscopic treatment of 321 ectopic pregnancies. *Fertil. Steril.*, **46**, 1093.

Reich, H., Freifeld, M. L., McGlynn, F. *et al.* (1987), Laparoscopic treatment of tubal pregnancy. *Obstet. Gynecol.*, **69**, 275.

Semm, K. and O'Neill-Freys (1989), Conventional operative laparoscopy (pelviscopy). In *Baillières Clinical Obstetrics and Gynaecology. International Practice and Research*, Vol. 3 (ed. C. J. G. Sutton), Tindall, London, pp. 451–85.

Sutton, C. J. G. (1989), Laser uterine nerve ablation. In *Laser Operative Laparoscopy and Hysteroscopy* (ed. J. Donnez), Nauwelaerts Printing, Leuven, pp. 43–52.

Tadir, Y., Kaplan, I., Zuckerman, Z. and Ovadia, J. (1981), Laparoscopic CO_2 laser sterilization. In *Human Reproduction*, (eds K. Semm and L. Mettler), Excerpta Medica, Amsterdam, p. 429.

7 *Neodymium-YAG laser laparoscopy*

STEPHEN L. CORSON

7.1 Basic science

The Nd-YAG is a solid-state laser in which the crystal (the YAG portion) is purposefully contaminated with neodymium ions which become the actual lasing medium. The most popular frequency has been a wavelength of 1.06 μm in the near infra-red portion of the spectrum, but other frequencies have been tried. A helium–neon aiming beam is needed since YAG laser energy is not in the visible spectrum. The energy is easily transmitted through optical fibres with high efficiency. The YAG laser can be used in a liquid environment which is the second major difference from CO_2 laser systems commonly used in gynaecology.

Somewhat colour seeking, although not to the extent of argon or KTP-532 lasers, YAG light is absorbed by all tissues to a depth of 3–5 mm, thus explaining the excellent haemostatic properties associated with its use. Its peculiar property is one of a high degree of backscatter which is not considered to be beneficial in most applications, with up to 40% of the energy being distributed in this fashion. This is another major difference from the CO_2 laser. The combination of red seeking and backscatter dictates use of special protective glasses when using the YAG laser. A lens which has a slight green filter with an optical filtration factor of 5 is needed. If surgery is performed through a video system using a camera **without** a beam splitter the glasses are not needed.

Because the YAG laser has only a 2% generating efficiency, high-pressure krypton or xenon arc lamps are necessary to pump the medium. This introduces the need for an efficient heat transfer system since the power to the lamp is in the neighbourhood of 5 kW. The newer units such as that made by Surgical Laser Technologies, Malvern, Pennsylvania, USA, are self-cooled by an internal water-cooled system obviating the need for special plumbing in the operating theater. A single phase 208–220 V powerline is needed.

In a pulsed mode, pulse trains of 5×10^{-9} s can be generated with megawatt power ranges. When high wattage is employed, a strong lens is necessary to focus the output and fibre diameters must also be increased. Most fibres used for gynaecologic application are 0.6 mm in diameter.

7.2 The sapphire probe

Although the scatter properties are excellent for destruction of volumes of tissue such as in a tumour bed, and for endometrial ablation via hysteroscopy, little laparoscopic use was forecast with this laser in the bare fibre mode. Lomano, (1985), however, described use of a bare YAG fibre to deliver light to destroy endometriotic implants via laparoscopy.

Development of the sapphire probes which attach to the optical fibre represents a quantum leap in Nd-YAG laser application (Joffe *et al.*, 1985). Firstly, the power requirements are drastically reduced since the energy is focused at the tip. Equal power densities are achieved at about 1/12 the wattage. Secondly, the objectional scatter is 90–95% reduced. Furthermore, the geometry of the probe determines the shape of the lesion and by modulating power output precise surgery can be performed in a tissue contact fashion obviating focusing of beams and concern about inadvertent tissue damage.

Early work, primarily by Joffe's group (Joffe, 1985; Joffe *et al.*, 1986) has demonstrated marked superiority of the contact probe in hepatic resection with tremendous reduction of power needs and blood loss compared with a bare fibre technique. Important for laparoscopy is an associated marked reduction in smoke plume formation. The probes have a high melting point (2030–2050°C) and are internally cooled via a conduit within the handle that allows for CO_2 or liquid as the cooling source.

Figure 7.1 depicts the relationship between the geometry of the probe and the shape of the lesion. Vaporization is best achieved with the rounded probe which is an excellent choice for endometrial implants on peritoneal surfaces and for destruction of cells lining the cyst wall of ovarian endometriomas. The flat probe is especially useful where coagulation is required. We have been able to completely seal intact blood vessels of 0.8 mm diameter using this probe at 20–22 W. The conical probe serves as a laser scalpel and can be used for lysis of adhesions and for incidental myomectomy.

The most versatile probe is the chisel tip. With this one can incise the ovarian tunica and shave off the cyst wall lining and vaporize the lining cells via laparoscopy with virtually no smoke production, no bleeding and no need for suturing. Pathologic tissue is destroyed *in*

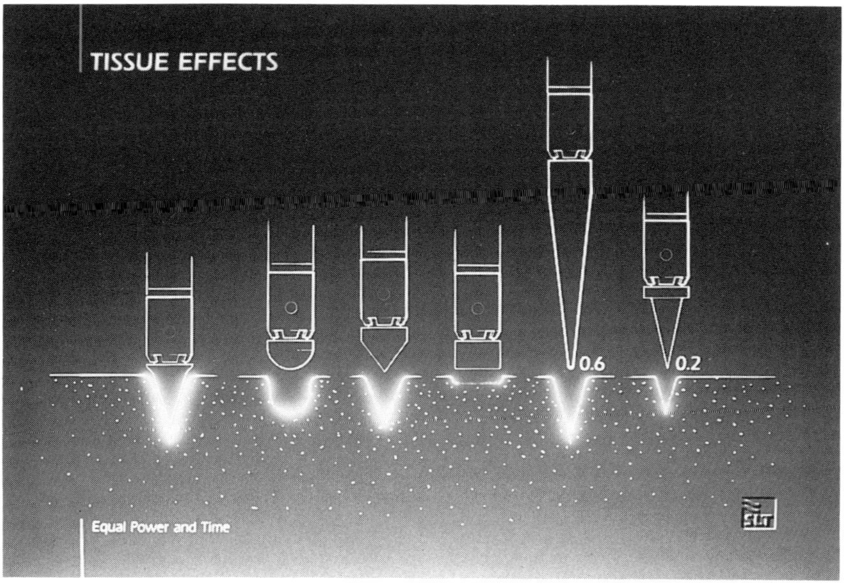

Figure 7.1 The geometry of the probe determines the shape of the lesion.

situ and nothing is removed except for purposes of histologic confirmation. This probe is also used for uterosacral sectioning when endometriosis posteriorly is associated with pelvic pain.

Figure 7.2 demonstrates the ability of the sapphire contact probe to modulate the depth of tissue necrosis while using reduced power output. Most surgeons are more comfortable with a touch technique. Energy levels drop off rapidly so that 1 cm past the tip there is virtually no tissue effect. Thus the propensity for inadvertent distal damage is almost nil.

Figure 7.3 shows the reduction of smoke production which is of great importance for the laparoscopist. Complicated methods for venting plume and smoke evacuation are not necessary. Figure 7.4 demonstrates the excellent haemostatic properties of a YAG contact scalpel used in the hepatic bed. Figure 7.5 shows that histologically the effect on tissue between the contact YAG and the CO_2 beam is virtually indistinguishable.

7.3 CO_2 vs YAG contact probe lasers

Table 7.1 summarizes the differences between the YAG contact probe system and the CO_2 beam system. Probably the chief advantage of the

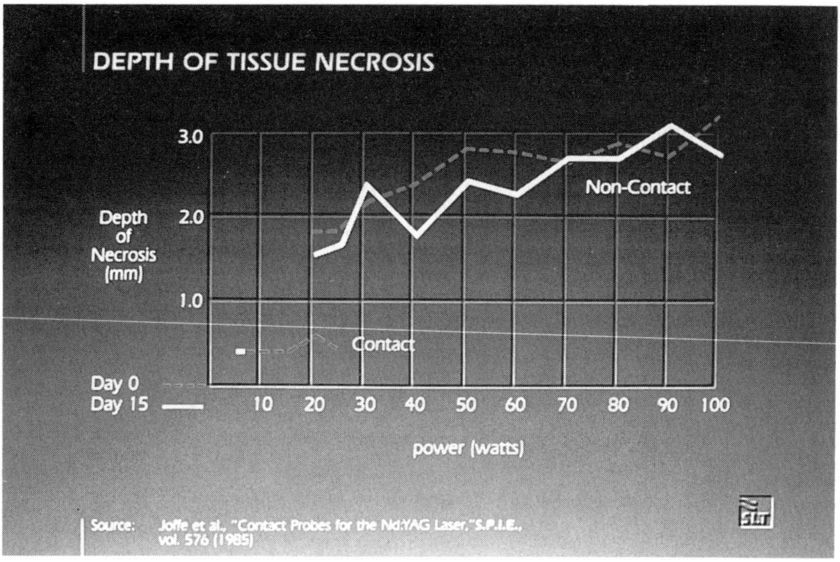

Figure 7.2 Reduced depth of tissue effect with the contact probe. Source: S. N. Joffe *et al.* (1985), Contact probes for the Nd:YAG laser. *S.P.I.E.*, **576**, 42–50.

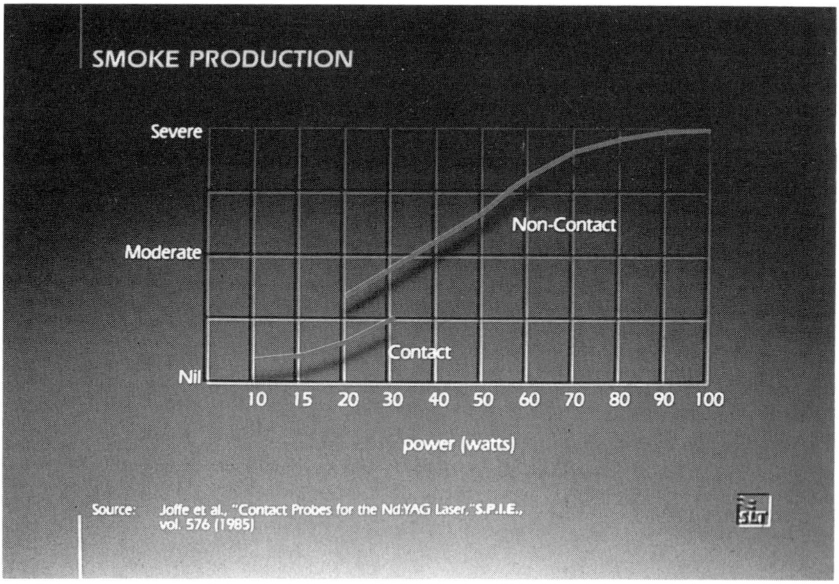

Figure 7.3 Reduction of smoke: contact vs bare fibre in the canine liver. Source: S. N. Joffe *et al.* (1985), Contact probes for the Nd:YAG laser. *S.P.I.E.*, **576**, 42–50.

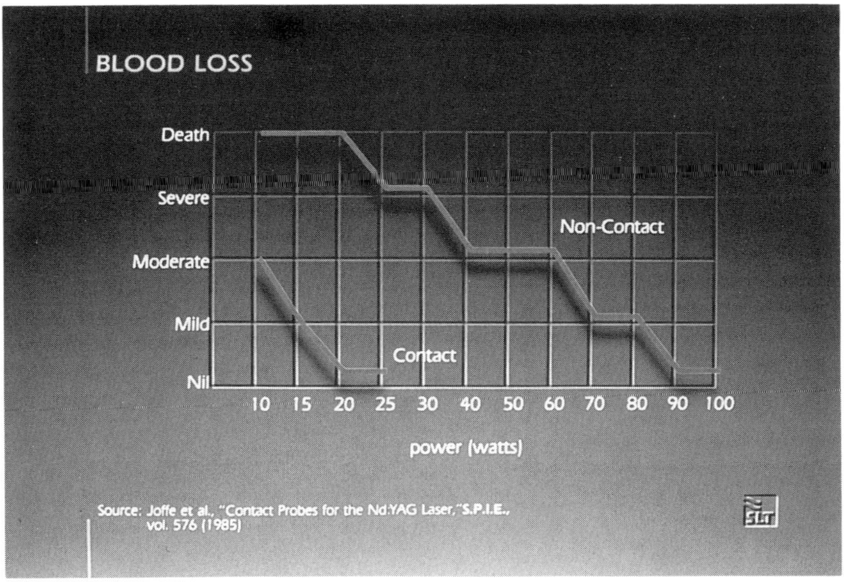

Figure 7.4 Blood loss. Source: S. N. Joffe *et al.* (1985), Contact probes for the Nd:YAG laser *S.P.I.E.*, **576**, 42–50.

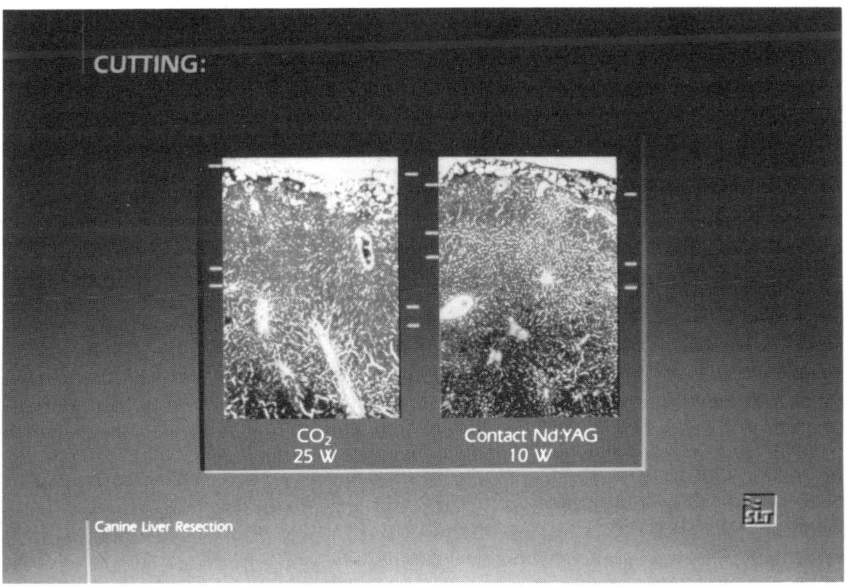

Figure 7.5 Section through tissue cut with the CO_2 laser and with the YAG laser. Canine liver resection. Source: S. N. Joffe *et al.* (1985), Contact probes for the Nd:YAG laser. *S.P.I.E.*, **576**, 42–50.

Table 7.1 Comparison of laser systems

	CO_2 laser	*Nd-YAG laser sapphire probe*
Delivery system	Rigid system	Flexible fibre
Absorption by water	Great	Small
Need for mirror alignment	Frequent	Rare
Production of smoke	Great	Small
Delivery	Focused beam	Touch
Vaporization	Great	Small
Coagulation	Small	Great
Propensity for tissue damage past intended target	Great	Small

YAG system is its 'user friendliness' with avoidance of the rigid arm delivery system associated with the CO_2 system and mandatory mirror focusing of the beam. In my experience no laparoscopic CO_2 laser coupler has been truly acceptable, and we usually spend 20 min of set-up time to perform 20 s of energy delivery. Reduction of smoke formation with the YAG laser is another endearing feature compared with the CO_2 units.

Since blood absorbs YAG output twice as well as avascular tissue, endometriotic lesions with pigmentation are better targeted for destruction, although this is not so important as with an argon beam. The inherent haemostatic qualities of the YAG system are in great contradistinction to those seen with the CO_2 laser which must be defocused to be an effective coagulator. Most important is the ability of the YAG to work in a liquid environment unlike the CO_2 laser whose energy is absorbed by water. This feature allows for use within an endometrioma cavity after it has been lavaged since fluid tends to accumulate in the most dependent portion.

The only real drawback to the contact YAG laser vs the CO_2 laser for laparoscopy is that the latter cuts better with less lateral tissue destruction. The YAG laser armed with the conical probe will not cut so well or so cleanly as the CO_2 beam. Clearly, no one laser system is ideal for every indication of application. Probably the CO_2 beam is superior for laparoscopic neosalpingostomy, but for linear salpingotomy for removal of an unruptured ectopic pregnancy the YAG scalpel is preferred because of the haemostatic effect even when dilute vasopressin is used.

All of this complex high technology becomes confusing to operating room personnel, especially if they do not use it on a regular basis. Therefore the touch-sensitive interactive console of the SLT unit is comforting to surgeon and nurse alike because it 'talks' one through the lamp warm-up cycle and fibre calibration procedures (Figure 7.6).

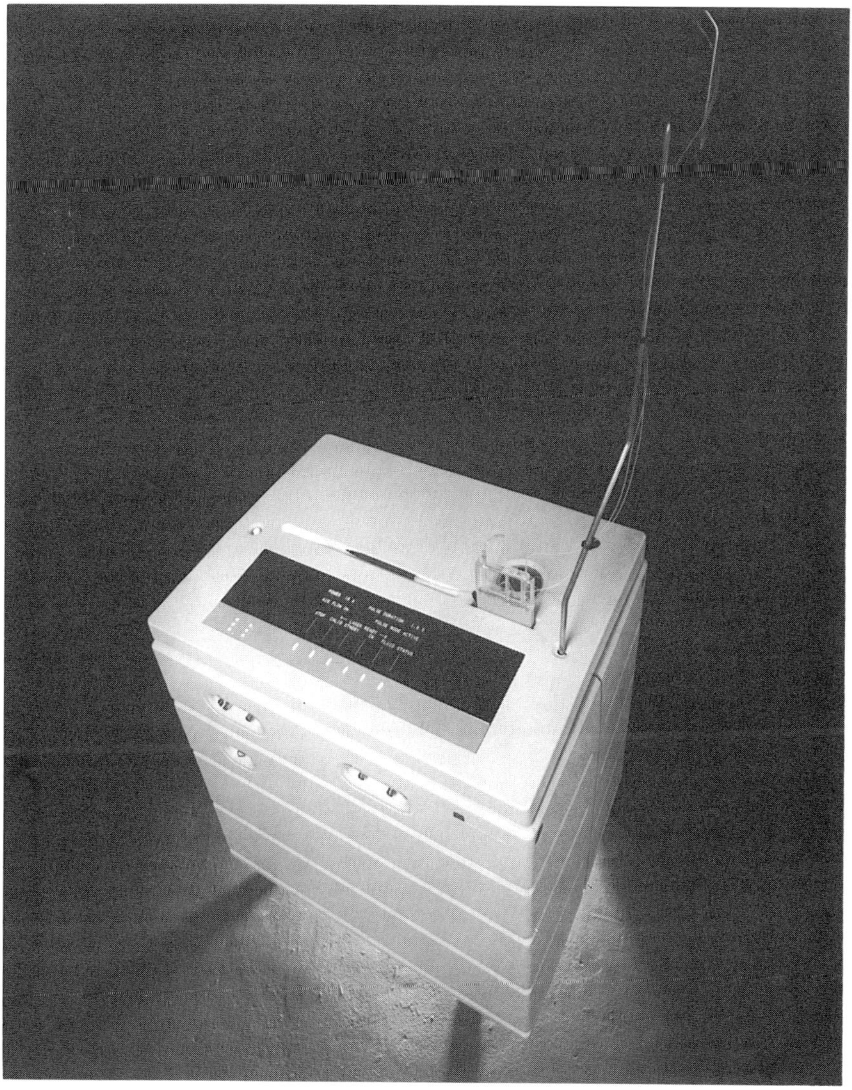

Figure 7.6 SLT YAG laser source.

Laser handles for laparoscopy are of various lengths and can be introduced via an operating laparoscopic sheath or 3 mm side sheath. The disposable handles are calibrated via a port on the laser generator so that the wattage selected is that which actually leaves the distal fibre, after automatic internal compensation for individual fibre energy transmission efficiency. The probe is cooled with CO_2 or a liquid cartridge

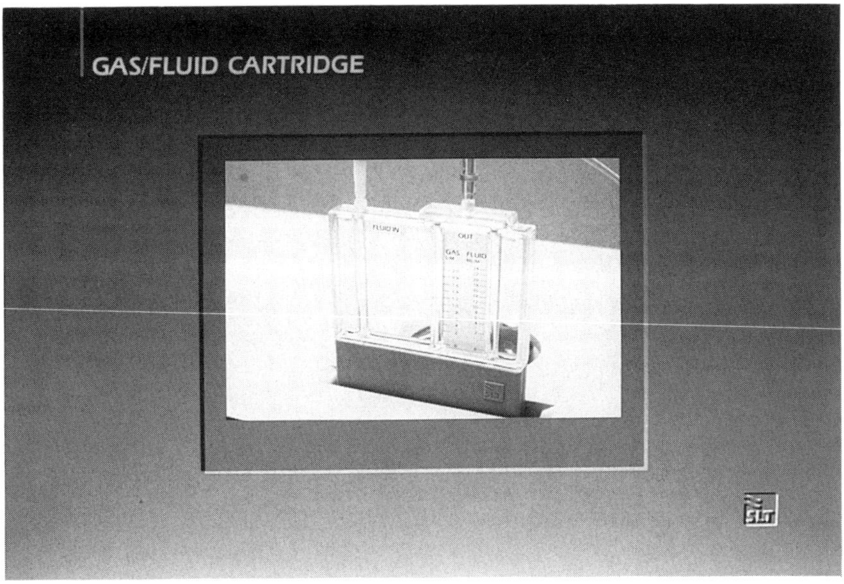

Figure 7.7 SLT liquid or gas cartridge for probe cooling.

(Figure 7.7). The CO_2 flow through the handle is quite safe for laparoscopy but is excessive for hysteroscopy and should never be used within the uterus. Almost any liquid can be employed as a coolant. Flow rates are adjustable over a wide range.

7.4 Laboratory experiments

In a laboratory experiment five adult New Zealand female rabbits were utilized in order to study the acute and chronic effects of the YAG laser on ovarian and uterine tissue. The contact sapphire 'chisel probe' was used at the usual clinical setting of 20 W. Lesions were made in the uterine wall and in the ovaries using continuous application of energy for 2–6 s. One ovary then was removed for acute studies, while the other was examined for 14–21 days. Width and depth of the lesion was measured microscopically after routine histologic preparation. Lesions made in the uterine horn showed a depth of 357–612 μm and a width of 612–816 μm with a 2-s pulse at 20 W (Figure 7.8). The acute ovarian lesions made with the same probe and settings had depths between 714 and 1112 μm and width between 1020 and 1122 μm and were less dependent on duration of probe–tissue contact than on angle of application and adequacy of contact (Figure 7.9).

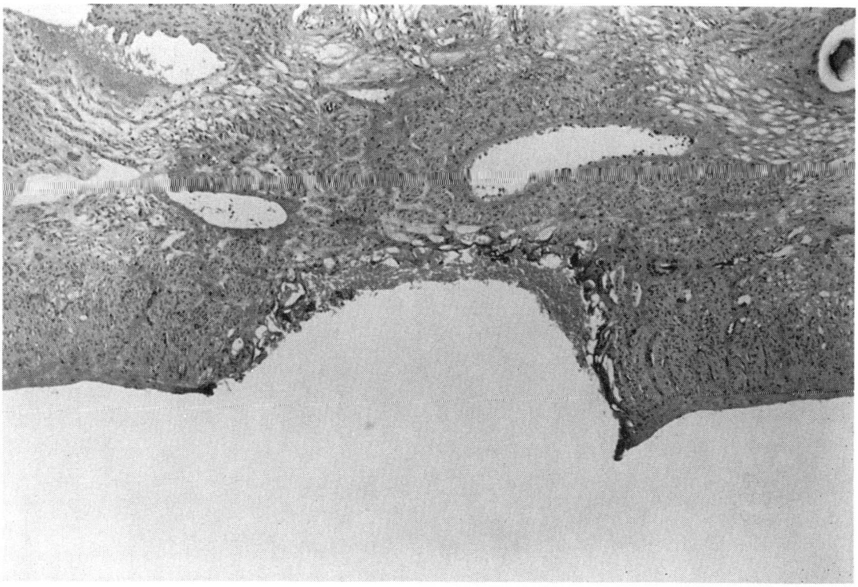

Figure 7.8 Acute uterine lesion (rabbit) with 2 s at 20 W with chisel probe (× 400).

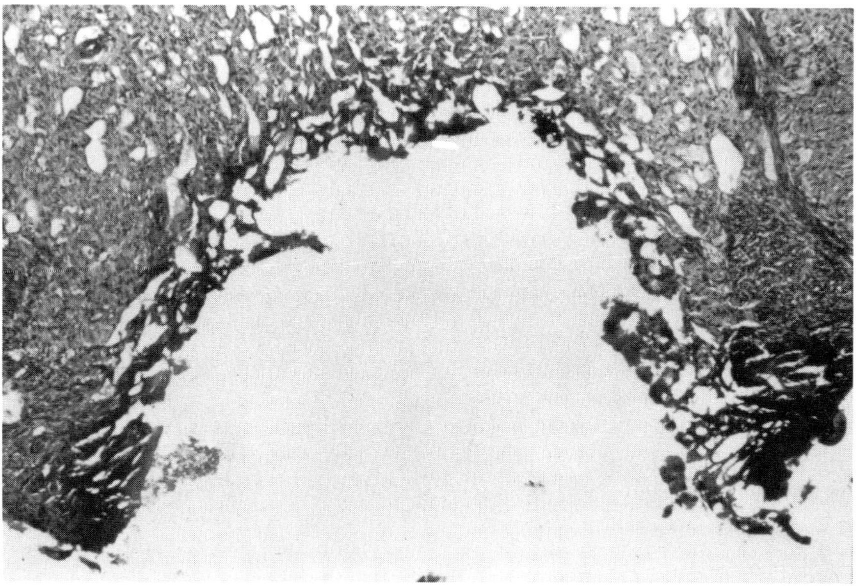

Figure 7.9 Acute ovarian lesion (rabbit) with 2 s at 20 W with chisel probe (× 400).

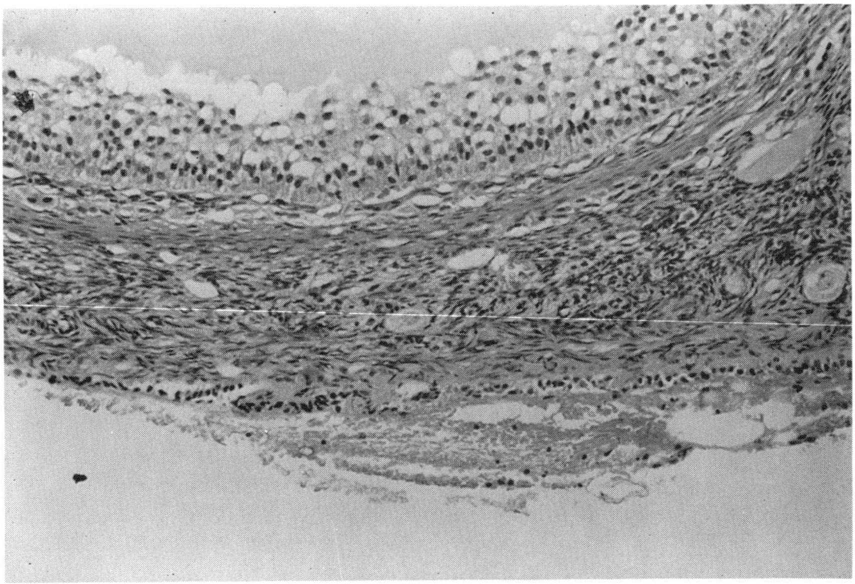

Figure 7.10 Rabbit ovary showing epithelial healing at 3 weeks (× 450).

The chronic study (Figure 7.10) shows that by 21 days the ovary is essentially completely healed with restoration of good epithelial covering.

7.5 Clinical applications

Any laparoscopic system will be compromised by its weakest member, and certainly use of a YAG laser or any other laser with antiquated or inadequate laparoscopic instrumentaton is inconsistent with both good medical practice and common sense. First, one needs a laparoscope and a light source capable of providing adequate light transmission and excellent resolution. This usually means a 10 mm telescope and xenon or halide light source.

Next one must be prepared for a four puncture technique: one for a diagnostic telescope (my preference); two for laparoscopic forceps to hold open the endometrioma cavity and one for the laser probe. A gas source capable of high flow (3–5 l/min) to compensate for loss of pneumoperitoneum is quite helpful. Since endometriomas are drained prior to ablation, one also needs a good irrigation system capable of delivering large volumes of warmed irrigants (lactated Ringer's is our choice) with rapid wall suction removal.

7.6 Description of technique

After laparoscopic exploration of the peritoneal cavity implants are targeted and destroyed with the appropriate contact probe. Reduced power and a light touch are necessary for lesions over the ureters, colon or bladder. If biopsy is desired this should be accomplished with a mechanical forceps prior to laser energy delivery.

Endometriomas are steadied with one or two laparoscopic forceps held by an assistant. Use of a video system is also mandatory under these circumstances so that the assistant can see what he or she should be doing to facilitate the procedure. No matter how large the screen some resolution is lost, and the operator may wish to use a beam splitter on the camera to allow for direct visualization through the telescope.

With the chisel probe used at a setting of 18–22 W the tunica is incised and spread open with the forceps. The irrigating cannula is substituted for one of the forceps and the cavity is vigorously flushed with 1–3 litres of irrigant depending on its size. The cul-de-sac is then cleared of the collection by suction. The ovary is steadied with two forceps while everting the cyst walls and the laser probe is used to 'paint' and destroy *in situ* the cyst wall. There is no attempt made to enucleate the cyst wall which usually is an arduous and often bloody procedure. After a final rinse the ovarian capsule collapses on itself and healing is quite rapid.

If uterosacral denervation is desirable, the chisel tip is used to section the ligament close to the uterus to a depth of 3–4 mm. This procedure, described by Doyle (1955) among others, seems to work best for pain relief when the posterior pelvic compartment and especially the uterosacral ligaments are involved with endometriosis. Results seem to be independent of the technique employed to create the lesion but laser lesions are probably safer than those made with unipolar electrosurgery because of the possibility of spread laterally to the ureter.

This is not the stage for a detailed discussion of the merits of laser therapy for endometriosis vs expectant management, but let us not forget that pregnancy rates with electrosurgical destruction (Sulewski *et al.*, 1980; Daniell and Christianson, 1981) are in the same range as those reported for CO_2 laser therapy of endometriosis (Martin, 1986; Nezhat, Crewgey and Gansen, 1986; Feste, 1987) and for therapy with the argon laser (Keye *et al.*, 1987). Comparisons of results among authors and techniques often have little meaning because of differences in staging systems and the distribution of the study groups within systems, concomitant therapy and follow-up durations.

What follows is a description of our first 100 patients with endometriosis who were treated with the contact YAG laser via laparoscopy.

Pelvic pain was recorded in 62, infertility in 70 and six presented with an asymptomatic mass. Pain had been present for a mean of 42.3 months and infertility for 50.4 months. American Fertility Society scores (1985) were distributed as Stage 1 (16), Stage 2 (21), Stage 3 (42) and Stage 4 (21). Previous surgery included laparoscopic procedures in 74, a laparotomy in 26 including oophorectomy in 14, danazol therapy in 50, progestin treatment in 26, and GnRH analogue therapy in three. Thirty-one patients had at least one endometrioma; the mean size was 4.8 cm with the largest 10 cm. Thus, this was a group of women who frequently had moderate to severe recrudescent endometriosis.

All laparoscopies were performed under general endotracheal anaesthesia with a total anaesthetic time of 46 min, standard deviation 14.9, range 20–91. The mean wattage used was 20.9 with 1864 J delivered to the pelvis ± 1247. Concomitant procedures include a lysis of adhesions (64), laparoscopic salpingostomy (5), hysteroscopic submucous myoma resection (2), uterosacral division (27) and gamete intrafallopian transfer (GIFT) (3).

Conception was achieved in 41.4% with a mean follow-up of 9.1 months. Some patients had additional therapy such as insemination and ovulation induction but this therapy had also been given (unsuccessfully) prior to surgery in most cases. The group followed for 11.4 months in which there had been pelvic pain did quite well. Relief of pain was total for 39 (63%), good in 18 (29%) requiring only occasional use of prostaglandin inhibitors, partial relief in four (7%) requiring stronger analgesics and one patient (1%) had no improvement. Thus, it was concluded that laparoscopic surgery with the contact sapphire probe of the YAG laser was efficacious for relief of pain as well as for restoration of fertility in a group of women with endometriosis sometimes of advanced stage and often recurrent and/or resistant to other therapies. Comparison with other laser studies was not performed for reasons cited previously.

7.7 Additional laparoscopic procedures

Huber, Hosman and Spona (1988) have described use of the YAG laser for laparoscopic ovarian wedge resection in polycystic ovarian syndrome for cases resistant to clomiphene citrate ovulation induction. Results were good in this small series. I have used the YAG laser for this indication infrequently since our first move in clomiphene citrate resistant patients is to switch to therapy with human gonadotrophins. Laparoscopy in these patients is employed as a general diagnostic measure, not specifically for establishment of the diagnosis of this syndrome based on the morphologic gross appearance of the ovary.

Diagnosis instead is one of an endocrine nature made by altered serum gonadotrophin ratios as well as testosterone levels and androstenedione concentrations. In any event, a drilling technique to unroof the multiple subcapsular cysts seems to work just as well, with less trauma to the ovary and less chance of adhesion formation. Only the outer layer of the cortex needs to be involved, and these little drill holes would seem to be less likely to cause adhesions than a deeper wedge type of procedure. The drilling technique with the laser is similar to the method described by Gjönnaess (1984) using electrocautery. Greenblatt and Casper (1987) used such a technique and also reported reversal of the abnormal endocrine profiles with four of six patients delivering.

As laparoscopic surgeons become more aggressive, some procedures hithertofore accomplished solely by laparotomy have fallen into the laparoscopic domain. I personally have destroyed a few small cystic teratomas *in situ* with the laser after drainage, lavage, and biopsy of the cyst wall. To date there have been no recurrences in a small number of patients followed at 6 month intervals with ultrasonography. These cysts were treated incidental to other laparoscopic procedures and all were less than 3 cm. One could also choose to enucleate the cyst and strip off the wall under laparoscopic guidance.

Procedures including salpingoophorectomy are now performed laparoscopically in many centres in Europe and North America using electrosurgical or laparoscopic ligation techniques for haemostasis. Salpingectomy may well lend itself to a YAG laser technique both for cutting and control of the vessels because of the great inherent haemostatic profile of this particular laser. Linear salpingotomy for removal of ampullary tubal pregnancy via laparoscopy is routine for us. This can be accomplished with a unipolar electric needle as well as with the conical point of the YAG-sapphire probe.

Finally, I confess to performing a few incidental myomectomies with the YAG laser via laparoscopy. These were stalked lesions of 2–5 cm coming off the fundus. Removal was done with a small colpotomy made under laparoscopic guidance after the lesion had been freed and placed into the cul-de-sac. I am not certain about the wisdom or necessity of this procedure unless one wants to make a case for prophylaxis against future growth. There are some laparoscopists who have considerable enthusiasm for incidental myomectomy, but the wisdom of this approach needs to be proven.

In summary, the YAG laser in its current configuration with contact sapphire probes has its greatest use laparoscopically for treatment of endometriosis. It is exceedingly safe because of the contact aspect of energy delivery. Like other lasers purchase is expensive but because it has great utilization in the lower generative tract – cervix and vulva – and can be used for hysteroscopic endometrial ablation, its overall cost effectiveness within an operating suite is excellent, especially given its use by other specialties such as urology, ophthalmology, and for respiratory tract surgery.

References

American Fertility Society (1985), Revised American Fertility Society classification of endometriosis. *Fertil. Steril.*, **43**, 351–2.

Daniell, J. Jr and Christianson, C. (1981), Combined laparoscopic surgery and danazol therapy for pelvic endometriosis. *Fertil. Steril.*, **35**, 521.

Doyle, J. B. (1955), Paracervical uterine denervation by transection of the cervical plexus for the relief of dysmenorrhea. *Am. J. Obstet. Gynecol.*, **70**, 1.

Feste, J. R. (1987), Advances in gynecologic endoscopic surgery: syllabus material, Maui, Hawaii, 14 July, pp. 162–3.

Gjönnaess, H. (1984), Polycystic ovarian syndrome treated by ovarian electrocautery through the laparoscope. *Fertil. Steril.* **41**, 20–5.

Greenblatt, E. and Casper, R. F. (1987), Endocrine changes after laparoscopic ovarian cautery in polycystic ovarian syndrome. *Am. J. Obstet. Gynecol.*, **156**, 279–85.

Huber, J., Hosmann, J. and Spona, J. (1988), Polycystic ovarian syndrome treated by laser through the laparoscope. *Lancet*, **2**, 215.

Joffe, S. N. (1985), The Neodymium:YAG laser in general surgery. *Contemp. Surg.*, **27**, 17.

Joffe, S. N., Brackett, K. A., Sankar, M. Y. and Daikuzono, N. (1986), Resection of the liver with the Nd:YAG laser. *Surg. Gynecol. Obstet.*, **163**, 437–42.

Joffe, S. N., Daikuzono, N., Osborn, J., Batra, P., Studer, R., Sankar, M. T. and Fisher, J. C. (1985), Contact probes for the Nd:YAG laser. *S.P.I.E.* **576**, 42–50.

Keye, W. R. Jr, Hansen, L. W., Astin, W. and Paulson, A. M. Jr (1987), Argon laser therapy of endometriosis: a review of 92 consecutive patients. *Fertil. Steril.*, **47**, 208.

Lomano, J. M. (1985), Photocoagulation of early pelvic endometriosis with the Nd:YAG laser through the laparoscope. *J. Reprod. Med.*, **30**, 77.

Martin, D. C. (1986), CO_2 laser laparoscopy for endometriosis associated with infertility. *J. Reprod. Med.*, **31**, 1089.

Nezhat, C., Crowgey, S. R. and Garrison, C. P. (1986), Surgical treatment of endometriosis via laser laparoscopy. *Fertil. Steril.*, **45**, 778.

Sulewski, J. M., Crucia, F. D., Brenitskey, C. *et al.* (1980), The treatment of endometriosis at laparoscopy for infertility. *Am. J. Obstet. Gynecol.*, **138**, 128.

8 *Ectopic pregnancy*

JÖRG KECKSTEIN

8.1 Introduction

Treatment of ectopic pregnancy has changed dramatically in the last decade. In the past, radical surgical procedures, in the form of salpingectomy or salpingo-oophorectomy, were the only method of treatment. With the development of sensitive beta-subunit human chorionic gonadotrophin (β-HCG) tests and improved ultrasound diagnosis, unruptured tubal pregnancies can be detected as early as the fifth to sixth week of gestation. Because of earlier diagnosis treatment is no longer determined by the immediate threat to the patient's life through tubal rupture with subsequent massive intraperitoneal haemorrhage.

It has been realized that ablative, radical surgery may not be required in all cases and that conservative surgical techniques might offer better prospects for future fertility (Skulj *et al.*, 1964; Langer *et al.*, 1972; Stromme, 1973; Bukowsky *et al.*, 1979; Sherman *et al.*, 1987). This is particularly true in patients with unruptured tubes who have an affected contralateral tube at operation or have suffered from previous infertility (Tuomivaara and Kauppla, 1988). In addition, clinical assessment and inspection alone at the time of treatment of an ectopic pregnancy does not accurately correlate with post-operative findings. Therefore, conservation of the Fallopian tube should be sought whenever possible (Mitchell *et al.*, 1987).

The first conservative operation for ectopic pregnancy was performed in 1953 by Stromme (1973), making an incision in the antimesenteric border of the tube just above the gestation site. Once the trophoblast was exposed by suction or by gentle digital expression, careful haemostasis was accomplished using a needle electrode or bipolar forceps. In some cases sutures had to be placed if coagulation was unsuccessful. Meanwhile linear salpingotomy had become a standard surgical technique for the treatment of unruptured ectopic pregnancy (Timonen and Nieminen, 1967).

Conservative management includes also segmental salpingectomy with or without anastomosis. This technique should be considered

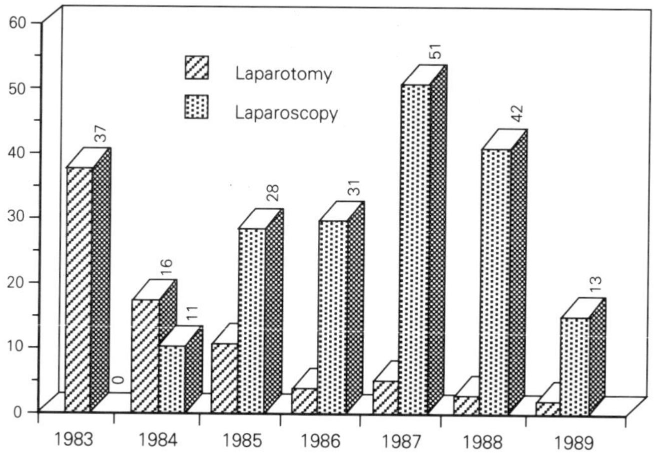

Figure 8.1 Changing trends of treatment of ectopic pregnancy since 1983 at the Department of Gynaecology and Obstetrics of the University of Ulm (laparotomy vs laparoscopy).

especially for isthmic ectopic pregnancy or heavily damaged tubes after rupture (Shapiro and Adler 1973). Gomel (1980) advocates segmental excision of the conceptus, whether or not it is ruptured, when the pregnancy is located in the isthmus or proximal half of the ampulla. End-to-end anastomosis may be undertaken later as an elective procedure if required.

Many procedures once performed with laparotomy are now accomplished with operative laparoscopy. Laparoscopy has long since been widely accepted as an effective tool for early diagnosis of tubal pregnancy; in the past few years it has also proved a valuable modality for its definitive treatment (Bruhat *et al.*, 1980; Loffer, 1986; Pouly *et al.*, 1986; Stangel, 1986; DeCherney and Diamond, 1987; Dubuisson, Aubriot and Cardane, 1987) (Figure 8.1).

Compared with laparotomy, this technique has several obvious advantages, particularly a lower morbidity rate and reduced formation of post-operative adhesions (Reich, Freifeld and McGlynn, 1987; Brumsted *et al.*, 1988). Additionally, laparoscopy is more cost-effective and the recovery period is shorter (Vermesh *et al.*, 1989). As the tube shows little change in the early stage of gestation, very delicate and precise instruments are required. Scalpels or microelectrodes used in microsurgery are not suited for laparoscopic surgery. Different instruments have been used to open the unruptured tube or to resect a portion of the tube.

8.1.1 ELECTROCAUTERY (Scissors, knife electrode, needle electrode ('Triton')) (Palmer, 1972; DeCherney, Romero and Naftolin, 1981; Cartwright, Herbert and Maxsen, 1986; Pouly *et al.*, 1986; Loffer, 1987).

Although laparoscopic cautery appears effective for treatment of tubal pregnancy, this technique still involves the danger of uncontrolled thermal damage to healthy neighbouring tissue caused by the size of instruments and strong coagulative effect of electric scissors (Bahig, 1968; Murphy, 1987). In our department we therefore no longer use either monopolar or bipolar instruments for laparoscopic procedures.

8.1.2 THERMAL COAGULATION

The endocoagulator recommended by Mecke, Semm and Lehmann-Willebroch (1989) and Semm and Mettler (1980) produces a large coagulation zone, which may interfere with secondary healing of the salpingotomy.

8.1.3 LASER

Introduction of the CO_2 laser into laparoscopic surgery facilitated more precise incisions due to the limited coagulation effect and controlled depth of penetration (Cartwright *et al.*, 1986; Johns and Hardie, 1986; Stangel, 1986; Loffer, 1987). Three other laser systems, the Nd-YAG laser with sapphire tips (Keckstein, Wolf and Steiner, 1987; Loffer, 1987), the argon laser, and the KTP-532 laser (Diamond and DeCherney, 1987; Daniell, 1989) increase the range of surgical effects achievable by laparoscopy while making surgery quicker and safer. Beam delivery by means of flexible fibreoptics makes these lasers very easy to use (Figure 8.2). These lasers have more coagulative properties, which makes them more effective in haemostatic control of ectopic pregnancy (Keckstein, Finger and Steiner, 1988). By altering the distance of the fibre from the tissue, or changing of sapphire tip, incision, vaporization and coagulation become possible with the same instrument (Kojiama *et al.*, 1988).

8.1.4 CHOICE OF OPERATIVE PROCEDURE

The basic principle of conservative treatment is to remove the ectopic conceptus and to preserve as much Fallopian tube as possible. The technique to be selected depends on the patient, the location of the pregnancy, and the experience of the surgeon. There are three different conservative techniques which may be performed through the laparoscope: (1) linear salpingotomy; (2) partial tubal resection and (3) aspiration.

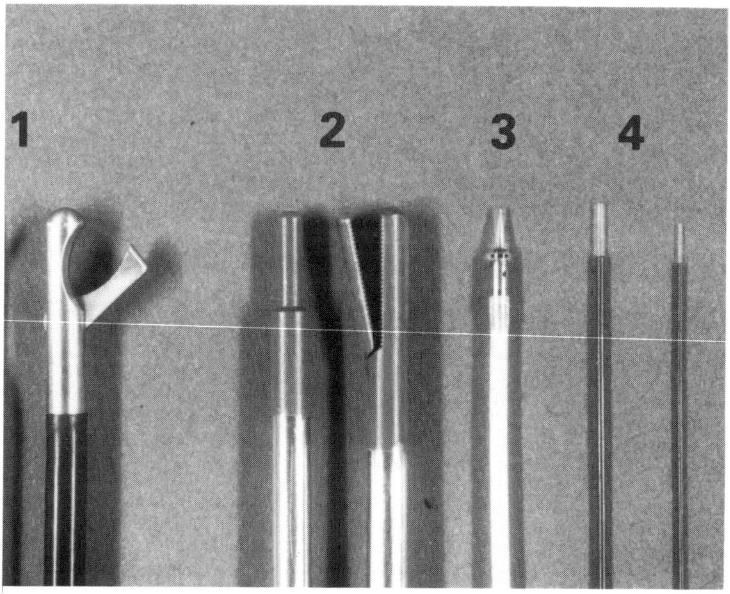

Figure 8.2 Instruments for laparoscopic surgery. Classic instruments (thermo-coagulation probe, scissors)(1 and 2). Nd-YAG contact sapphire tip attached to a 2.2 mm laser fibre(3) and 'bare fibre'(4) for argon and KTP-532 lasers. Note the remarkable difference in size between 'classic' and laser instruments.

8.2 Technical aspects

For laparoscopic treatment of tubal pregnancy the patient should be in a stable haemodynamic condition. Laparoscopy is accomplished by the use of the triple-puncture technique. A 10-mm Wolf laparoscope (Wolf, Knittlingen, Germany) is inserted through an intraumbilical incision. Forceps, suction and irrigation instruments are introduced through 5-mm trocar sheaths (Figure 8.3). All procedures are recorded with a video camera (Wolf, Knittlingen, Germany), which can be helpful when the multiple puncture technique is used.

8.2.1 LAPAROSCOPIC SALPINGOTOMY

After aspiration of the haemoperitoneum Vasopressin (2.5 IU diluted in 20 ml saline) is injected into the mesosalpinx (Semm and Mettler, 1988). This leads to a decreased blood flow to the involved segment of the tube and minimizes bleeding during the operative procedure.

The tube is manipulated with an atraumatic 5 mm grasping forceps. The ischaemic tube is opened over the pregnancy using one of the laser

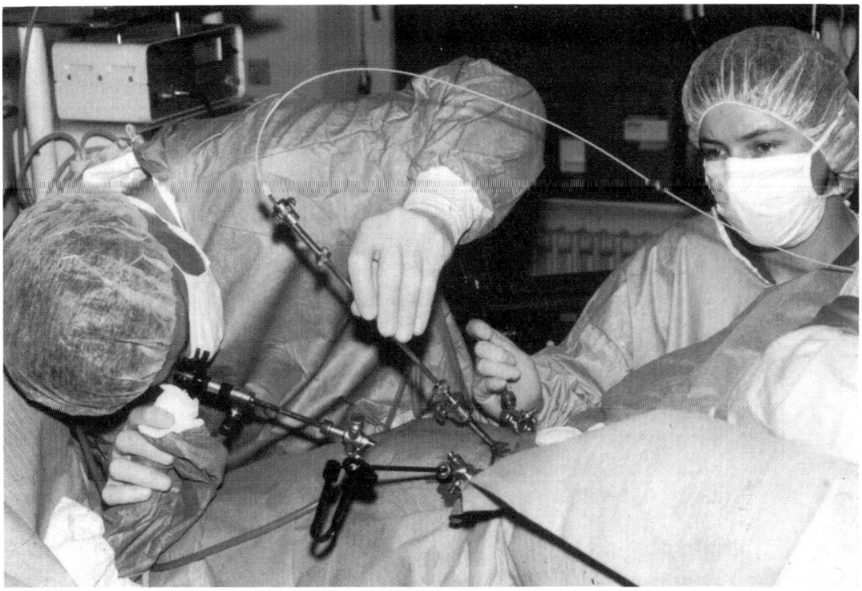

Figure 8.3 Laser laparoscopy using the fibreoptic laser. The laser beam passes through a flexible quartz fibre. A special laser fibre steering device allows deflection of the fibre tip.

systems (Figure 8.4). The incision should be done along the proximal portion of the ectopic gestation. Initial rinsing into the tubal opening mobilizes the trophoblast and blood clots which are then aspirated or extracted by forceps (Figure 8.4). Next, the tube is inspected and any remaining trophoblastic tissue is removed. In contrast to Diamond and DeCherney (1987), we advocate removal of all material, in order to avoid problems arising from persistent trophoblastic tissue. Bleeding from the wound margins or from the implantation site, seen more frequently in intact tubal pregnancies, can be controlled by the different laser systems or by the thermocoagulation probe. The tubal incision is left open and allowed to heal by secondary intention. An intraperitoneal drain is introduced into the pouch of Douglas through the second trocar sheath and is left in place for 4 to 24 hours, depending on the amount of sero-sanguinous fluid in the collecting system.

8.2.2 SEGMENTAL SALPINGECTOMY

This technique should be considered particularly for ectopic pregnancies located in the isthmic portion of the tube since linear salpingotomy

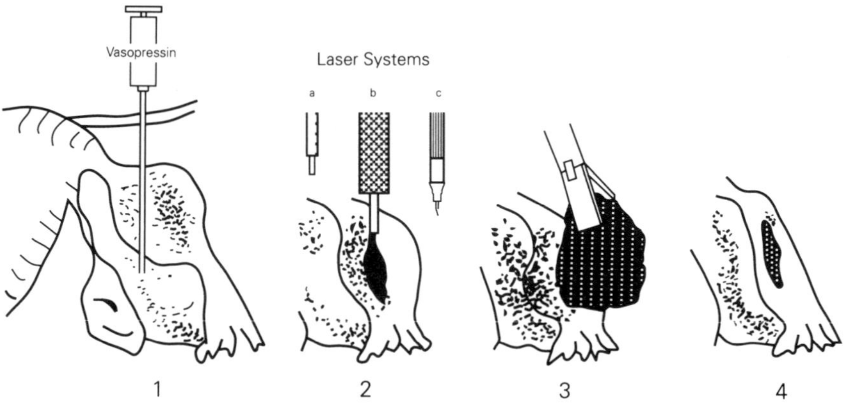

Figure 8.4 Treatment of unruptured tubal pregnancy by linear salpingotomy. (1) Injection of vasopressin into the mesosalpinx. (2) Linear incision of the distended tube on the anti-mesenteric side (a, 'bare-fibre'; b, CO_2 laser probe; c, sapphire tip). (3) Removal of the trophoblast and blood clots. (4) Salpingotomy wound left open.

may be less effective here due to the danger of uncontrollable bleeding and the high post-operative occlusion rate.

Although resection of the tubal segment can be done easily with the use of endoloop sutures we use fibreoptic lasers to excise the segment (Figure 8.5) to preserve as much of the tube as possible. Evacuation of the tube prior to resection, leading to a reduction of tubal size may be very helpful. The advantage of using lasers for this procedure is that they allow both precise incision and coagulation without the need to change instruments. After coagulation of the vessels underlying the Fallopian tube and the mesosalpinx by the non-contact technique, the tissue is then excised accurately and that portion of the tube removed. Microsurgical tubal anastomosis may be performed later, if necessary. This procedure should also be considered when the tube has already ruptured or if bleeding will not stop after salpingotomy.

8.2.3 ASPIRATION

Fimbrial evacuation or 'milking out' of a distal ampullary or infundibular pregnancy by laparotomy (Sherman *et al.*, 1987), or aspiration by laparoscopy has been suggested as a possible alternative to salpingotomy. Due to the danger of persistent trophoblastic tissue (Rivlin, 1985), recurrent ectopic pregnancies (Timonen and Nieminen, 1967), and possible formation of adhesions (Keckstein, 1989), careful selection of the patients is necessary when this technique is used.

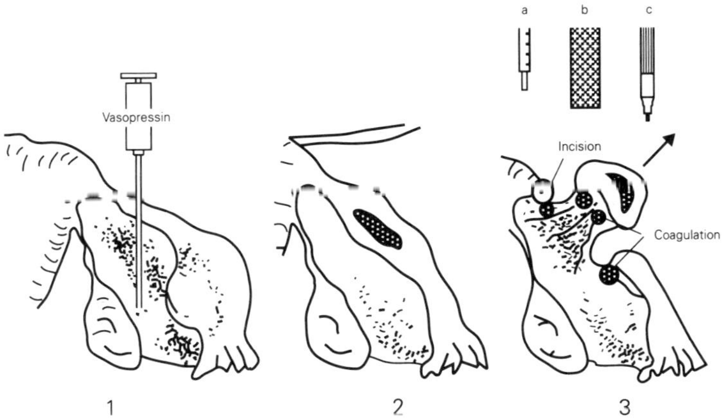

Figure 8.5 Segmental salpingectomy. (1) Injection of vasopressin into the mesosalpinx. (2) Evacuation of the distended tube. (3) Coagulation of the vessels underlying the Fallopian tube and mesosalpinx, and resection of the tubal segment by lasers.

8.2.4 LASERS AND DELIVERY SYSTEMS

(a) CO_2 laser

The CO_2 laser 'Heracure' LS 500 (Fa. Heraeus, Hanau, Germany) is used through the operative channel of the laparoscope or through a special laparoscopic laser probe which is introduced through a 5-mm trocar sheath.

The laser power is set at 10–20 W on continuous mode. For linear salpingotomy, the laser beam is focused with a spot size of 0.4 mm (Plate 7a+b). Due to vaporized blood and tissue an excessive amount of laser plume may be generated, hampering visualization. This is eliminated by a special laser-plume filtering system (Fa. Wolf, Knittlingen, Germany) without any loss of intraperitoneal gas pressure. Significant bleeding is controlled by the defocused laser beam or with additional instruments such as a thermocoagulation probe.

The disadvantages of this technique lie in its unwieldiness due to the rigid arms of the delivery system, the large amount of smoke generated during the operation, and the minimal haemostatic effect of the CO_2 laser.

(b) Fibreoptic lasers (Nd-YAG, argon, KTP-532)

In contrast to the CO_2 laser, energy from fibreoptic lasers may be delivered through a flexible system to the tissue and have more effective haemostatic properties (Keckstein *et al.*, 1988). The laser fibre is passed either through the operating channel of the laparoscope or through a special laser steering instrument (Wolf Instruments, Knittlingen, Germany) into the abdomen (5-mm trocar sheath). This allows deflection of the fibre tip during the operation (Plate 8). It is particularly helpful in patients where severe peritubal adhesions have to be lysed before salpingotomy can be performed. Suction and irrigation is also possible through this instrument.

Nd-YAG laser

For delivering Nd-YAG laser light (1060 nm) sapphire tips (SLT, Surgical Laser Technologies, Malvern PA, USA) are fixed to a standard optical fibre. Differently shaped endoprobes (Figure 8.6) enable power variability for each procedure. During operation the sapphire tips are cooled by continuous CO_2 gas flow.

Incision is made with the conical sapphire probe MRTP 5® (tip diameter 0.2 mm) (Figure 8.6 and Plate 9a). The initial power is 8–12 W. With the commencement of tissue vaporization, power input is lowered to 7–8 W. Exact layer-by-layer incision is possible due to the special properties of the endoprobes (Plate 9b,c). Small-vessel haemorrhage is controlled by using the flat probe or even the sidewall of the conical sapphire tip. Maximum laser power is 12 W.

Argon laser/KTP-532 laser

Argon (wavelength 488 and 515 nm) and KTP-532 (532 nm) lasers generate visible light. In order to protect the operator's eyes and improve visibility during the procedure, it is necessary to work with safety filters, incorporated into the laparoscope.

For the delivery of the argon laser light (Model 20 Surgical Laser System, HGM, Salt Lake City, USA) a 300 μm fibre is used either with the non-contact or contact technique. Focusing tips are not necessary for this laser. With the bare fibre a 5–20 mm incision is made by directly touching the tissue (Plate 10a,b). The procedure is performed with a power of 3–6 W. Small-vessel haemorrhage may be controlled by using the laser with the non-contact technique. For this purpose the laser fibre is positioned 1–2 mm from the bleeding site producing a decrease in power density. Thus, the desired coagulation effect is achieved.

The KTP laser energy delivered through a 400 or 600 μm fibre can be used in the same way. Due to similarity of these lasers in wavelength, the tissue effects are comparable.

There are, however, three problems facing the user of fibreoptic lasers: (1) the change of transmission rate of quartz fibres due to high temperatures generated during the 'bare-fibre' contact method; (2) the

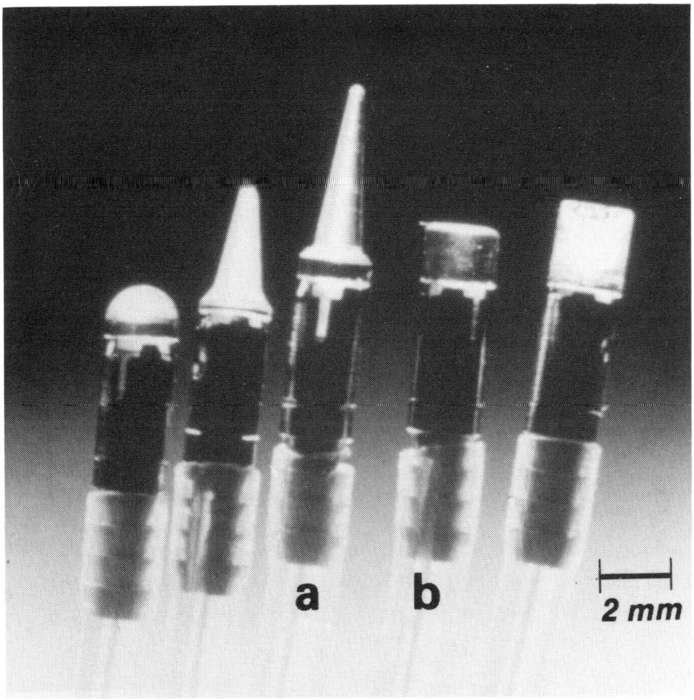

Figure 8.6 Different types of sapphire endoprobes (SLT, Surgical Laser Technologies, Malvern, PA, USA) which are screwed into a metal universal connector attached to the tip of the quartz fibre (a, conical probe for incision; b, flat probe for coagulation).

failure-prone connection between fibre and sapphire tip and (3) the need for eye protection filters which interfere with visual acuity whenever the laser is activated.

8.3 Experimental and clinical studies

Feasibility and efficacy of the three different laser systems mentioned above have been compared in a clinical and experimental study at the Department of Gynaecology and Obstetrics of the University of Ulm.

8.3.1 ANIMAL EXPERIMENTS

In an animal study, the different characteristics of the three laser systems for linear salpingotomy have been evaluated. We performed 'salpingotomies' using the laser on the uterine horns of rabbits which are roughly similar to human Fallopian tubes in terms of size and tissue structure. Thus, the experimental conditions approximated to those existing in early unruptured tubal pregnancy.

Twenty-two New Zealand female white rabbits were randomly divided into three groups, six to have laser incision (0.5–1.5 cm of length) of cornua uteri (Figure 8.7a) by CO_2 laser, seven by Nd-YAG contact laser and seven by argon laser. The incision was made under magnification with the laser technique as mentioned above. Haemostasis at the site of the salpingotomy was also obtained with the various laser systems. The incision was left to heal by secondary intention. Four weeks after the original procedure, all 22 animals were killed. To compare the various tissue effects of the lasers, such as coagulation, vaporization, healing process and post-operative condition of the uterine horn, we used both macroscopic (Figure 8.7b) and histologic criteria.

Our observations in this animal model showed no significant differences in post-operative formation of adhesions, fistulas or stenoses. The histological criteria (Figure 8.8) for cicatrization also showed similar findings for all three systems.

8.3.2 CLINICAL STUDY

One hundred and seventy-six patients with tubal pregnancy were treated by way of laparoscopy in the Department of Gynaecology and Obstetrics at the University of Ulm. In 108 cases the ectopic pregnancy was located in the ampullary portion and in seven cases in the isthmic part of the tube. Four different instruments were used for linear salpingotomy in 115 patients.

1. Conventional technique (thermocoagulation) $n = 49$

Laser

2. CO_2 laser $n = 13$
3. Nd-YAG laser $n = 22$
4. Argon laser $n = 31$

8.4 Results and discussion

8.4.1 COMPLICATIONS

We did not have any intraoperative complications necessitating laparotomy. Due to secondary bleeding from the wound margins in the

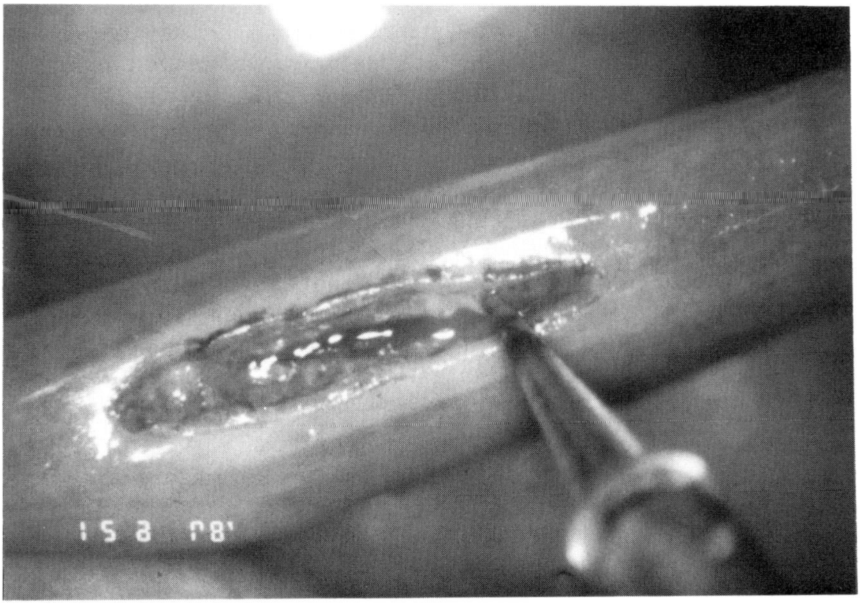

(a)

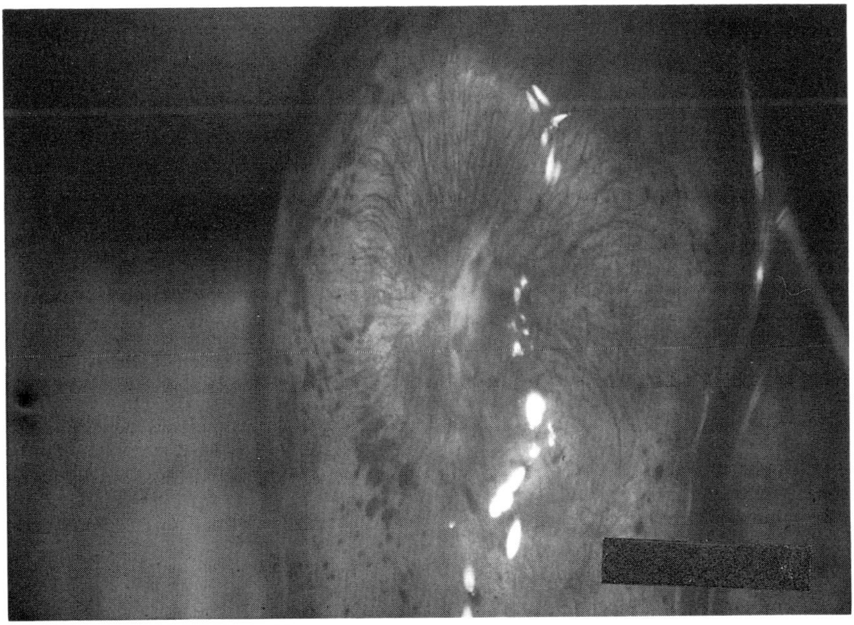

(b)

Figure 8.7 (a) Incision of the rabbit uterine horn with the Nd-YAG contact laser probe. There is only a minimal coagulation zone and mild degree of carbonization. (b) Same uterine horn 6 weeks after laser incision.

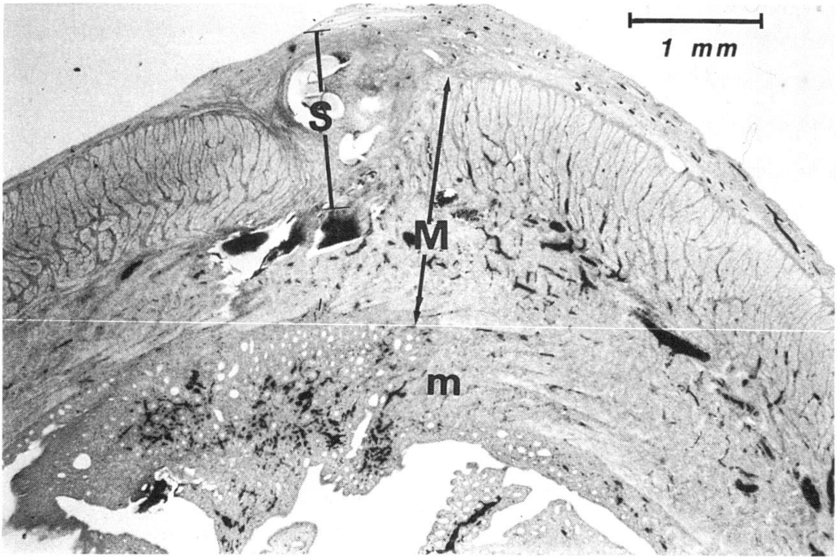

Figure 8.8 Photomicrograph of a cross-section through the rabbit uterine horn 6 weeks after laser incision (Figure 8.7). There is only mild scarification (S). The main part of the muscle layer (M) is still intact. The mucosal layer (m) is not affected at all.

post-operative period second laparoscopy ($n = 2$) or laparotomy ($n = 1$) was required in three cases. Interestingly, salpingotomy had been done with the CO_2 laser in all three cases. Therefore, additional instruments have to be used occasionally for haemostasis (Johns and Hardie, 1986). Persistently high β-HCG levels and suspicious clinical signs after salpingotomy called for repeat laparoscopy in two patients (see below).

8.4.2 TUBAL STATUS

Since evaluation of post-operative fertility after conservative treatment of tubal pregnancy is of limited value with regard to tubal status, we used the parameters of tubal patency and formation of adhesions as a means to judge the value of this new technique. Fifty-three (47%) patients underwent a hysterosalpingography ($n = 15$) or second-look laparoscopy ($n = 38$).

(a) Patency test

Results of patency tests by hysterosalpingography (HSG) or laparoscopic dye studies are shown in (Figure 8.9). After laser treatment a higher

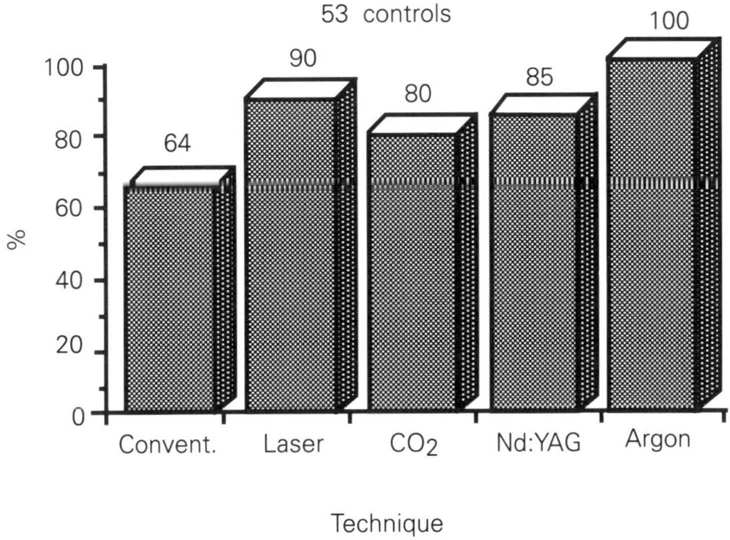

Figure 8.9 Patency test after salpingotomy in 53 controls (hysterosalpingography, second-look laparoscopy).

patency rate (90%) was achieved in comparison to that after conventional technique using thermocoagulation and scissors (64%).

Inspection and chromopertubation during second-look laparoscopy revealed one tubal fistula (Plate 11). The ectopic pregnancy in this patient was the largest in the series and the salpingotomy had to be extended to 3.5 cm for evacuation of the trophoblast. In this patient the fistula was welded with the argon laser by non-contact technique at the time of second-look laparoscopy.

(b) Adhesion formation (Plate 12)

In our study, the incidence of post-operative formation of adhesions was evaluated in 38 (34%) patients. The evaluation was performed by the scoring system described by Mage *et al.* (1986), which considers both the extent and severity of adhesion formation. Since many of the patients have had adhesions at the time of ectopic pregnancy, only *de novo* adhesions were scored. Results are shown in Figure 8.10.

Formation of adhesions at the site of salpingotomy is less likely than with other tubal surgical procedures. We found a significantly higher rate of tubal occlusion and formation of adhesions after the use of the

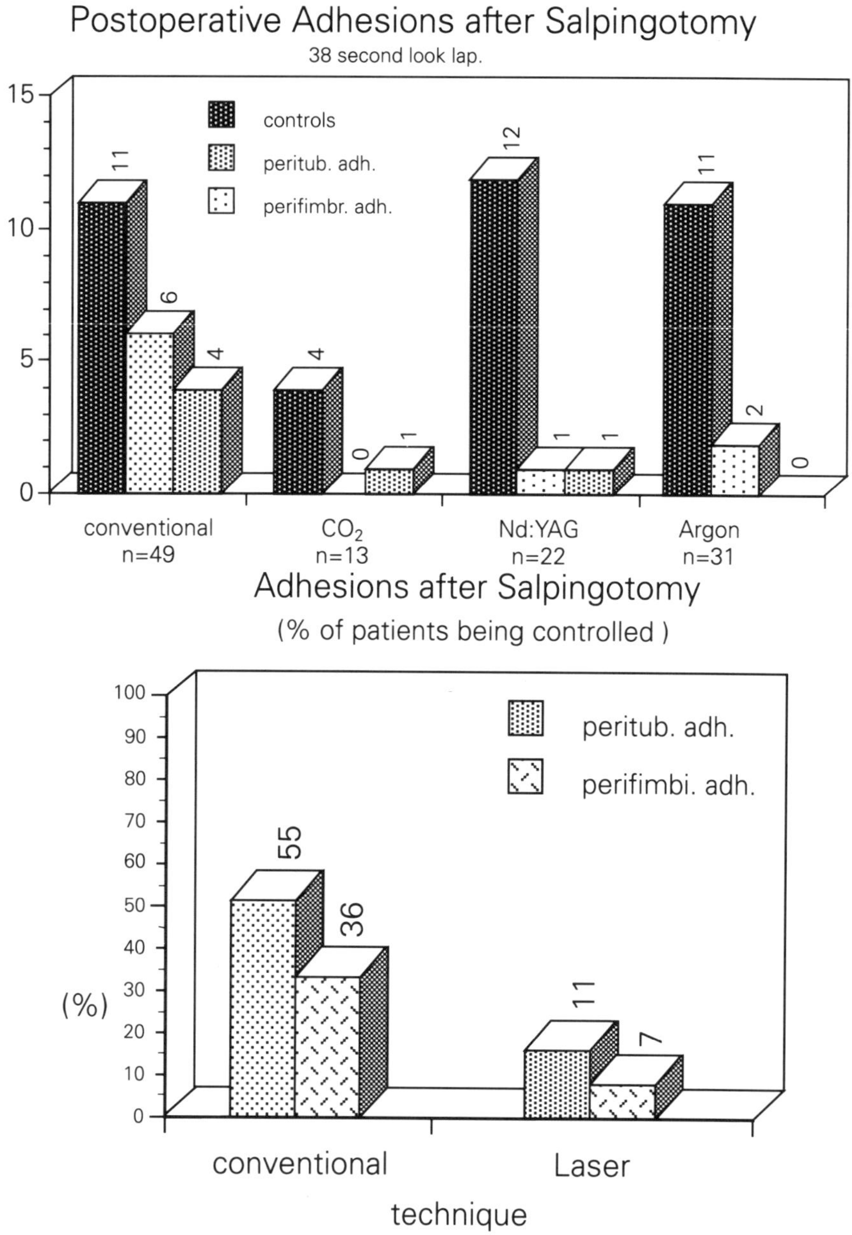

Figure 8.10 Formation of adhesions after salpingotomy in unruptured tubal pregnancy. Thirty-eight second-look laparoscopies were performed for evaluation of adhesions covering the incision site (peritubal) or the distal part of the tube (perifimbrial). Conventional techniques are compared with different laser techniques.

thermocoagulation probe compared to laser techniques. We started to perform linear salpingotomy by this conventional technique. Therefore a learning process may partly account for this result. However, adhesion formation may also be caused by the extensive damage to tubal tissue after thermocoagulation. In contrast lasers minimize tissue damage as seen in our animal experiments and clinical study.

To avoid post-operative adhesions some surgeons have suggested closure of the linear salpingotomy to achieve better haemostasis along the incisional margins and to reduce the raw surface (Mettler and Semm, 1987; Mecke *et al.*, 1989). In contrast, incisions by lasers are very precise with sufficient haemostatic effect, especially with fibreoptic lasers. Studies by others have shown no advantage of primary tubal closure compared to secondary healing. McComb and Gamel (1984) even observed advantages associated with secondary closure of the tube (Nelson, Magara and Winston, 1986) and it is now our practice to leave the salpingotomy incision open. Other important factors influencing post-operative healing results, include tubal size, status of pregnancy (intact?), tubal rupture and previous tubal surgery.

8.4.3 PERSISTENT TROPHOBLASTIC TISSUE AFTER CONSERVATIVE TREATMENT

Persistent ectopic pregnancy results from proliferation of trophoblast remaining in the abdominal cavity (Rivlin, 1985). Trophoblastic tissue may be located within the tubal lumen, in the muscular layer, or between the muscularis and serosa. Kelly, Martin and Strickler (1979) were the first to report on one patient in whom delayed intraperitoneal haemorrhage occurred 18 days after removal of a tubal pregnancy by salpingostomy.

In our series of 176 patients we had four women with rising ß-HCG levels after conservative treatment of ectopic pregnancy. In Figure 8.11 ß-HCG levels of six patients are shown. In two patients the pregnancy was located in the ampullary portion of the tube. Therefore the gestation was removed out at the terminal end of the tube, obviously incompletely. In one of the remaining two cases part of the trophoblastic tissue was rinsed out of the tube after salpingotomy and reimplanation occurred into the omentum close to the liver (Plate 13). In all cases trophoblastic tissue was present at the time of repeat laparoscopy. Treatment of persistent trophoblast has included salpingectomy (Bell, Awadalla and Mattox, 1987; DiMarchi *et al.*, 1987), methotrexate therapy (Higgins and Schwartz, 1986), and expectant management (Kamrava *et al.*, 1963; Cartwright *et al.*, 1986). In our series, conservative surgical management was performed in all patients with rising ß-HCG levels.

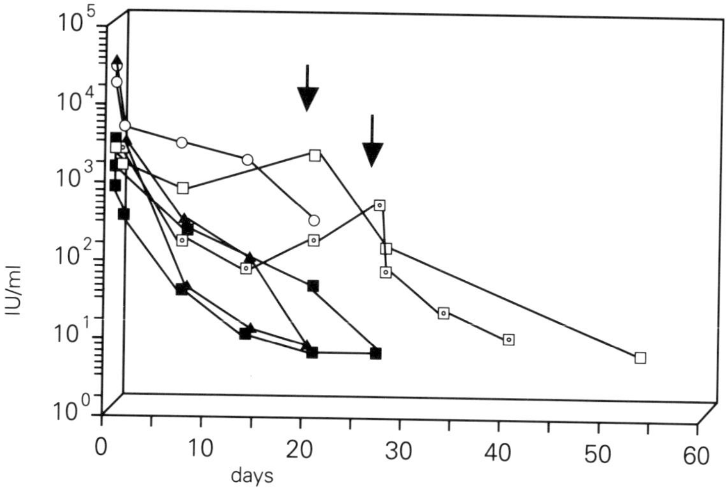

Figure 8.11 Follow-up of ß-HCG values in six patients after linear salpingotomy. Arrows indicate increase of ß-HCG concentration in two patients with persistent trophoblastic tissue.

8.4.4 POST-OPERATIVE FERTILITY

In our study the overall fertility rate of 44% following conservative operation is comparable to that reported by other authors (Palmer, 1972; Sherman *et al.*, 1982; Pouly *et al.*, 1986), describing intra-uterine pregnancy rates of between 20 and 83%. The considerable rate variance can be explained by additional risk factors. It has been demonstrated that in a high percentage of patients with tubal pregnancy the contralateral tube also is affected by disease. In our group we found evidence of chronic inflammation in 40% of the cases. The incidence of recurring ectopic pregnancy on the ipsi- or contralateral side is directly linked to these factors. Pouly *et al.* (1986) reported a subsequent extra-uterine gestation (EUG) rate of 22%. In our study, 8% had a second EUG in the same tube and 14% in the contralateral tube. A comparison of the different techniques for this purpose is of limited value, because of the different follow-up periods ranging from 2 to 55 months.

8.5 Conclusion

For therapy of early diagnosed ectopic pregnancy laparoscopic treatment has become more important as a conservative and less traumatic form of therapy. For many years, electrocautery was the only laparoscopic method capable of both coagulation and incision. Due to undesirable characteristics of electrocautery, such as the unpredictable coagulation effect and resulting danger to neighbouring healthy tissue, new instruments were developed. The introduction of various laser systems into laparoscopic surgery offers the surgeon more precise and easier control of the incision.

Opening of the unruptured tube or resection of tubal segments by the use of these laser systems are both safe and simple procedures. Closure of the linear salpingotomy incision is neither necessary nor desirable. Post-operative healing after laser incision seems to be better when compared to conventional techniques (Plate 14). Unfortunately, the high purchase cost of laser systems has so far precluded laser technology from gaining general acceptance and widespread use for the treatment of ectopic pregnancies.

References

Bahig, C. S. (1968), Electrosurgical burn injuries and their prevention. *JAMA*, **204**, 1025–7.

Bell, O. R., Awadalla, S. G. and Mattox, J. H. (1987), Persistent ectopic syndrome: A case report and literature review. *Obstet Gynecol.*, **69**, 521–3.

Bruhat, M. *et al.* (1980), Treatment of ectopic pregnancy by means of laparoscopy. *Fertil. Steril.*, **33**, 411–14.

Brumsted, J. *et al.* (1988), A comparison of laparoscopy and laparotomy for the treatment of ectopic pregnancy. *Obstet. Gynecol.*, **71**, 889–92.

Bukowsky, I. *et al.* (1979), Conservative surgery for tubal pregnancy. *Obstet. Gynecol.*, **53**, 709–11.

Cartwright, P., Herbert, C. and Maxson, W. (1986), Operative laparoscopy for the management of tubal pregnancy. *J. Reprod. Med.*, **31**, 589–91.

Daniell, J. (1989), Fibreoptic laser laparoscopy. In *Baillière's Clinical Obstetrics and Gynecology* (ed. C. J. G. Sutton), Baillière Tindall, London, pp. 545–62.

DeCherney, A. and Diamond, M. (1987), Laparoscopic salpingostomy for ectopic pregnancy. *Obstet. Gynecol.*, **70**, 948–50.

DeCherney, A., Romero, R. and Naftolin, F. (1981), Surgical management of unruptured ectopic pregnancy. *Fertil. Steril.*, **35**, 21–24.

Diamond, M. and DeCherney, A. (1987), Surgical techniques in the management of ectopic pregnancy. *Clin. Obstet. Gynecol.*, **30**, 200–9.

DiMarchi, J. M. *et al.* (1987), Persistent ectopic pregnancy. *Obstet. Gynecol.*, **70**, 555–8.

Dubuisson, J. B., Aubriot, F. X. and Cardone, V. (1987), Laparoscopic salpingectomy for tubal pregnancy. *Fertil. Steril*, **47**, 225–8.

Gomel, V. (1980), Clinical results of infertility microsurgery. In *Microsurgery in Female Infertility* (eds B. Crosignani and B. Rubin).

Higgins, K. A. and Schwartz, M. B. (1986), Treatment of persistent trophoblastic tissue after salpingostomy with methotrexate. *Fertil. Steril.* **45**, 427–8.

Johns, D. A. and Hardie, R. P. (1986), Management of unruptured ectopic pregnancy with laparoscopic carbon dioxide laser. *Fertil. Steril.*, **46**, 703–5.

Kamrava, M. *et al.* (1983), Disappearance of human chorionic gonadotropin following removal of ectopic pregnancy. *Obstet. Gynecol.*, **62** 486–7.
Keckstein, G. (1989), Secondary implantation of trophoblastic tissue after linear salpingotomy through the laparoscope.
Keckstein, J., Finger, A. and Steiner, R. (1988), Laser application in contact- and noncontact procedures; Sapphire tips in comparison to 'bare-fiber', argon laser in comparison to Nd:YAG laser (in German). *Laser Med. Surg.*, **4**, 158–62.
Keckstein, J., Wolf, A. and Steiner, R. (1987), The use of contact laser probe in gynaecological endoscopy. Proceedings of the 7th Congress International Society for Laser Surgery and Medicine, Munich, pp. 267–72.
Kelly, R., Martin, S. and Strickler, R. (1979), Delayed haemorrhage in conservative surgery for ectopic pregnancy. *Am. J. Obstet. Gynecol.*, **133**, 225–6.
Kojiama, E. *et al.* (1988), Nd:YAG laser endoscopy. *J. Reprod. Med.*, **33**, 907–11.
Langer, R. *et al.* (1982), Conservative surgery for tubal pregnancy. *Fertil. Steril.*, 427–30.
Loffer, F. (1986), Surgical settings and incision for the management of ectopic pregnancies. *J. Reprod. Med.*, **31**, 94–7.
Loffer, F. D. (1987), Outpatient management of ectopic pregnancies. *Am. J. Obstet. Gynecol.*, **156**, 1467–72.
McComb, P. F. and Gomel, V. (1984), Linear ampullary salpingotomy heals better by secondary versus primary closure. *Fertil, Steril.*, **41**, 45 S.
Mecke, H., Semm, K. and Lehmann-Willebrock, E. (1989), Results of operative pelviscopy in 202 cases of ectopic pregnancy. *Int. J. Fertil.*, **34**, 93–100.
Mettler, L. and Semm, K. (1987), Diagnostik und konservierende Behandlung der Tubargravidität per pelviscopiam in Vergleich zur Laparotomie. *Geburtshilfe Frauenheilk*, **47**, 717–20.
Mitchell, D. E. *et al.* (1987), Hysterosalpingographic evaluation of tubal patency after ectopic pregnancy. *Am. J. Obstet. Gynecol.*, **157**, 618–22.
Murphy, A. A. (1987), Operative laparoscopy. *Fertil. Steril.*, **47**, 1–18.
Nelson, L. M., Magara, R. A. and Winston, R. M. L. (1986), Primary and secondary closure of ampullary salpingotomy compared in the rabbit. *Fertil. Steril.*, **45**, 292–5.
Palmer, R. (1972), Resultats et indications de la chirurgie conservatrice au cours de la grossesse extrauterine. *C. R. Soc. Fr. Gynecol.*, **42**, 317–19.
Pouly, J. *et al.* (1986), Conservative laparoscopic treatment of 321 ectopic pregnancies. *Fertil. Steril.*, **46**, 1093–7.
Reich, H., Freifeld, M. and McGlynn, F. (1987), Laparoscopic treatment of ectopic pregnancy. *Obstet. Gynecol.*, **69**, 275–9.
Rivlin, M. (1985), Persistent ectopic pregnancy: Complication of conservative surgery? *Int. J. Fertil.*, **30**, 10–14.
Semm, K. and Mettler, L. (1980), Technical progress in pelvic surgery via operative laparoscopy. *Am. J. Obstet. Gynecol.*, **138** 121–7.
Semm, K. and Mettler, L. (1988), Local infiltration of Ornithin 8-Vasopressin (POR 8) as a vasoconstrictive agent in surgical pelviscopy (applied to myoma enucleation, salpingotomy in cases of tubal pregnancy and peripheral salpingostomy). *Endoscopy*, **20**, 298–304.
Shapiro, H. I and Adler, D. H. (1973), Excision of an ectopic pregnancy through the laparoscope. *Am. J. Obstet. Gynecol.*, **117**, 290–4

Sherman D. *et al.* (1982), Improved fertility following ectopic pregnancy. *Fertil. Steril.*, **37**, 497–502.

Sherman, D. *et al.* (1987), Reproductive outcome after fimbrial evacuation of tubal pregnancy. *Fertil. Steril.*, **47**, 420–4.

Skulj, V. *et al.* (1964), Conservative operative treatment of tubal pregnancy. *Fertil. Steril.*, **15**, 634–9.

Stangel, J. (1986), Conservative surgical procedure for tubal pregnancy. *J. Reprod. Med.*, **31**, 103–7.

Stromme, W. (1973), Conservative surgery for ectopic pregnancy: A twenty year review. *Obstet. Gynecol.*, **41**, 215–23.

Timonen, S. and Nieminen, U. (1967), Tubal pregnancy: Choice of operative method of treatment. *Acta Obstet. Gynecol. Scand.*, **46**, 327–39.

Tuomivaara, L. and Kauppila, A. (1988), Radical or conservative surgery for ectopic pregnancy? A follow-up study of fertility of 323 patients. *Fertil. Steril.*, **50**, 580–3.

9 *Neodymium-YAG laser hysteroscopy: total endometrial ablation*

MILTON H. GOLDRATH

The advent of hysteroscopic laser surgery has provided an alternative to hysterectomy in women with menorrhagia refractory to other forms of treatment. This procedure has been used with considerable success to reproduce the signs and symptoms of Asherman's syndrome. Experience in 335 patients treated hysteroscopically with a Nd-YAG laser has demonstrated that excellent results (amenorrhoea or limited spotting) were achieved in 97% of cases. All 46 patients with clotting disorders did well following surgery. The major complications associated with this procedure have included fluid overload, profuse bleeding, post-operative urinary tract infection, and post-operative haematometra, all of which have been successfully controlled.

9.1 Introduction

More than 600 000 hysterectomies are performed annually, making this the most common major surgery performed in the United States today (Cole and Berlin, 1977). Approximately 20–25% of these procedures are for the relief of menorrhagia, defined as excessive menstrual bleeding in ovulatory women in the absence of significant gynaecologic pathology.

Menorrhagia represents a widespread clinical problem, and is the leading cause of elective hysterectomy in women with a normal uterus (D'Esopo, 1962; Parrot, 1971; Cole and Berlin, 1977; Dyck *et al.*, 1977). Various methods are used to treat this condition, including dilatation and curettage (D&C), hormone therapy, ergot derivatives, antifibrinolytic agents, and non-steroidal anti-inflammatory drugs (Nilsson and Goran, 1971). While oral contraceptives appear to be the most effective approach to treatment, their usefulness is limited by side effects and contraindications to therapy.

Until recently, women who did not respond to pharmacologic intervention were limited to one of two options: hysterectomy or continued cycles of heavy menstrual bleeding. With the advent of hysteroscopic laser surgery in 1979, women with menorrhagia refractory to other methods of therapy were offered an alternative to hysterectomy (Goldrath, Fuller and Segal, 1981). For the first time, it was possible to destroy the abnormal endometrial tissue without making any incision. Laser ablation has also been employed in recent years to treat patients with moderate-sized fibroids. Thus, the number of patients for whom this procedure is potentially beneficial is quite sizeable.

This chapter describes the use of hysteroscopic laser surgery in the treatment of menorrhagia in women pretreated with danazol (Danocrine), a 2,3-isoxazole derivative of 17-ethinyl testosterone. Danazol is an effective inhibitor of normal follicular maturation, and thus inhibits endogenous oestrogen production. It has been widely used for the treatment of endometriosis, and has been shown to suppress menstrual bleeding (Greenblatt *et al.*, 1971; Chimbira *et al.*, 1979, 1980; Luciano, 1982; Fraser, 1985; Lamb, 1987).

9.2 Methods

The primary objective of laser surgery is to limit uterine bleeding and produce amenorrhoea – in essence, replicating Asherman's syndrome. First described by Fritch in 1894, Asherman identified this syndrome in 1948 as a condition involving uterine synechiae, which usually result from post-abortal or post-partum uterine curettage (Asherman, 1948). The syndrome is associated with amenorrhoea and infertility.

It soon became apparent that any technique capable of reproducing Asherman's syndrome might be used to correct excessive uterine bleeding. In subsequent years, a variety of chemical and physical methods were used for this purpose, the majority of which proved unsuccessful. While radium and cryocoagulation were both associated with some limited success, radium is no longer used in the absence of malignancy, and the cryocoagulation procedure described by Droegemueller (Droegemueller, Makowski and Macsalka, 1971; Droegemueller, Greer and Makowski, 1971) was abandoned because of the potential for producing painful haematometra. More recently, DeCherney and Polan (1983) have successfully destroyed the endometrium and produced amenorrhoea through the use of a high-frequency coagulating current.

With the development of optical fibres capable of transmitting laser energy, lasers have steadily gained acceptance over the last decade for use in performing endoscopic and hysteroscopic surgical procedures. One such laser, the Nd-YAG, is particularly well suited to photocoagulation of the endometrium as a result of its high power and transmission through fibreoptics. Its deep-tissue penetration (up to 4 mm beneath the surface) and extensive heating distinguish it from the CO_2 and argon lasers.

Only a small percentage of the power of the Nd-YAG laser is absorbed by the tissue, the majority being diffused backwards (30–40%) and forwards (25–30%) as the laser energy scatters. Because of the danger posed to the surgeon from backscatter after tissue impact, use of special safety lenses or a protective filter over the eyepiece of the hysteroscope is essential.

The human uterus is characterized by a relatively thick myometrium (usually >1.5 cm) and thin endometrium (usually <1 mm), thus providing an ideal environment for laser surgery. The fact that only about 5% of the uterine thickness must be ablated in order to destroy the endometrium, provides a substantial safety factor.

Five per cent dextrose in physiological saline is currently used to distend the uterus and has proven an excellent visualizing medium. Previous experience with dextran (Hyskon) demonstrated that its high viscosity was associated with large bubbles that obscured vision. In addition, it discoloured with the intense heat of the laser. Gaseous distending mediums may be useful for diagnostic purposes, but should **never** be used as a medium for therapeutic hysteroscopic surgery because of the risk of fatal gas emboli.

The procedure is performed with the patient under general or spinal anaesthesia. A continuous-flow hysteroscope is used. The fluid flows in by gravity only and is removed by low suction to provide a constant flow of fluid at low pressure. This is important not only for the removal of blood and gas bubbles from the operative field, but also for the prevention of earlier problems with excess fluid absorption.

Endometrial photovaporization and photocoagulation are performed under direct visualization using a power output of 50 W continuous wave. The entire endometrial lining is treated, commencing in the cornual area and extending across the fundus and down the anterior and posterior walls to the isthmus, terminating 4 cm from the external cervical os. To avoid treating the endocervix, the level of the internal os (4 cm) is marked on the sheath of the hysteroscope. Care is also taken to avoid perforation near the tubal ostia, the thinnest portion of the uterus.

Endometrial ablation results in pitting and charring of the treated areas. After a long healing period, synechiae develop that are similar to those described by Asherman (1948). This procedure takes 30–40 min in a normal-sized uterus, longer in a larger uterus.

Danazol was initially used in an attempt to duplicate the hormonal state of patients who developed Asherman's syndrome (Goldrath *et al.*, 1981). Since post-abortal or post-partum endocrine activity is negligible, it was believed that by placing a patient on danazol for 3 weeks prior to surgery and for 2 weeks following surgery, healing might occur before the endometrium had an opportunity to regenerate.

It has subsequently been discovered that healing takes up to 6 months following the procedure. Thus, Danazol is no longer used post-operatively. However, the pre-operative use of danazol greatly facilitates ablation of the endometrium, since the steroid decreases the thickness of the endometrial lining.

At present, 324 women aged 12–53 years have undergone 335 hysteroscopic laser procedures for the treatment of menorrhagia. More than 50% of the patients (n = 176) had fibroids, most of which were submucous fibroids or adenomyosis. The criteria for patient selection includes: (1) excessive and disabling bleeding; (2) inability or unwillingness to use other therapies; (3) candidacy for hysterectomy; (4) future childbearing not desired; and (5) D&C within 6 months of the surgical procedure to rule out adenocarcinoma of the endometrium or cancer precursors.

Most patients have fared extremely well post-operatively. The procedure is usually performed on an ambulatory basis, with the patients discharged 2–3 h later. Although severe cramping typically occurs for the first 2 h following surgery, it has recently been noted that the use of bupivicaine hydrochloride (Marcaine) 0.25% with epinephrine (adrenalin) 1:200 000 as a paracervical block upon completion of the procedure greatly reduces the post-operative pain. Overall, the post-operative symptoms resemble those associated with a D&C. All patients have experienced varying degrees of serosanguinous discharge that lasts for approximately 4 weeks. None of the patients has become febrile.

9.3 Results

Overall, the results have been excellent in 292 patients, 50% of whom became amenorrhoeic and the remainder of whom experienced only a few days of spotting per cycle. Seven patients reported good results, meaning they were satisfied with treatment and experienced what they considered to be normal menstrual bleeding. Of the 22 patients who had poor results, 10 of 11 who were retreated are currently amenorrhoeic and one had a hysterectomy. The remaining 10 patients underwent hysterectomy and were not retreated. One patient elected to put up with her symptoms.

Forty-five of the patients had clotting disorders, all of whom did well following surgery. Eighteen of the patients were receiving warfarin (Coumadin) therapy; 10 had von Willebrand's disease; five were renal transplant patients; four had immunologic thrombocytopenic purpura; three were dialysis patients; an additonal three had storage-pool disease, a platelet disorder; and one had Bernard–Soulier syndrome. One was a symptomatic haemophilia carrier.

Out of a total of 19 hysterectomies, eight were laser successes and eight laser failures. In three, laser use was terminated because of complications, e.g. the presence of large, submucous myomas (two) or cervical bleeding (one). The latter complications deserve special comment. At the time, it was our practice to continue administering danazol for 2 weeks after the procedure. The patient was taking warfarin. Ten days following surgery, excessive, uncontrollable bleeding occurred, necessitating hysterectomy. It has since been published that the dose of warfarin must be reduced in patients receiving danazol therapy (Goulbourn and Macleod, 1981). This underscores an important precaution in the prescribing of danazol: coadminister with warfarin with great care. Danazol potentiates the action of warfarin, greatly increasing the prothrombin time. If the two drugs must be administered concomitantly, the warfarin dosage should be reduced by half. It is also advisable to monitor prothrombin times every 3 days through the course of combination therapy. Of the early failures, one had large submucous myomas, two had adenomyosis, and one failed for unknown reasons. Among the late failures, one involved a significantly enlarged fibroid, and three had adenomyosis. Thus, five of the eight hysterectomies that failed had adenomyosis.

Because of the possibility that adenomyosis was associated with endometrial regeneration, it was decided to administer a single 150 mg dose of medroxyprogesterone acetate (Depo-Provera®) to patients with suspected adenomyosis or fibroids on the day of surgery. Sixty-nine per cent of the patients treated with medroxyprogesterone acetate became amenorrhoeic, as compared with only 37% of those who did not receive treatment. This difference was highly significant ($P < 0.00001$). Quite possibly, the use of danazol for 4–5 months following surgery might also inhibit endometrial regeneration, but this requires additional study.

9.4 Complications

The major complication observed with this procedure has been fluid overload, which led to frank pulmonary oedema in two cases. However, it should be noted that this problem occurred early when a 'push' infusion method was used to distend the uterus. We now use a continuous irrigation technique that involves gravity feed of fluid into the uterus and active suction out of the uterus, with the rate of flow adjusted to distend the uterus and control any bleeding.

Following surgery, profuse bleeding developed in 13 patients after withdrawal of irrigating pressure. The bleeding was controlled by balloon tamponade using a Foley catheter inserted into the uterus (Goldrath, 1983). Three patients had post-operative urinary tract infections related to the catheter drainage. In one patient endomyometritis developed 1 week post-operatively. Although asymptomatic, she was hospitalized for 2 days and treated with intravenous antibiotics. The purulent discharge immediately stopped.

All patients are followed 1 and 3 months post-operatively by suction curettage; if haematometra is found, suction curettage is performed weekly until the condition resolves. Experience suggests that if haematometra has not developed within 3 months following hysteroscopy, it will not develop subsequently. Routine suction curettage revealed 12 cases of post-operative haematometra.

Three patients had allergic reactions to danazol. The reaction was mild in two cases, and therapy was continued. Only one patient had to discontinue treatment because of a severe allergic reaction.

Laser ablation was not completed in one patient due to an instrument-related uterine perforation. The patient returned to the hospital 2 months later, at which time the laser procedure was completed.

9.5 Conclusion

The data accumulated over the last decade suggest that hysteroscopic laser surgery offers a highly viable alternative to hysterectomy in patients with menorrhagia who are not good candidates for other forms of treatment. Our current experience indicates that this procedure is remarkably safe and effective and involves minimal post-operative morbidity and discomfort. The pre-operative use of danazol to enhance endometrial atrophy has greatly facilitated the success of this endoscopic intervention.

While the use of hysteroscopic laser surgery in other applications is somewhat more limited at present, preliminary evidence suggests that this technique may be used for removal of uterine septae and synechiae, as well as for hysteroscopic resections of submucous myomas. The outcome of these procedures is also enhanced by pre-treatment with danazol. Based on this initial experience, it appears that the future applications of hysteroscopic laser surgery will be numerous and diverse.

References

Asherman, J. G. (1948), Amenorrhoea traumatica (atretica). *J. Obstet. Gynecol. Br. Emp.*, **55**, 23–30.

Chimbira, T. H., Anderson, A. B. M., Naish, C. *et al.* (1980), Reduction of menstrual blood loss by danazol in unexplained menorrhagia: lack of effect of placebo. *Br. J. Obstet. Gynaecol.*, **87**, 1152–8.

Chimbira, T. H., Cope, E., Anderson, A. B. M. *et al.* (1979), The effect of danazol on menorrhagia, coagulation mechanisms, haematological indices and body weight. *Br. J. Obstet. Gynaecol.*, **86**, 46–50.

Cole, P. and Berlin, J. (1977), Elective hysterectomy. *Am. J. Obstet. Gynecol.*, **129**, 117–23.

DeCherney, A. and Polan, M. L. (1983), Hysteroscopic management of intra-uterine lesions and intractable uterine bleeding. *Obstet. Gynecol.*, **61**, 392.

Droegemueller, W., Greer, B. and Makowski, E. (1971), Cryosurgery in patients with dysfunctional uterine bleeding. *Obstet. Gynecol.*, **38**, 256–8.

Droegemueller, W., Makowski, E. and Macsalka, R. (1971), Destruction of the endometrium by cryosurgery. *Am. J. Obstet. Gynecol.*, **110**, 467–9.

Dyck, F. J., Murphy, F. A., Murphy, J. K. *et al.* (1977), Effect of surveillance in the number of hysterectomies in the Province of Saskatchewan. *N. Engl. J. Med.*, **296**, 1326–8

D'Esopo, D. A. (1962), Hysterectomy when the uterus is grossly normal. *Am. J. Obstet. Gynecol.*, **83**, 113–22.

Fraser, I. S. (1985), Treatment of dysfunctional uterine bleeding with danazol. *Aust. N.Z. J. Obstet. Gynaecol.*, **25**, 224–5.

Goldrath, M. H. (1983), Uterine tamponade for the control of acute uterine bleeding. *Am. J. Obstet. Gynecol.*, **147**, 869–72.

Goldrath, M. H., Fuller, T. A. and Segal, S. (1981), Laser photovaporization of endometrium for the treatment of menorrhagia. *Am. J. Obstet. Gynecol.*, **140** 14–19.

Goulbourne, I. A. and Macleod, D. A. D. (1981), Interaction between danazol and warfarin: Case report. *Br. J. Obstet. Gynaecol.*, **88**, 950–1.

Greenblatt, R. B., Dmowski, W. P., Mahaesh, V. B. *et al.* (1971), Clinical studies with an antigonadotropin danazol. *Fertil. Steril.*, **22**, 102–12.

Lamb, M. P. (1987), Danazol in menorrhagia: A double blind placebo controlled trial. *J. Obstet. Gynaecol.*, **7**, 212–16.

Luciano, A. A. (1982), A guide to managing endometriosis. *Contemp. Obstet. Gynecol.*, **19**, 211–34.

Nilsson, L. and Goran, R. (1971), Treatment of menorraghia. *Am. J. Obstet. Gynecol.*, **110**, 713–20.

Parrot, M. (1971), Elective hysterectomy. *Am. J. Obstet. Gynecol.*, **113**, 531–7.

10 *Laser hysteroscopic surgery and focal ablation of the endometrium*

JACQUES DEQUESNE

10.1 Introduction

10.1.1 ND-YAG LASER THERAPY OF DYSFUNCTIONAL UTERINE BLEEDING

Until recently dilatation and curettage (D&C) was the most usual operation in the diagnosis and surgical therapy for benign endometrial lesions. In the treatment of menorrhagia for instance, the usual sequence was prostaglanclin synthetase inhibitors (PGSIs), progestogen substitution, antifibrinolytic agents and D&C. When these procedures failed hysterectomy was performed and the number of these operations has increased in such a way that it is now one of the most frequently performed operations in the Western world.

In 1948, Asherman described a syndrome of amenorrhoea, infertility and intra-uterine synechiae. This was usually caused by vigorous post-partum curettage. For many years gynaecologists have had the idea of reproducing this syndrome in some patients suffering from menorrhagia as an alternative to hysterectomy. Chemical and physical methods have been used, and in 1947, Rongy suggested that radium be introduced into the uterus to induce endometrial atrophy (Rongy, 1947). Droegmueller suggested that the endometrium could be destroyed by cryosurgery (Droegmueller, Greer and Makowski, 1971a; Droegmueller, Makowski and Macsalka, 1971b). In 1973, Shenker and Polishuk instilled chemical agents such as quinacrine into the uterus (Shenker and Polishuk, 1973). Most of these methods have fallen into disrepute due to side effects and poor success rate.

Hysteroscopy was first introduced in 1970, but needed certain optical and technical improvements before this method of examination became practical and efficient. Diagnosis was improved by this technique and surgery under direct vision started first with mechanical instruments, such as scissors, but this procedure was quite bloody. Later on surgery was undertaken with the electrodiathermy resectoscope. A drawback to this technique was that the electric current can spread out and can cause damage (burning) to proximal organs.

Laser intra-uterine surgery was first performed by Milton Goldrath in Detroit, Michigan. He attempted to create Asherman's syndrome by performing total endometrial ablation through a rigid hysteroscope (Goldrath, Fuller and Segal, 1981). The aim of the operation was to achieve complete amenorrhoea by destroying all the endometrial tissue. For this purpose, Goldrath chose the Nd-YAG laser, because of the photo-coagulation effect and deep tissue penetration. The technique is described in detail by Professor Goldrath in Chapter 9. This procedure is efficient (94% amenorrhoea), but the equipment required is expensive and the operation itself tends to be long and tedious. An alternative technique pioneered by Neuwirth (1978) employed electrodiathermy resection to ablate the endometrium. In Europe many patients prefer the restoration of normal menstruation and at the same time the possibility of pregnancy.

Since 1985 in the Clinic Cecil in Lausanne, Switzerland, we have attempted focal laser therapy to the areas of the endometrium which are actively bleeding, allowing the possibility for the women to return to a normal menogram and normal trophicity of the uterine cavity. To avoid cervical damage, we avoid dilatation, using a flexible thin (4.9 mm) hysteroscope.

10.2 Focal ablation of the endometrium

10.2.1 PATIENTS

One hundred and sixty-eight women were selected for focal laser therapy. All had excessive uterine bleeding resistant to conventional treatment and they were referred originally for hysterectomy. All patients with carcinoma, hormonal abnormalities or infections were excluded from the study. All the patients studied had undergone diagnostic curettage within the previous 6 months and cervical cytology had been performed within the previous year.

Since 1988, we have performed an office hysteroscopy and curettage 3–4 months pre-operatively to provide samples for histological examination. The patients ages ranged from 26 to 63 years (median 34). Sixty-five had fibroids with or without associated adenomyosis and 52 had polyps. Trophoblastic remnants were found in six well-vascularized synechiae in five and in 11 cases no lesion was found. In this last group of patients, six were treated with anticoagulant, two had coagulation disorders, one had an IUD and two were HIV positive.

Another group of 34 patients preferred to undergo total ablation of the endometrium (Goldrath's technique) because of high anaesthetic risks or because they wanted amenorrhoea. At the present time we have also performed total ablation when results with focal therapy were poor.

10.2.2 INSTRUMENTS AND IRRIGANT FLUID

We use a flexible hysteroscope (CHFP 20 Olympus), modified with a rigid eyepiece. This instrument is usually used for choledochoscopy. The outer diameter of 4.9 mm permits operative hysteroscopy at the same time as diagnostic hysteroscopy, which would be impossible with a rigid device without dilatation of the cervix and changing the operating sheath. The advantage lies in its flexibility (bending 160° up and 130° down) which makes the procedure less traumatic for the endocervix and the mobility of the tip allows thorough examination and surgical accessibility of the uterine cavity.

Glycine is used to distend the uterine cavity and to clear any debris. We prefer this to CO_2 gas insufflation, because of the risks of gas embolism described by Baggish and Daniell (1989), and because liquid perfusion allows cooling of the laser tip and avoids the problem of smoke evacuation. Initially we used Hyskon, but stopped after the Maillard Effect (caramelization) was described by Schmidt in a lecture in 1987.

We have not found it necessary to sterilize patients with Yoon rings because we carefully measure inflow and outflow during surgery and never allow more than 1 litre to remain inside the patient during the procedure (overloading prevention). We collect the irrigant fluid in a calibrated urologic extra-vaginal pouch.

The glycine perfusion is placed 0.5 m above the level of the operating table. Less perfusion pressure is necessary because of the small diameter of the optical hysteroscope, which allows outflow around the device and allows the possibility to suction blood and debris by a special suction switch on the new device (CHFP 20).

The laser used was the Nd-YAG laser (MBB, Medilas, Germany), which produced a power output up to 100 W. This allowed destruction of solid lesions such as fibroid, septae, and also provided more effective penetration of the endometrium. We used a modified gastroenterological laser fibre, made from quartz (400–600 μm diameter) and covered by a Teflon protective sheath (Figure 10.1). The Nd-YAG wavelength of 1.06 μm is invisible, so a helium–neon aiming beam was incorporated into the system. The power, duration, number of shots and total energy were measured at the end of the fibre. The laser was controlled by a foot-switch interlocked with an audible signal during laser activation.

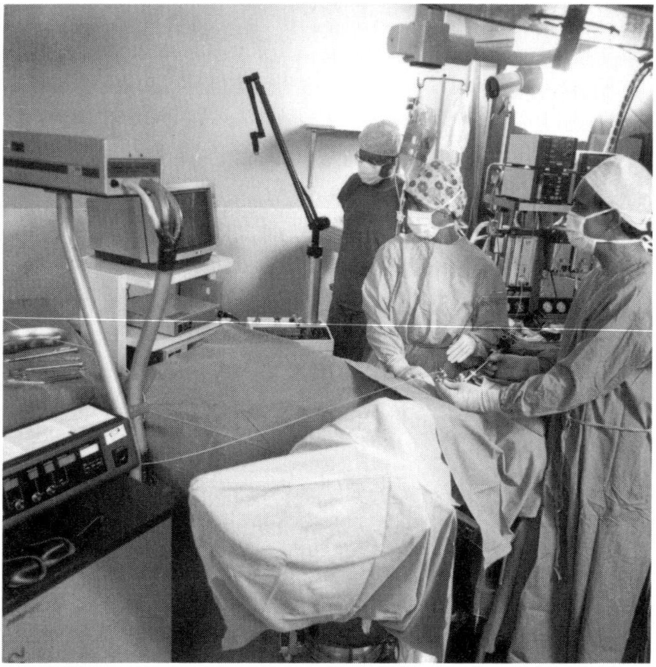

Figure 10.1 Laser hysteroscopic surgery using a modified gastroenterological laser fibre.

10.3 Practical aspects of the procedure

Paracervical block was used with 20 ml of carbocaine hydrochloride injected 5 min before the procedure. In our series, 25% had general anaesthesia because they also required a laparoscopy.

The cervix was grasped with a Pozzi forceps. No cervical dilatation was performed, except when the endocervical channel had been damaged by previous surgery. The glycine infusion was connected to the irrigation channel of the hysteroscope (2.2 mm), after introduction of the laser fibre with tip protection, to avoid damage during transit of the endoscope channel. Before insertion into the cervix, this protection was removed. The television camera was fixed on the eyepiece of the instrument, and the focus and the colour balance adjusted before endoscopy. Diagnostic endoscopy was then performed with the laser fibre in place and without prior dilatation.

The patient, the staff and the surgeon can follow the procedure on the monitor. Protective goggles are worn only in case of surgery. Protection of the eyes is very important, because the Nd-YAG laser energy is absorbed by the retina and can destroy the macula permanently. All the staff and the patient must wear protective goggles in case of fibre breakage on the way from the laser to the endoscope. The backscattering danger is avoided because surgery is performed via the television camera on the eyepiece.

In focal therapy we avoid total ablation of the endometrium and resultant amenorrhoea by focusing the energy on the lesion causing bleeding or possible infertility. The haemorrhagic areas are treated and all visible vessels are photo-coagulated before the lesions responsible for the bleeding are resected or vaporized. Polyps are coagulated by using a laser power of 30–40 W, in continuous mode, and are then removed by using the bare laser fibre, biopsy forceps or scissors.

Fibroids are treated by coagulating the surrounding area and vessels, prior to treating the tumour itself. The fibroid is usually vaporized or, if very large, removed by dissection with the laser at high power (80–100 W). Adenomyosis is treated by coagulation of the surrounding vessels and crypts to a depth of 6–7 mm, by using a laser power of 30 W. Treated areas change colour from pink to brown, brown–black on the lesions and white around and on the vessels.

Care must be taken to avoid perforation. The region of the tubal ostia is the thinnest portion of the myometrium and the uterine wall is particularly thin in post-menopausal patients. In case of large lesions, 2 mm of the lesion is left in place to ensure success and this usually disappears after 6 weeks.

A second-look hysteroscopy is performed 8 weeks after focal therapy to ensure that the hypertrophic vessels are absent and the lesions responsible for the bleeding have disappeared. With large lesions like fibroids and septae further corrective surgery is sometimes necessary. Histological examination of biopsy material taken at this time showed that treated areas had returned to normal endometrium and there were no carbon particles or foreign-body giant cell reaction.

10.4 Results

Table 10.1 shows follow-up data after 8–56 months, indicating that 78% of patients had a return to normal menses following hysteroscopic surgery. Menstrual blood loss was not measured but we considered a normal menstruum to be of 3–4 days' duration without flooding or the passage of clots. Seven patients required a repeat procedure because the initial results were poor. On this occasion total endometrectomy was performed and all had a successful result. Eleven patients (7%) continued to have menorrhagia and underwent hysterectomy and a further 12 were lost to follow-up.

Table 10.1 Hysteroscopic treatment of abnormal bleeding with Nd-YAG laser. Long-term results (8–56 months)

Focal surgery		*No. of patients*	%
Normal menogram		131	78
Lost to follow-up		12	7
Hysterectomy		11	7
Treatment of recurrences			
Good results (focal surgery)		6	3
Good results (total endometrectomy)		8	5
Diagnosis of 168 cases:	Fibroids		41
	Polyps		30
	Adenomyosis		17
	Trophoblastic remnants		3
	Synechiae		3
	No lesion		6
Total endometrectomy		34	
Good results		29	85
Lost to follow-up		3	8
Hysterectomy		2	7
Dysmenorrhoea		51	
Complete relief		33	65
Partial relief		10	20
No relief		8	15

In a separate series 34 patients were treated with total endometrial ablation. Twenty-nine (85%) had an excellent result (amenorrhoea or monthly spotting), three were lost to follow-up and two (7%) underwent hysterectomy. The results of the treatment of recurrences with the Nd-YAG laser are shown in Figure 10.2.

10.4.1 TREATMENT OF DYSMENORRHOEA INFERTILITY

In our preliminary study (Dequesne, 1987), out of 45 patients treated for abnormal bleeding using the Nd-YAG laser as well as in the following group of 168 patients reported here, we obtained a number of unexpected effects in addition to the restoration of normal menses. The first was an effect on dysmenorrhoea, which is shown in Table 10.1.

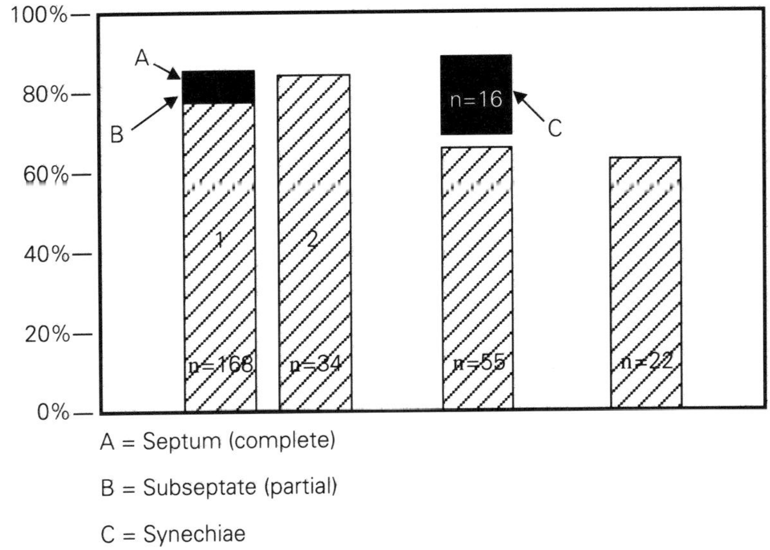

Figure 10.2 Treatment of recurrences with the Nd-YAG laser. Long-term results (8–56 months). ■ One-step surgery: 1, Focal surgery; 2, Total endometrium surgery. ■ Two-step surgery.

Out of a group of 51 dysmenorrhoeic women, 65% had total relief and a further 20% had partial relief of dysmenorrhoea.

The other unexpected, and surprising effect was on infertility. Several patients found themselves unexpectedly pregnant after the ablation of intra-uterine lesions, especially sub-mucous fibromas, polyps or endocervical or endo-uterine synechiae. As our experience of intra-uterine laser surgery increased our detection of hysteroscopic abnormalities associated with infertility has currently risen to around 20–25%.

10.4.2 INTRA-UTERINE SEPTAE AND SYNECHIAE

For the diagnosis and treatment of these lesions, hysteroscopy is the modus operandi par excellence. For thin synechiae, we perform adhesiolysis with the end of the fibre hysteroscope with subsequent coagulation of the areas of insertion. For large synechiae, we prefer to use the Nd-YAG laser by a contact technique, either with the bare fibre or with artificial sapphire tips, so as to limit the inflammatory effect and tendency of recurrence.

For this type of operation, we use a paracervical anaesthetic which enables us to evaluate the proximity to the uterine serous peritoneum. If the Nd-YAG laser energy encroaches on this sensitive surface pain sensation is felt by the patient and the laser is inactivated. The ability of the conscious patient to signify pain sensation is an important safety factor in this type of surgery.

As far as the therapy of septae is concerned, it is desirable to perform simultaneous laparoscopy, so as to know if the uterus is bicornuate or if a single septum is involved. For these procedures, a hysterosalpingogram and hysteroscopic examination are performed exactly 8 weeks after the first procedure and small corrective surgery can be performed at the same time.

As far as after-care is concerned we have abandoned the practice of inserting a Fowler probe or an intra-uterine device in the cavity. The oral contraceptive pill is given for two cycles immediately after surgery. The post-operative course of metroplasties is very similar to focal ablative therapy. The patients have a sero-sanguinous discharge for 1–3 days, very little pain, and no effect on subsequent vaginal delivery. Like similar procedures with electrosurgery and mechanical scissors, the uterine musculature seems to have normal strength and there is no need for delivery by Caesarean section which would be necessary if conventional uterine reconstructive surgery had been performed. A particular form of synechiae or intra-cavity irregularity is associated with the post-Caesarean scar. We have treated several swellings on the internal surface of the scar which, in some cases, went as far as the formation of synechiae.

10.4.3 RESULTS IN INFERTILITY

The results of our preliminary study on 75 infertile women are summarized in Table 10.2. There were six pregnancies in women with cornual pedunculate fibroids and intracavity polyps; five pregnancies in women with septae and 19 pregnancies in women with 36 synechiae.

No complications were found at the time of delivery but particular care must be taken following correction of isthmic stenosis after Caesarean section which tends to induce weakness of the Caesarean scar.

10.5 Alternatives to the Nd-YAG laser in hysteroscopic surgery

In order to test the effectiveness of the Nd-YAG laser we have also treated this type of lesion with the electrodiathermy resectoscope and the argon laser (5 W).

Table 10.2 Hysteroscopic treatment of infertility. Long-term results (8–30 months)

	No. of patients	*Normal cavity*	*Two-step surgery*	*Pregnancies*	*Abortions*	*Lost to follow-up*
Septae	14	11	7	5	1	3
Subseptae	11	10		4	2	1
Synechiae	36	30	6	19	4	5
Asherman	4	2	1	0		
Cornual lesions	6	6	2	3		1
Intracavity lesions	4	4	2	3	1	1

10.5.1 ELECTRODIATHERMY RESECTION

The diathermy resectoscope already tested by Neuwirth (1978) and DeCherney and Polan (1983), with an outside diameter of 21 mm including an inflow and outflow channel, is similar to the one used in urology for transurethral resection of the prostate. The wire loop diathermy operating up to 400 W facilitates the treatment of fibroids and polyps and enables us to coagulate areas of adenomyosis. Our patients were treated with focal therapy in contra-distinction to electrosurgical resection employed by Neuwirth (1978) and Hamon and Salat-Baroux (1982). We feel that the haemostatic effect is not as good as with the Nd-YAG laser but to some extent this can be compensated by changing the electrodiathermy loop to the roller-ball. Our results are shown in Figure 10.3. The success rate with the Nd-YAG laser was considerably better than that achieved with the argon laser or electrodiathermy resection.

10.5.2 SANDWICH TECHNIQUE

At the present time we use electrodiathermy in patients with large fibroids and polyps or for multiple lesions. The sandwich technique involves: (1) coagulation of the pedicle of the fibroid with the Nd-YAG laser, (2) removal of the remainder of the lesion with the electrodiathermy loop and (3) coagulation of the base of the lesion with the Nd-YAG laser. The micro-resector (24 mm) is used in patients wishing further pregnancies and a larger resector (28 mm) is used in patients who wish no further pregnancies.

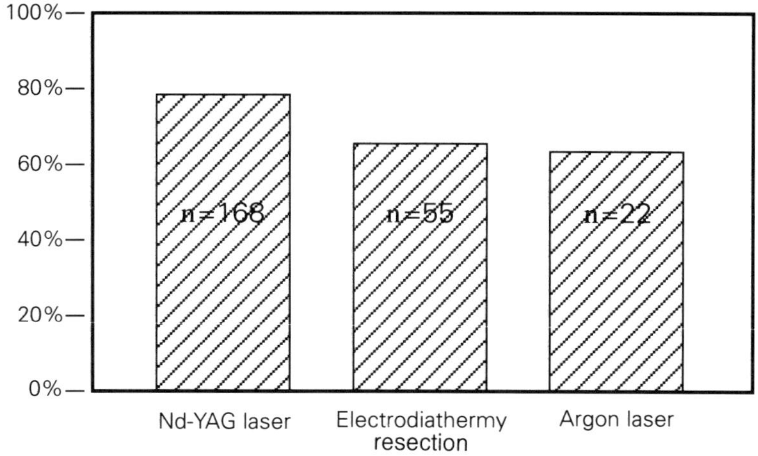

Figure 10.3 Comparative long-term results (8–56 months) of focal treatment. ■ Good results indicated by normal menogram.

Table 10.3 Argon laser. Long-term results (8–56 months)

	No. of patients	%
Normal menogram	14	63.5
Poor results	8*	36.5

* Two mucous polyps, three fibroids and three adenomyosis.

10.5.3 ARGON LASER

The argon laser (5 W) has been used in hysteroscopy with flexible endoscopes but as shown in Table 10.3 the procedure was ineffective in the treatment of bleeding, except in cases with pedunculated polyps or small areas of adenomyosis. Further clinical trials should be conducted with higher power argon lasers (20 W) and with KTP-532 lasers to evaluate the real effectiveness of visible light lasers.

10.6 Complications and side effects

Most patients tend to have a brown discharge for 1 week after surgery, sometimes lasting up to 5 weeks (11 patients out of 168). In these 11 patients, seven had large uterine fibroids, and the other four had endometritis caused by anaerobic bacteria and required 5 days of antibiotic treatment. Uterine contractions, lasting 3–5 min, occurred sometimes after the first attempt at sexual intercourse. One patient developed a haematometra with an enlarged uterus which resolved after 15 days of antibiotic therapy.

Four patients had signs of fluid overload with facial oedema and excessive diuresis the following day. No patient had electrolyte imbalance except one who absorbed more than 1.5 litres of fluid. In spite of this the electrolyte imbalance corrected itself spontaneously. In the event of significant absorption during the procedure (more than 1 litre), the fluid is removed by suction through the flexible endoscope before terminating the procedure. The use of a small diameter endoscope allows an adequate fluid outflow around the hysteroscope, without prior dilatation and this limits the inflow pressure. It is very important to photo-coagulate all the vessels around the lesions, before cutting or vaporizing. Otherwise the surgeon needs to increase the inflow pressure to control blood loss and to maintain clear vision and this can give rise to increased fluid absorption.

One patient had a uterine perforation during dilatation before hysteroscopy. Three post-menopausal women complained of pain during surgery in the cornual area. For this reason we prefer to perform hysteroscopic laser procedures under local anaesthesia except in treatment of septae, and large sub-mucous fibroids.

10.7 Conclusion

Focal hysteroscopic laser surgery can avoid hysterectomy in patients with abnormal bleeding and avoid uterotomy in the treatment of infertility due to septae, synechiae and intra-uterine lesions. The advantage of focal therapy lies in the ability to treat those women with menorrhagia who may still wish to have further children.

References

Asherman, J. G. (1948), Amenorrhea traumatica (atretica). *J. Obstet. Gynaecol. Br. Emp.*, **55**, 23–30.

Baggish, M. S. and Daniell, J. F. (1989), Death caused by air embolism associated with Nd:YAG laser surgery and artificial sapphire tips. *Am. J. Osbtet. Gynecol.*, **161**, 877–8.

DeCherney, A. and Polan, M. L. (1983), Hysteroscopic management of intrauterine lesions and intractable uterine bleeding. *Obstet. Gynecol.*, **61**, 392.

Dequesne, J. (1987), Hysteroscopic treatment of uterine bleeding with the Nd-YAG laser. *Lasers Med. Sci.*, **2**, 73.

Droegmueller, W., Greer, B. and Makowski, E. (1971a), Cryosurgery in patients with dysfunctional uterine bleeding. *Obstet. Gynecol.*, **38**, 256–8.

Droegmueller, W., Makowski, E. and Macsalka, R. (1971b), Destruction of the endometrium by cryosurgery. *Am. J. Obstet. Gynecol.*, **110**, 467–9.

Goldrath, M. H., Fuller, T. A. and Segal, S. (1981), Laser photovaporization of endometrium for the treatment of menorrhagia. *Am. J. Obstet. Gynecol*, **104**, 14.

Hamou, J. and Salat-Baroux, J. (1982), Hysteroscopie et microchirurgie. *Encycl. Med. Chir. (Paris)*, **72**, 1710.

Neuwirth, R. S. (1978), A new technique for an additional experience with hysteroscope resection of submucous fibroids. *Am. J. Obstet. Gynecol.*, **131**, 91.

Rongy, A. J. (1947), Radium therapy in benign uterine bleeding. *J Mt Sinai Hosp.* **14**, 569–75.

Shenker, J. G. and Polishuk, W. Z. (1973), Regeneration of rabbit endometrium following intra-uterine instillation of chemical agents. *Gynecol. Invest.*, **4**, 1–13.

11 *Laser treatment of cervical and vaginal intraepithelial neoplasia*

NIGEL SAUNDERS, FRANK SHARP and JOSEPH A. JORDAN

11.1 Historical aspects of cervical intraepithelial neoplasia

The epithelial lining of the cervix is derived from two separate embryological precursors, the junction of which occurs typically in the vicinity of the external os. The vaginal aspect of the cervix is covered by stratified squamous epithelium, whereas the endocervical canal is lined by a single layer of mucus-secreting columnar cells up to the level of the internal os. The canal and its lining epithelium communicates directly with clefts or crypts which dip down into the substance of the cervical stroma.

The original position of the squamocolumnar junction (SCJ) is determined during embryological development and during postnatal life. The position of this junction is modified by the process of squamous metaplasia whereby columnar epithelium exposed to the vaginal environment may undergo transformation into a squamous type of epithelium. The metaplastic process proceeds in a *cephalad* direction and results in a new SCJ separated from the old SCJ by a field of metaplastic epithelium. This area of change is known by colposcopists as the transformation zone for obvious reasons.

Although the exact origin of the metaplastic cells is still under debate there is little doubt that the actual stimulus to metaplasia is the acid pH of the vagina and it appears that a pH of below 7.4 favours the presence of squamous epithelium (Coppleson and Reid, 1967). During periods of rising oestrogen production such as puberty and pregnancy, volume changes in the cervix promote eversion of the columnar epithelium causing previously unexposed areas of the endocervical mucosa to be involved in the metaplastic process.

Although metaplasia is a common physiological event it appears that under certain circumstances, possibly in response to some mutagenic stimulus, the process proceeds in an atypical fashion with the formation of potentially neoplastic areas of epithelium within the transformation zone.

Intraepithelial cancer was first described at the margin of an invasive cervical lesion by Williams (1888), and in the early part of the 20th century several other workers described similar cases. Rubin (1910) reported two cases in which the cervical epithelium possessed the morphological characteristics of carcinoma but appeared to lack an invasive component. The significance of these findings was uncertain but Rubin quite correctly suggested that they represented the 'beginning formation of carcinoma'; and furthermore that the diagnosis could be made solely on cytological characteristics of the epithelium. Given that invasion was at that time the fundamental criterion of malignancy, intraepithelial carcinoma was seen as a contradiction in terms. As a result of this conceptual problem a plethora of different labels were applied to the same morphological changes, each term reflecting to some extent the perceived biological significance of this histological variant. Schiller was perhaps the first to understand that the invasive potential of these lesions might not be realized for months or years but that they nevertheless constituted an early phase in the development of frank carcinoma (Schiller, 1933).

Gradually the term 'carcinoma *in situ*' introduced by Broders (1932) gained general acceptance, and to the present day is still used in some quarters to denote the most marked forms of epithelial atypia. The histological diagnosis of carcinoma *in situ* was not however exact, being based on the subjective assessment of the morphology of individual cells and the relationship of those cells one to another. By convention full thickness epithelial abnormalities were designated as carcinoma *in situ* and lesser changes as dysplasia. This system may be considered unsatisfactory as inconsistencies frequently occur in allocating lesions to one or other diagnostic category (Cocker, Fox and Langley, 1968) and the use of separate nomenclature implies differences in biological behaviour between severe dysplasia and carcinoma *in situ* which now do not appear to exist.

The concept of epithelial atypia as a disease continuum encompassing all grades of abnormality was therefore suggested by several groups of workers. Richart (1964), holding a similar viewpoint, introduced the terms cervical intraepithelial neoplasia (CIN) grades I, II and III which have to a large extent replaced the older terminology. Recently it has been suggested that even this classification is not always reproducible and a more sensible approach would be to describe lesions merely as being high or low grade (Robertson *et al.*, 1989).

Assessment of the true malignant potential of intraepithelial neoplasia has proven extremely difficult. The first attempts to demonstrate progression of carcinoma *in situ* to invasive disease were made retrospectively. By reviewing the previous cervical biopsy specimens of patients presenting with invasive cancer it was possible to identify some instances where carcinoma *in situ* had been present many years beforehand but the significance of the changes had been overlooked at the time of the original biopsy. The first such case was described by Smith and Pemberton (1934) and many similar reports followed. All these reports were flawed by the fact that it was generally impossible to know whether or not an invasive component had co-existed with the intraepithelial elements at the time of the original biopsy, but had not been sampled, or equally that the intraepithelial abnormality had been completely removed by the biopsy and the subsequent development of cancer was an unrelated event.

Prospective studies were undertaken in an attempt to gain a clearer understanding of the rate of malignant transformation of intraepithelial disease. Such studies have demonstrated to the satisfaction of most physicians that the risk of invasive progression is great enough to warrant reasonably prompt intervention. The most often quoted works of Peterson (1958) and more recently McIndoe *et al.* (1984) both show a consistent trend towards invasive transformation with time. Earlier reports refuting or minimizing the potential dangers of carcinoma *in situ* were based on an inadequate length of follow-up (Green, 1970) and failure to appreciate the effect of biopsy on the natural history of the disease. CIN may resolve following biopsy thus introducing a variable into the behaviour of the disease which cannot be quantified. As Richart (1967) has said, 'a small lesion totally removed by biopsy is equivalent, from the stand-point of observing the lesion, to a hysterectomy'. In the absence of biopsy it appears that regression of higher grade CIN appears to be infrequent enough to justify treatment in all patients (Campion *et al.*, 1986).

Premalignant disease of the cervix is not associated with any characteristic signs or symptoms and practical screening for preclinical cervical disease did not become a reality until Papanicolaou and Traut published their cytology method in 1941, demonstrating that malignant cells exfoliating from the cervix could be sampled and recognized microscopically. The introduction of population screening with this method had a profound impact on clinical practice as thousands of asymptomatic women were found to have abnormal cervical cytology and clinicians were faced with the dilemma of how to manage these patients. Gynaecologists responded to this challenge with an impressive array of alternative therapies. Radical treatment in the form of extended hysterectomy and lymphadenectomy or radiotherapy was initially predominant in the United States and Britain (Corscaden, 1950; Way *et al.*, 1968). It is likely that the terminology, i.e. carcinoma *in situ*, was partially responsible for this radical approach, since it was a commonly held view that cancer was cancer and should be treated as such. The situation was further confused by the interpretation of the distribution of CIN, which has a propensity to involve the epithelium of the cervical crypts to a variable depth, but usually no greater than 5 mm (Anderson and Hartley, 1980). This frequent phenomenon of 'gland involvement' was erroneously labelled as invasion by some authors (Galvin and Telinde, 1949) and probably contributed to the use of radical treatment methods. Such treatment, however, was not without its own risks and this in combination with the gradual recognition that true intraepithelial disease was not associated with metastases prompted a more conservative approach. Simple hysterectomy thus became the treatment of choice for CIN III in the 1960s and 1970s (Brudenell, Cox and Taylor, 1973).

As less radical therapy was introduced for CIN III it became essential to exclude the possibility of co-existent invasive disease before embarking upon simple hysterectomy. A minority of authors suggested that random cervical punch biopsy would suffice for this purpose but there have been many reports of invasion overlooked by this method. All studies with comparative data favour conization over random biopsy, which thus became the preferred diagnostic method in women presenting with an abnormal cervical smear.

Hysterectomy, although effective therapy for most cases of intraepithelial disease, inevitably produced sterility and this fact stimulated a move towards more conservative therapy for young women wishing to retain their fertility. In 1933 Schiller had reported the apparent cure of carcinoma *in situ* following amputation of the cervix, and it was also well recognized that histological examination of hysterectomy specimens would often fail to reveal residual cervical disease if performed after diagnostic conization. This phenomenon did not occur frequently enough for many to countenance clinically evident recurrent or persistent disease following therapeutic conization were low enough for the procedure to become gradually accepted into general gynaecological practice. It is now clear that conization is adequate treatment for the majority of patients with CIN III and Jordan (1976), in reviewing the results of seven large series of conizations, noted that only 22 of 2326 patients so managed went on to develop subsequent invasive disease.

11.2 Conservative trends in management

Moves towards yet further conservatism in the management of CIN were driven by concerns about the morbidity of conization coupled with an increasing appreciation of the value of colposcopy in both delineating the distribution of the disease and allowing directed biopsy of the transformation zone. Whereas random biopsy of the cervix carries the very real risk of overlooking invasive disease many authors have reported colposcopically directed biopsy to be a reliable diagnostic technique upon which decisions concerning therapy may be safely based providing that the entire transformation zone is visible (Fowler and Shingleton, 1971; Donohue and Merriwether, 1972).

After colposcopy and directed biopsy has provided a diagnosis of intraepithelial neoplasia local ablation of the abnormal transformation zone may be undertaken. The use of local ablative therapy is based on the principle that following the destruction of abnormal epithelium healthy tissue will regenerate to cover the cervix. The exact treatment modality requires destruction in depth and cryosurgery, diathermy and laser vaporization have all been applied with good effect. Not all patients are suitable for local ablative therapy and most authors are agreed that diagnostic conization is still mandatory if the entire transformation zone cannot be visualized because of endocervical extension, if there is a suspicion of microinvasive disease, glandular neoplasia or a major discrepancy between the cytological and colposcopic findings.

If endocervical curettage is part of the colposcopy protocol a positive result should be an indication for conization in order to enable a firm diagnosis to be made (Drescher, Peter and Roberts, 1983), although some may argue that primary conization is a better option in all situations where endocervical curettage is likely to be positive, the transformation zone extends into the canal, no lesions are visible, and there is a discrepancy between cytology and colposcopic biopsy (Benedet, Anderson and Boyes, 1985).

11.3 Available treatment methods

Presently CIN may be treated by a range of techniques varying from local ablative methods such as cryotherapy or laser vaporization, excisional procedures such as laser or knife cut cone biopsy and even hysterectomy. The most frequently used methods will be described and their advantages and disadvantages discussed.

11.3.1 CRYOTHERAPY

One of the original forms of local ablative therapy introduced in the 1960s, cryotherapy has enjoyed considerable popularity in the United States for the treatment of CIN. A range of suitably shaped probes are available through which refrigerant gas is channelled. The probe is placed against the transformation zone of the cervix and an ice ball is created on the cervix which produces epithelial necrosis and thereby the destruction of intraepithelial neoplasia. Heat transfer may be improved by coating the cervix with a layer of water-soluble lubricant. It has been reported that a freeze–thaw–freeze cycle is more effective than a single freeze technique (Creasman, 1984). No anaesthesia is required and patient discomfort is minimal. Many patients suffer a watery vaginal discharge for several weeks following treatment. After the cervix has healed the SCJ is often found to be inside the endocervical canal which could hinder colposcopic and cytological surveillance.

Reports comparing the cure rates following cryotherapy or laser vaporization modalities (Townsend and Richart, 1983; Jobson and Holmesley, 1984; Kirwan, Smith and Naftalin, 1985; Berget, 1987) indicate success rates in the region of 90% following one treatment, although it appears that laser may be more effective in dealing with large lesions or those that extend into the endocervix.

Reports of invasive cancer subsequent to the use of conservative treatment modalities, especially cryotherapy (Townsend *et al.*, 1981) may be due in no small part to failure to follow accepted assessment protocols before embarking on treatment. Such errors include reliance on blind biopsy and concurrent therapy at the time of diagnostic biopsy.

11.3.2 ELECTRODIATHERMY

This method of ablative therapy has been pioneered by Australian workers (Chanen and Hollyock, 1974). Using needle diathermy the epithelium of the cervical crypts is destroyed by numerous insertions of the electrode until the entire transformation zone has been covered. Diathermy proceeds until mucus no longer bubbles up from the cervix. Any remaining superficial epithelium is then destroyed using a ball electrode. The treatment is painful and a general anaesthetic is usually required which is one of the main disadvantages of this method, although recently the use of local anaesthesia with the method has been described (Chanen, 1984/5, 1989). The columnar epithelium of the lower centimetre of the cervical canal is intentionally destroyed as this is said to increase the success rate of this approach, but as with cryotherapy, the SCJ may recede into the endocervical canal after treatment thus impeding follow-up. The reported cure rates of over 97% are very impressive given the low incidence of secondary haemorrhage (1.4%) and cervical stenosis (0.6%). In a paper comparing cryotherapy and electrodiathermy there was no statistically significant difference between the cure rates of the two procedures (O'Shea, Need and Pomeroy, 1986).

11.3.4 COLD COAGULATION

This method has some features in common with cryocautery and electrodiathermy. Teflon-coated thermosounds are heated to around 100°C and applied to the transformation zone. The epithelium is blistered off and the underlying stroma is destroyed to a depth of 3–4 mm (Duncan, 1983). The probe is held in contact with the cervix for 20 s and approximately five applications of the instrument are required to cover the entire transformation zone. Complications are infrequent although patients may notice some vaginal discharge or light bleeding in the first weeks following treatment. General anaesthesia is not required and as with other conservative treatment methods, cure rates of over 90% may be achieved with one treatment.

11.3.5 LASER VAPORIZATION

The CO_2 laser produces radiant energy which may be focused and applied to the cervix in a precise manner by means of a micromanipulator. Light energy is converted to heat and tissue is vaporized as intracellular water is rapidly heated to boiling point. The power density of the laser beam will determine the rate at which vaporization occurs. Thermal damage to adjacent tissues is related to the duration of exposure and can be minimized by selecting high-power densities ($>1000\ W/cm^2$) resulting in rapid vaporization.

Although the laser was first used on the cervix to treat benign disease (Kaplan, Goldman and Ger, 1973) its potential in eradicating premalignant epithelium was soon recognized (Stafl, Wilkinson and Mattingly, 1977).

Early attempts at laser vaporization were associated with rather high failure rates due to an inadequate depth of tissue destruction. Removal of the entire transformation zone to a depth of 5–7 mm (including any disease in cervical crypts) has produced much better results (Stanhope *et al.*, 1983; Townsend and Richart, 1983; Wright, Davies and Riopelle, 1983). Laser vaporization cone may be performed on an out-patient basis and side effects are minimal. Patient discomfort may be almost totally abolished by local anaesthetic infiltration, and the only problem which occurs with any frequency is secondary haemorrhage from the cone bed, but this is rarely a significant clinical problem and usually responds to conservative measures. Cervical stenosis is very unusual following treatment and pelvic inflammatory disease is rare, although it may occur in patients with an intra-uterine contraceptive device in place. It would appear sensible to consider removal of such a device prior to treatment. The healed cervix shows minimal distortion and the new SCJ is characteristically visible at the external os which may be an advantage in terms of colposcopic and cytological follow-up.

11.3.6 COLD KNIFE EXCISIONAL CONE BIOPSY

Knife excisional cone biopsy was at one time the standard diagnostic procedure for women with abnormal cervical cytology. With the acceptance of colposcopy and directed biopsy to provide a diagnosis the operation is nowadays performed much less frequently. At present only 15–20% of patients with abnormal cytology will ultimately undergo diagnostic conization (Singer and Walker, 1982). The traditional knife excisional conization is performed under general anaesthetic and haemostasis is usually obtained through the use of cervical sutures. The operation carries a higher rate of morbidity than almost any other gynaecological procedure. Although the risk of operative mortality is low, as is the incidence of subsequent invasive cancer, the short- and long-term complications of the procedure include primary and secondary haemorrhage, pelvic infection, cervical stenosis and increased obstetric morbidity in subsequent pregnancy. The complication rate is increased when a large cone specimen is taken (Lieman, Harrison and Robin, 1980; Luesley *et al.*, 1985). Recently the microcolpohysteroscope has been used to determine the distribution of endocervical disease so that the cone biopsy may be tailored to allow removal of the minimum volume of cervical tissue compatible with complete disease excision (Fenton *et al.*, 1984).

11.3.7 LASER EXCISIONAL CONE BIOPSY

The first attempts at laser excisional conization were by Taoff (1976) with a hand-held CO_2 laser. Access to the cervix was poor and the technique was improved by Dorsey and Diggs (1979) who mounted the laser on a colposcope. The laser beam was focused to a spot size of 1.5 mm and moved across the cervix by means of a micromanipulator. As the CO_2 laser has the ability to seal blood vessels up to 1.0 mm in diameter with minimal thermal damage to neighbouring tissue (Hall, Hill and Beach, 1971) it is an appropriate cutting modality for conization. The haemostatic effect has been confirmed in comparative studies of laser vs knife excisional cone biopsy (Larsson, Grunberg and Grundell, 1983; Bostoffe *et al.*, 1986; Fenton *et al.*, 1986) and primary haemorrhage is less frequently seen with its use.

Secondary haemorrhage and cervical stenosis is also less common when the laser is employed to cut the cone specimen. Recent work has suggested that haemostatic suturing (required for knife but not laser excisional cone biopsy) may be responsible for this phenomenon (Gilbert *et al.*, 1989). The cure rate of CIN after laser excisional cone is very impressive (97%) (Baggish, Dorsey and Adelsen, 1989). It is interesting that in the treatment of CIN the best results have been obtained with techniques which destroy or remove at least the distal 1 cm of endocervical mucosa (i.e. electrodiathermy or laser excisional cone). It may be, therefore, that with less extensive treatment measures some recurrences arise from transformed but colposcopically normal endocervical mucosa.

Early invasive cancer may be overlooked even by an experienced colposcopist and with this problem in mind, laser excisional cone biopsy has been recommended in order to provide tissue for histological diagnosis in patients whom many would consider suitable for local ablative therapy (Bekassy *et al.*, 1983; Partington *et al.*, 1989) and the laser excisional procedure may eventually replace vaporization for this reason (McIndoe *et al.*, 1989).

11.3.8 LARGE LOOP EXCISION OF THE TRANSFORMATION ZONE

The haemostatic qualities of surgical diathermy were utilized by Hyam (1928) and Crossen (1935) when they introduced electrodes designed to excise cervical tissue. Whilst this was perhaps acceptable for the management of benign disease, thermal damage to the pathological specimen made this technique inappropriate for the diagnosis of CIN. Recently there has been a resurgence of interest in the use of the diathermy loop excision of CIN generated by the work of Rene Cartier of Paris (Cartier, 1984; Atkinson, 1984). Modifications to the thickness of the diathermy wire and alterations in the current have allowed cutting diathermy with minimal thermal artefact to the histological specimen. Under local anaesthetic the entire transformation zone may be removed with the instrument. Using a pure cutting current of around 30 W the loop is moved through the cervix and the resected portions of the cervix are available for histological assessment. Bleeding may then be controlled with a ball probe and coagulating current. This technique has many of the attractions of laser excisional cone but as yet no randomized comparative studies exist to assess the relative advantages and disadvantages of the two methods.

11.3.9 HYSTERECTOMY

The use of hysterectomy in the management of CIN may be appropriate for older parous patients with co-existing gynaecological disease, such as fibroids. Prior to operation it is still essential to exclude invasive cervical disease by colposcopy and directed biopsy. Any vaginal extension of intraepithelial disease may also be identified in this way and the operation thus modified to include the removal of a cuff of vaginal epithelium.

11.4 Techniques of laser vaporization and excisional conization

11.4.1 LASER VAPORIZATION CONE

The technique may be performed on an out-patient basis in most cases although very anxious patients and those with large lesions extending onto the vagina may benefit from general anaesthesia. Local anaesthesia is appreciated by most patients although it is not essential. A mixture of lignocaine and vasopressin injected with a fine gauge needle and a dental syringe is suitable for this technique. Submucosal injection at several sites around the transformation zone is more effective than paracervical block. Non-reflective speculae are desirable when using laser in the upper genital tract to avoid the risk of inadvertent reflection of the beam onto the patient or operator. Effective smoke evacuation equipment is essential to maintain a satisfactory view of the cervix during treatment, and for health and safety reasons.

After colposcopic examination has confirmed the original findings and demonstrated that the entire transformation zone is visible, treatment may begin. The cervix is stained with Lugol's iodine to highlight the transformation zone and using a spot size of 1–2 mm and a power output of around 20 W the cervix is lasered 2–3 mm peripheral to the transformation zone to outline the area. The depth of tissue destruction in this peripheral border is deepened to around 5–6 mm which will reduce the blood supply to the central cervix and will lessen the likelihood of haemorrhage during the subsequent vaporization. It is then convenient to destroy the transformation zone by quadrants, starting on the posterior aspect of the cervix until the desired depth of tissue destruction has been achieved. Depth can be measured using a specially designed dip stick or even a simple cotton-tipped swab. The main problem encountered during treatment is one of haemorrhage and this may be dealt with in a variety of ways: defocusing the laser beam and reducing the power output of the laser will generate more heat during vaporization and may produce the desired coagulative effect. Arterial bleeding is best treated by lasering around the vessel until it is isolated from the surrounding cervical stroma at which point the beam is directed onto the vessel itself. Simple pressure, vasoconstrictor injection or even cervical suture may be helpful in some cases.

11.4.2 LASER EXCISIONAL CONIZATION

This procedure again may be performed under local anaesthesia. Small spot size and high power densities ensure a rapid vaporizing (cutting effect). The lesion is outlined as with the vaporization procedure but the incision is deepened to 1.0–1.5 cm at which point the laser is directed towards the endocervical canal and a cone or cylinder of tissue 1.5–2.0 cm in depth is eventually removed. The beam is directed in the appropriate manner by a combination of manipulation of the cervix with specially designed instruments and alteration of the position and angle of the colposcope and micromanipulator. Some operators cut the apex of the cone with a knife or scissors to reduce thermal artefact at this point.

11.4.3 COMBINATION PROCEDURE

For larger lesions which cover the ectocervix and enter the endocervical canal the combination procedure of peripheral vaporization and central conization of the acquired transformation zone is well suited to allow eradication of disease with minimal destruction of the cervix. The peripheral visible portion of the cervix is assessed as usual by colposcopically directed biopsy before treatment. If there are no features of invasive disease on colposcopic or histological examination then this part of the cervix is vaporized to destroy the full thickness of the epithelium. The central inaccessible portion of the transformation zone is removed as in the laser excisional procedure.

11.5 Problems of vaginal intraepithelial neoplasia

Vaginal intraepithelial neoplasia (VAIN) demonstrates similar histological features to those seen in CIN although it is a much less common disease. The natural history of the disorder is uncertain but it is assumed that like CIN it has significant malignant potential. It is known that the transformation zone may extend onto the vaginal vault in some 10% of the normal population and it may be that atypical metaplasia of the transformation zone in this subgroup is the mechanism whereby most VAIN originates.

The disease may come to light in patients with CIN in whom the vaginal component is merely an extension of the cervical disease. Similarly patients with a history of CIN treated by hysterectomy may subsequently be found to have VAIN. It is likely that in many of such patients the vaginal component was present at the time of original therapy but was overlooked due to inadequate colposcopic assessment.

In a small proportion of patients the vaginal disease is part of multifocal intraepithelial neoplasia affecting also cervical, vulval and even perianal skin and such patients may have evidence of iatrogenic or idiopathic immune dysfunction (Sillman *et al.*, 1984).

Colposcopy allows the distribution of VAIN to be delineated in most cases, and following appropriate diagnostic biopsies, laser provides an ideal method of treatment in patients who have not been subjected to previous surgery. Control of the depth of tissue destruction is precise and many authors have reported satisfactory cure rates with the technique (Petrilli *et al.*, 1980; Jobson and Homesley, 1983; Stuart *et al.*, 1988). A much shallower depth of destruction (2 mm) is required compared to the cervix. Full thickness epithelial destruction is signalled by the occurrence of tissue fluid weeping from the stroma. General anaesthesia is preferred during the treatment of large lesions. Scarring is minimal and re-epithelialization is usually complete within weeks.

In patients with a history of previous hysterectomy it appears that laser therapy of disease involving the vault suture line is much less likely to produce a cure due to the presence of buried or inaccessible atypical epithelium. There is also a danger of overlooking invasive disease at the vault resection line in such patients (Barclay, 1979; Jordan and Sharp, 1986; Ireland and Monaghan, 1988) and vault excision is probably a better option than laser vaporization.

11.6 Advantages of laser

Despite the disadvantages of cost, the CO_2 laser has several major points in its favour in the context of therapy for lower genital tract intraepithelial neoplasia, especially of the cervix. Most treatment can be performed on an out-patient basis, under local anaesthesia. Treatment can be applied to the required location and depth with great precision, cervical healing is rapid, side effects infrequent and the cure rates are high. It is the ideal method of therapy for patients with extensive disease and is likely to remain so for the foreseeable future.

11.7 Organization of a colposcopic laser service

As previously described there are several cheap and effective alternatives to laser therapy in the management of the straightforward patient with CIN. Not all units may be able to justify the expenditure required to purchase a CO_2 laser, particularly if the referral rate for abnormal cervical cytology to their unit is not great. On the other hand, in hospitals with busy colposcopy clinics the advantages of laser therapy in selected patients will almost certainly justify the financial cost. Most laser therapy will be performed in the colposcopy clinic in an outpatient setting although a minority of patients will require general anaesthetic. One laser may be moved between the clinic and operation room but this frequent movement may result in a loss of efficiency from the laser due to misalignment of reflective mirrors and ideally there should be a separate laser for each setting. Most laser surgery can be readily performed with machines that have a power output of 25–40 W, although for excisional work and particularly to control blood loss in haemorrhagic cases, higher power output is an advantage.

Before purchasing a laser several factors should be borne in mind. It is important to determine whether the hospital will be able to provide an effective service for routine in-house maintenance of the machine and the exact maintenance contracts should be negotiated with individual laser manufacturers as the level of back-up in this area is important. Some of the costs of purchasing and maintenance may be shared with other specialties in the hospital, e.g. ENT, and this point should be discussed before purchase. Individual tastes may vary in the preferred type of colposcope and micromanipulator used in association with the laser and it is advisable to request that the laser companies provide a demonstration of the laser and ancillary equipment before making a final choice.

References

Anderson, M. C. and Hartley, R. B. (1980), Cervical crypt involvement by intraepithelial neoplasia. *Obstet. Gynecol.*, **55**, 546–50.

Atkinson, K. (1984), Diathermy loop excision. *Colp. Gynecol. Laser Surg.*, **1**, 285–9.

Baggish, M. S., Dorsey, J. H. and Adelson, M. (1989), A ten year experience treating cervical intraepithelial neoplasia with the CO_2 laser. *Am. J. Obstet. Gynecol.*, **161**, 60–8.

Barclay, D. L. (1979), Carcinoma of the vagina after hysterectomy for severe dysplasia or carcinoma *in situ* of the cervix. *Gynecol. Oncol.*, **8**, 1–11.

Bekassy, Z., Alm, P., Grundsell, H., Larsson, G. and Astedt, B. (1983), Laser miniconization in mild and moderate dysplasia of the uterine cervix. *Gynecol. Oncol.*, **15**, 357–62.

Benedet, J. L., Anderson, G. H. and Boyes, D. A. (1985), Colposcopic accuracy in the diagnosis of microinvasive and occult invasive cancer. *Obstet. Gynecol.*, **65**, 557–62.

Berget, A. (1987) Outpatient treatment of CIN. The CO_2 laser versus cryotherapy: A randomised trial. *Acta Obstet. Gynecol. Scand.*, **66**, 531–6.

Bostoffe, E., Berget, A., Falkk, L., Pedersen, P. H. and Rank, F. (1986), Conization by CO_2 laser or cold knife in the treatment of cervical intraepithelial neoplasia. *Acta Obstet. Gynecol. Scand.*, **65**, 199–202.

Broders, A. C. (1932), Carcinoma *in situ* contrasted with benign penetrating epithelium. *JAMA*, **99**, 1670–4.
Brudenell, M., Cox, B. S. and Taylor, C. W. (1973), The management of dysplasia carcinoma *in situ* and microcarcinoma of the cervix. *J. Obstet. Gynaecol. Br. Emp.*, **80**, 673–9.
Campion, M. J., McCance, D. J., Czick, J. and Singer, A. (1986), Progressive potential of mild cervical atypia: Prospective cytological, colposcopic and virological study. *Lancet*, **i**, 237–40.
Cartier, R. (1984), *Practical Colposcopy*. Laboratoire Cartier, Paris.
Chanen, W. (1984/5), Symposium on cervical neoplasm III, electrocoagulation diathermy. *Colp. Gynecol. Laser Surg.*, **1**, 281–5.
Chanen, W. (1989), The efficacy of electrocoagulation diathermy performed under local anaesthesia for the eradication of precancerous lesions of the cervix. *Aust. N.Z. J. Obstet. Gynaecol.*, **29**, 189–92.
Chanen, W. and Hollyock, V. E. (1974), Colposcopy and the conservative management of cervical dysplasia and carcinoma *in situ*. *Obstet. Gynecol.*, **43**, 527–34.
Cocker, J., Fox, H. and Langley, F. A. (1968), Consistency in the histological diagnosis of epithelial abnormalities of the cervix uteri. *J. Clin. Pathol.*, **21**, 67–70.
Coppleson, M. and Reid, B. (1967), *Preclinical Carcinoma of the Cervix Uteri*, Pergamon Press, Oxford, pp. 93–136.
Corscaden, J. A. (1950), The treatment of early carcinoma of the cervix uteri. *Am. J. Obstet. Gynecol.*, **59**, 272–84.
Creasman, W. T. (1984), Symposium on cervical neoplasia II, cryosurgery, colposcopy and gynecologic laser surgery. *Colp. Gynecol. Laser Surg.*, **1**, 275–9.
Crossen, R. J. (1935), New electrode for conization of the cervix. *J. Miss. State Med. Assoc.*, **32**, 125.
Donohue, L. R. and Merriwether, W. (1972), Colposcopy as a diagnostic tool in the investigation of cervical neoplasms. *Am. J. Obstet. Gynecol.*, **113**, 107–10.
Dorsey, J. H. and Diggs, E. S. (1979), Microsurgical conization of the cervix by the carbon dioxide laser. *Obstet. Gynecol.*, 505–70.
Drescher, C. W., Peter III, W. A. and Roberts, J. A. (1983), Contribution of endocervical curettage in evaluation of abnormal cervical cytology. *Obstet. Gynecol.*, **62**, 343–7.
Duncan, I. D. (1983), The Semm cold coagulator in the management of cervical intraepithelial neoplasia. *Clin. Obstet. Gynecol.*, **26**, 996–1000.
Fenton, D. W., Soutter, W. P., Sharp, F. and James, C. (1986), A comparison of knife and CO_2 laser excisional cone biopsies. In *Gynaecological Laser Surgery*. (eds F. Sharp and J. A. Jordan), Perinatology Press, New York, pp. 77–84.
Fenton, D. W., Soutter, W. P., Sharp, F. and Mann, M. (1984), Preliminary experience with microcolpohysteroscopically controlled cone biopsies. *Colp. Gynecol. Laser Surg.*, **1**, 167–72.
Fowler, W. C. and Singleton, H. (1971), Impact of dysplasia clinic on cervical conization rates. *Obstet. Gynecol.*, **38**, 609–12.
Galvin, G. A. and Telinde, R. W. (1949), The present day status of non-invasive cervical carcinoma. *Am. J. Obstet. Gynecol.*, **57**, 15–36.
Gilbert, L., Saunders, N. J. S., Stringer, R. and Sharp, F. (1989), Hemostasis

and cold knife cone biopsy: A prospective randomised trial comparing a suture versus non-suture technique. *Obstet. Gynecol.*, **74**, 640–3.

Green, G. H. (1970), Cervical carcinoma *in situ*. *Aust. N.Z. J. Obstet. Gynaecol.*, **10**, 41–8.

Hall, R. R., Hill, D. W. and Beach, A. D. (1971), A carbon dioxide surgical laser. *Ann. R. Coll. Surg. Engl.*, **48**, 181–9.

Hyam, S. M. N. (1928), A new instrument for excision of diseased endocervix with surgical diathermy. *New York J. Med.*, **28**, 646–8.

Ireland, D. and Monaghan, J. M. (1988), The management of the patient with abnormal vaginal cytology following hysterectomy. *Br. J. Obstet. Gynaecol.*, **95**, 973–5.

Jobson, V. W. and Homesley, H. D. (1983), Treatment of vaginal intraepithelial neoplasia with the carbon dioxide laser. *Obstet. Gynecol.*, **62**, 90–3.

Jobson, V. W. and Holmesley, H. D. (1984), Comparison of cryosurgery and carbon dioxide laser ablation for treatment of CIN. *Colp. Gynecol. Laser Surg.*, **1**, 173–80.

Jordan, J. A. (1976), Diagnosis and management of premalignant condition of the cervix. *Clin. Obstet. Gynecol.*, **3**, 295–315.

Jordan, J. A. and Sharp, F. (1986), CO_2 laser treatment of vaginal intraepithelial neoplasia. In: *Gynaecological Laser Surgery* (eds F. Sharp and J. A. Jordan), Perinatology Press, New York, pp. 181–8.

Kaplan, I., Goldman, J. and Ger, R. (1973), The treatment of erosions of the uterine cervix by means of the CO_2 laser. *Obstet. Gynecol.*, **41**, 795–6.

Kirwan, P. H., Smith, I. R. and Naftalin, N. J. (1985), A study of cryosurgery and the CO_2 laser in treatment of CIN III of the uterine cervix. *Gynecol. Oncol.*, **22**, 195–200.

Larsson, G., Grunberg, B. and Grundell, H. (1983), A comparison of complications of laser and cold knife conization. *Obstet. Gynecol.*, **62**, 213–17.

Leiman, G., Harrison, N. A. and Robin, A. (1980), Pregnancy following conization of the cervix: Complications related to cone size. *Am. J. Obstet. Gynecol.*, **136**, 14–18.

Luesley, D. M., McCrum, A. M., Terry, P. B. *et al.* (1985), Complications of cone biopsy related to the dimensions of the cone and the influence of prior colposcopic assessment. *Br. J. Obstet. Gynecol.*, **92**, 158–64.

McIndoe, G. A. J., Robson, M. S., Tidy, J. A., Mason, W. P. and Anderson, M. C. (1989), Laser excision rather than vaporisation: The treatment of choice for cervical intraepithelial neoplasia. *Obstet. Gynecol.*, **74**, 165–8.

McIndoe, W. R., McLean, M. R., Jones, R. W. and Mullins, P. R. (1984), The invasive potential of carcinoma *in situ* of the cervix. *Obstet. Gynecol.*, **64**, 451–8.

O'Shea, R. T., Need, J. A. and Pomery, G. J. (1986), Cryotherapy versus electrocoagulation diathermy for cervical intraepithelial neoplasia – A prospective randomised trial. *Colp. Gynecol. Laser Surg.*, **2**, 159–61.

Papanicolaou, G. N. and Traut, H. F. (1941), The diagnostic value of vaginal smears in carcinoma of the uterus. *Am. J. Obstet. Gynecol.*, **42**, 193–206.

Partington, C. K., Turner, M. J., Soutter, W. P., Griffiths, M. and Krausz, T. (1989), Laser vaporisation versus laser excision conization in the treatment of cervical intraepithelial neoplasia. *Obstet. Gynecol.*, **73**, 775–8.

Peterson, O. (1958), Spontaneous course of cervical precancerous conditions. *Am. J. Obstet. Gynecol.*, **72**, 1063–71.

Petrilli, E. S., Townsend, D. E., Morrow, C. P. and Nakao, C. Y. (1980), Vaginal intraepithelial neoplasia: Biological aspect and treatment with topical 5-Fluorouracil and the carbon dioxide laser. *Am. J. Obstet. Gynecol.*, **138**, 321–8.

Richart, R. M. (1964), Observations on the biology of cervical dysplasia. *Bull. Sloane Hosp. Women, New York*, **10**, 170–4.

Richart, R. M. (1967), Natural history of cervical intraepithelial neoplasia. *Clin. Obstet. Gynecol.*, **10**, 748–84.

Robertson, A. J., Anderson, J. M., Swanson-Beck, J. *et al.* (1989), Observer variability in histopathological reporting of cervical biopsy specimens. *J. Clin. Pathol.*, **43**, 231–8.

Rubin, I. C. (1910), The pathological diagnosis of incipient carcinoma of the uterus. *Am. J. Obstet. Gynecol.*, **62**, 668–76.

Schiller, W. (1933), Early diagnosis of carcinoma of the cervix. *Surg. Gynecol. Obstet.*, **56**, 210–22.

Sillman, F., Stanek, A., Sedlis, A. *et al.* (1984), The relationship between human papilloma virus and lower genital tract neoplasia in immunosuppressed women. *Am. J. Obstet. Gynecol.*, **150**, 300–8.

Singer, A. and Walker, P. (1982), What is the optimal treatment of cervical premalignancy? *Br. J. Obstet. Gynecol.*, **89**, 335–7.

Smith, G. and Pemberton, F. A. (1934), The picture of very early carcinoma of the uterine cervix. *Surg. Gynecol. Obstet.*, **54**, 1–8.

Stafl, A., Wilkinson, E. J. and Mattingly, R. F. (1977), Laser treatment of cervical and vaginal neoplasia. *Am. J. Obstet. Gynecol.*, **128**, 128–36.

Stanhope, C. R., Phibbs, G. D., Stuart, G. C. *et al.* (1983), Carbon dioxide laser surgery. *Obstet. Gynecol.*, **61**, 624–7.

Stuart, G. C. E., Flagler, E. A., Nation, J. G., Duggan, M. and Robertson, D. I. (1988), Laser vaporisation of vaginal intraepithelial neoplasia. *Am. J. Obstet. Gynecol.*, **158**, 240–3.

Taoff, R. (1976), The carbon dioxide laser in gynaecological surgery. In *Laser Surgery III* (ed. I. Kaplan), Jerusalem Academic Press, Jerusalem, pp. 129–32.

Townsend, D. E. and Richart, R. M. (1983), Cryotherapy and CO_2 laser management of CIN: A controlled comparison. *Obstet. Gynecol.*, **61**, 75–8.

Townsend, D. E., Richart, R. M., Marks, E. and Neilson, J. (1981), Invasive cancer following out-patient evaluation and therapy for cervical disease. *Obstet. Gynecol.*, **57**, 145–9.

Way, S., Hennigan, M., Wright, V. C. (1968), Some experiences with preinvasive and microinvasive carcinoma of the cervix. *J. Obstet. Gynaecol. Br. Emp.*, **75**, 593–602.

Williams, J. (1888), *Cancer of the Uterus.* Harveian lectures for 1886. H. K. Lewis, London, pp. 8–13.

Wright, V. C., Davies, E. and Riopelle, M. A. (1983), Laser surgery for cervical intraepithelial neoplasia – Principles and results. *Am. J. Obstet. Gynecol.*, **145**, 181–4.

12 *Laser surgery on the vulva*

RICHARD REID

12.1 Basic treatment philosophy

Sexually transmitted human papillomavirus (HPV) infections are now accepted as having a major role in the aetiology of lower genital tract neoplasia (Lorincz and Reid, 1989). Nonetheless, clinicians must remember that progression to cancer is both rare and predictable. Moreover, although oncogenic human papillomaviruses (HPVs) involving the entire lower tract generally induce a 'field infection', neoplastic sequelae within the stable squamous epithelia of the vagina and vulva are at least 100-fold less common than malignant change within the metaplastic epithelium of the cervical transformation zone. Hence, principles of management differ according to the anatomical sites affected. It would be clearly inappropriate to destroy the entire anogenital epithelium in every patient with an abnormal smear. Rather, the therapeutic objective is to ablate the transformation zone by the most conservative method possible and thereafter follow the patient for life (Reid, 1989a). In contrast, the treatment of most HPV-associated lesions of the vulva and vagina is undertaken primarily for the control of this sexually transmitted disease, rather than as a prophylaxis against eventual gynaecological malignancy.

Although sexually transmitted HPV infections are remarkably common, disease expression appears to be the exception rather than the rule. When disease expression does occur, differences in host susceptibility produce enormous variability in clinical outcome. Lesions may be unicentric or multicentric, and severity ranges from minute to massive. Clinical course varies from trivial and self-limiting to extensive and refractory. Because simple problems should have simple solutions, it is reasonable to expect that the majority of patients will be managed by office methods.

Soaking with 5% acetic acid will usually produce prominent acetowhitening of skin that had appeared normal to naked eye examination. In women without obvious condylomas, the true clinical significance of acetowhite changes and vestibular micropapillae is presently shrouded

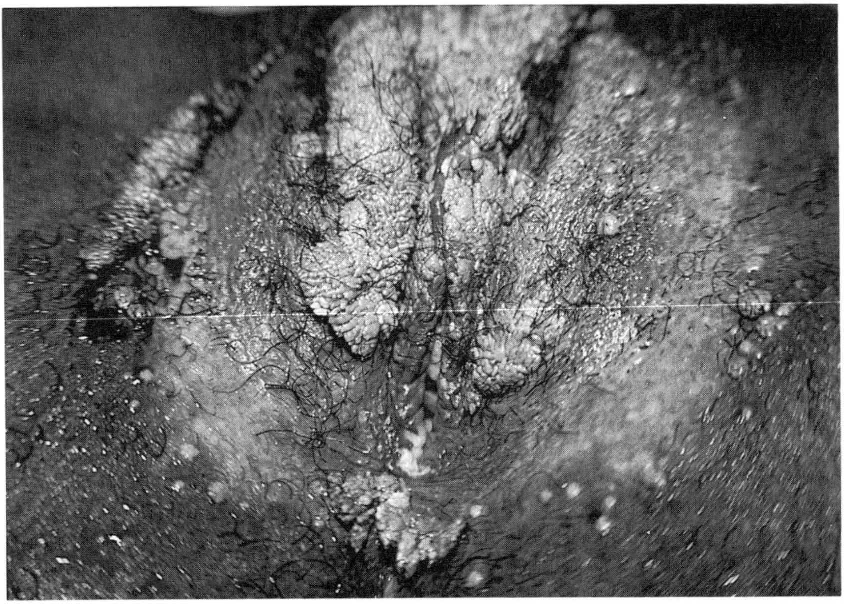

Figure 12.1 A colpophotograph 9 weeks after surgery, showing condylomata formation along the distal margin of extended laser vaporization.

in confusion. Although biopsies from such areas will usually show low-grade koilocytotic atypia, papillomaviral genomes are not generally detectable within these tissues (Reid *et al.*, 1988).

In contrast, Southern blot hybridization of samples taken from acetowhite epithelium at the margins of exophytic condylomas or high-grade dysplasias identified the same type of HPV DNA as found within the principal biopsies (Reid *et al.*, 1987). Ferenczy *et al.* (1985) correlated the risk of treatment failure with the presence of detectable HPV DNA at the lesion margin. Moreover, the Koebner phenomenon (new warts arising at the treatment margins) is a well-recognized manifestation of the proclivity for latent HPV infection to convert to active expression during tissue regeneration (Figure 12.1). Hence, there is little doubt that, in patients who present with classical disease stigmata, these adjacent areas of acetowhite epithelium represent an important viral reservoir.

Experience gained in the treatment of large decorative tattoos on non-genital skin has shown that large expanses of epidermis can be safely removed by a rapid brushing technique, such that healing will occur by outgrowth from the underlying skin appendages rathr than by ingrowth from the wound edges (Reid and Muller, 1980). Clinical judgement suggested that, in difficult cases, the best hope for a resurgence of host immune dominance lay with the simultaneous destruction of both the macroscopic papillomas and the entire field of colposcopically recognizable HPV infection. Hence, in 1983, the author began treating difficult-to-manage patients by extended laser ablation (Reid, 1985a). Over the succeeding 7 years, 160 of the 1000 women referred with HPV-associated vulvar disease were found to have problems severe enough to warrant treatment in the operating room, using a surgical technique that would have a 2–3 week recovery time (Reid *et al.*, 1990).

With optimal equipment in the hands of a skilled surgeon, extended laser ablation offers a highly effective method for destroying any volume of HPV-associated vulvar or vaginal disease under precise depth control. Morbidity is low, and the risk of scarring is negligible. Hence, the aggressive use of the CO_2 laser offers a means of removing large condylomatous aggregations (especially in pregnancy) (Schwartz *et al.*, 1987), of simultaneously debulking the entire viral load and of destroying any foci of dysplastic epithelium to an appropriate depth. The biggest weakness of extended laser ablation is that, literally from the time the laser is switched off, reactivation of the viral reservoir is out of the surgeon's control. Hence, this technique would be well complemented by the availability of an effective adjuvant regimen.

12.2 Principles of effective laser surgery

Laser usage has expanded enormously over the last decade, and there is a widespread belief that surgical success is essentially guaranteed by the technical sophistication of the CO_2 laser. Unhappily, but not unexpectedly, such beliefs are ill-founded. Lasers are like violins: the potential for harmonious melody will rapidly degenerate into a rude cacophony, if placed in the hands of the unskilled. Obtaining a good result with the CO_2 laser has two fundamental requirements: the ability to limit non-specific heat conduction to surrounding tissues, and the ability to control the actual laser beam as it impacts the operative site (Reid and Dorsey, 1990a). In reality, these two objectives depend upon different physical principles (Reid, 1987).

12.2.1 STRATEGIES TO LIMIT LATERAL HEAT CONDUCTION

(a) *Rapid superpulse and chopped wave*

In molecular terms, lateral heat conduction is a relatively slow event. For example, it takes about 600 μs to heat dermis (a collagen matrix, suspended within an aqueous solution) to the critical temperature (65°C) for thermal denaturation. Hence, if laser energy is supplied in pulses that are of shorter duration than this thermal relaxation time, the zone of coagulation at the crater base can be restricted to 70 μm or less. In contrast, if pulse duration is allowed to equal or exceed the thermal relaxation time of the target tissue, then the zone of coagulation necrosis will increase dramatically (e.g. 170 μm for a 2 ms pulse, 750 μm for a 1/20 s pulse). To capitalize on this fact, modern lasers are now designed to operate in more sophisticated temporal modes, such as rapid superpulse or chopped wave.

Rapid superpulse is a major advance in laser technology and has two important features. First, laser energy is delivered in a series of high energy pulses, each with a peak power some 5–7 times higher than the output attainable from this laser tube, if used in the continuous wave mode (Figure 12.2). Second, by keeping the pulse repetition rate at below 300 pulses per second (normally termed 300 Hz), the surgeon allows enough time for the impact site to cool between pulses (by convection and radiation back into the atmosphere, and through heat dispersed by tissue circulation). Given a superpulsed laser of adequate fluence, emitting pulses shorter than the thermal relaxation time and interspersed by sufficient cooling intervals, thermal damage is a function of the optical properties of the incident energy as defined by Beer's law. That is to say, absorption of the delivered energy occurs at the impact surface, resulting in maximal photovaporization and negligible photocoagulation. Unfortunately, rapid superpulse has one major disadvantage: the choice of a narrow pulse and low pulse frequency will reduce available power by about two-thirds. Such a diminution in power output makes it impractical to treat large volumes of diseased epithelium with this temporal mode. Hence, in practice, the ideal form of superpulse is generally reserved for treating small disease volumes that require maximum precision.

A handy compromise between the high precision of rapid superpulse and the high power output of continuous wave is obtained from the chopped mode, in which the laser tube is electrically pulsed so as to produce broad, flat pulses and a shortened interpulse interval (Figure 12.2). Consider, for example, the electrical pulse of a 120 W laser tube, governed such that the ratio of on:off time (the duty cycle) will never exceed 5:1. When used at the highest duty cycle, maximal output would be 100 W (i.e. 120 × 5/6). In contrast, selecting a 1:9 duty cycle would produce an output of only 12 W (i.e. 120 × 1/10). Because the peak power of each pulse is not amplified (as in the rapid superpulse mode), such an electrically pulsed laser tube will not have a refractory phase. Hence, when a laser is used in the chopped mode, repetition rate can be increased to virtually any frequency. However,

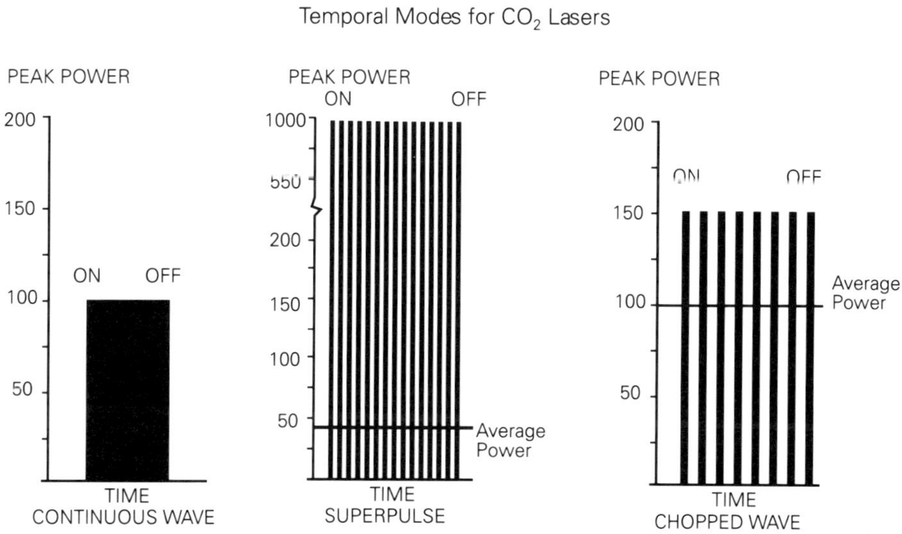

Figure 12.2 The differences between continuous wave, rapid superpulse, and chopped wave. (From Reid, 1987, with permission.)

optimal performance is obtained at a duty cycle of about 1:1 (providing 60 W of power in this instance), while still preserving about half of the interpulse cooling time. If the duty cycle is allowed to exceed 2:1, excessive heat will accumulate at the laser impact site between pulses. Thermal diffusion will occur, and the clinical effect will resemble that of a continuous wave laser.

(b) High power outputs

To minimize the duration of any lateral heat conduction, the necessary energy dose should be delivered in the shortest possible time. Specifically, the faster the rate of energy supply, the shorter the duration of surgery (Figure 12.3). Hence, the use of a high power output will reduce the duration of any heat conduction to the skin appendages. This is crucial to vulvar surgery, because epithelial regeneration from the non-injured appendages is the only mechanism by which satisfactory healing will occur. Surgeons who do extensive vulvar laser surgery at low powers (less than 40 W of continuous wave) are in great danger of producing a third-degree burn (Reid and Dorsey, 1990a).

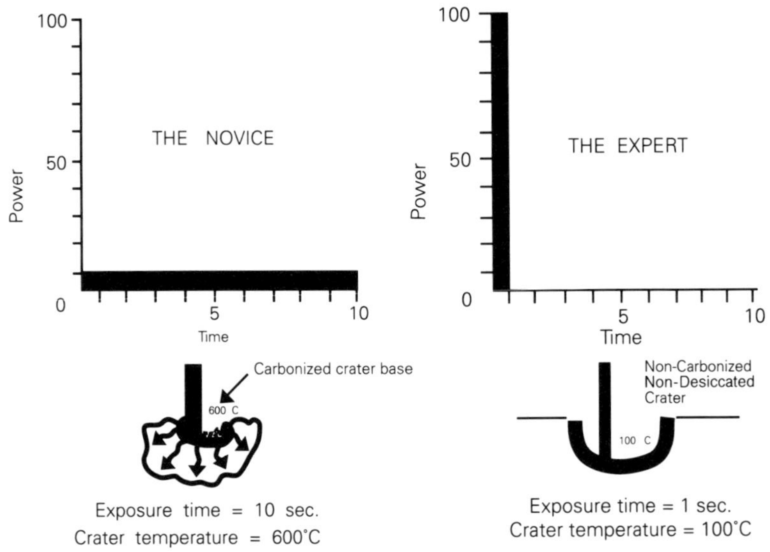

Figure 12.3 Diagram showing how novice laser surgeons erode the potential advantages of the CO_2 laser through the use of slow rates of energy delivery, resulting in both prolonged durations of lateral heat conduction and higher crater temperatures. Even used with average skill (meaning power densities high enough to avoid carbonization of the crater base), failure to maximize energy delivery rates results in more thermal conduction than desired. Only the expert, using maximal rates of energy delivery, is successful in minimizing thermal injury to adjacent tissues. (From Reid, 1986, with permission.)

(c) Maintaining average power density above carbonization levels

Irrespective of power settings and temporal mode, average power density within the focal spot must be kept above carbonization levels (750 W/cm^2). Tissues irradiated at relatively low rates of irradiance (power density) tend to desiccate before the threshold for actual photovaporization is reached. Such desiccation produces areas of anhydrous protein, which will carbonize, just as witnessed in the barbecuing of a steak. Continued irradiance of a carbonized impact surface will raise crater temperatures from 100°C to more than 600°C, thereby increasing the conduction gradient (Reid and Dorsey, 1990a).

Aside from causing excessive thermal damage, such slow rates of vaporization can cause steam formation within underlying blood vessels, thereby aerosolizing viable tissue fragments into the laser plume (the 'popcorn effect'). Hence, in the long run, one might anticipate that evolutionary selection will eventually eradicate poor laser surgeons.

12.2.2 STRATEGIES TO AID SURGICAL CONTROL

Surgeons must not try to control a laser by simply turning the power output down to a lower setting, because such low power outputs and low power densities will cause excessive thermal damage to adjacent tissues (Reid and Dorsey, 1990a). Moreover, turning down the laser output is a relatively ineffective strategy. Instead, the surgeon must control the physical variables that determine tissue interaction within the focal spot. Fortunately, these control strategies are as easy to apply to high powered beams, as to low powered emissions.

(a) Choice of a comfortable power density

Surgeons must not confuse power output and power density. *Power output* refers to the wattage generated within the laser tube and emitted as a 'raw beam' (i.e. power output is a quality-related variable, but has little effect on beam control). In contrast, *power density* (or 'irradiance') refers to the average power within the focused beam, and is therefore primarily a surgical control strategy. Surgeons must keep power density greater than 750 W/cm^2 (the level needed to avoid undue carbonization). Within the range of irradiance levels that are surgically practicable, small changes in average power density will have very little effect on the degree of non-specific thermal injury in the adjacent tissues. Rather, heat avoidance depends upon pulse duration and rate of energy delivery (Reid *et al.*, 1990).

In contrast, speed of vaporization (and hence the speed at which the joystick or handpiece must be moved) is a function of effective power within the focal spot, but is essentially independent of power output within the 'raw beam'. Hence, surgical control depends upon an appropriate titration of spot size against power output, so as to produce a power density to suit the operating speed of the individual surgeon. The author typically uses a power density of about 1500 W/cm^2. As explained under the next principle, power density is adjusted by turning the microslad to a comfortable point of defocus (Reid and Dorsey, 1990a). This point would have a spot diameter of about 1.7 mm for a 40 W beam and about 2.7 mm at 100 W of power output.

(b) Adjusting beam geometry to produce a crater of an appropriate shape

Because of the emphasis placed upon the concept of average power density, there is a tendency to think of a given irradiance level as being widely representative of energy intensity throughout the impact crater. In reality, energy intensity changes markedly from point to point within the focal spot, depending upon the degree of focus/defocus. Since crater shape mirrors the intensity profile of the incident energy,

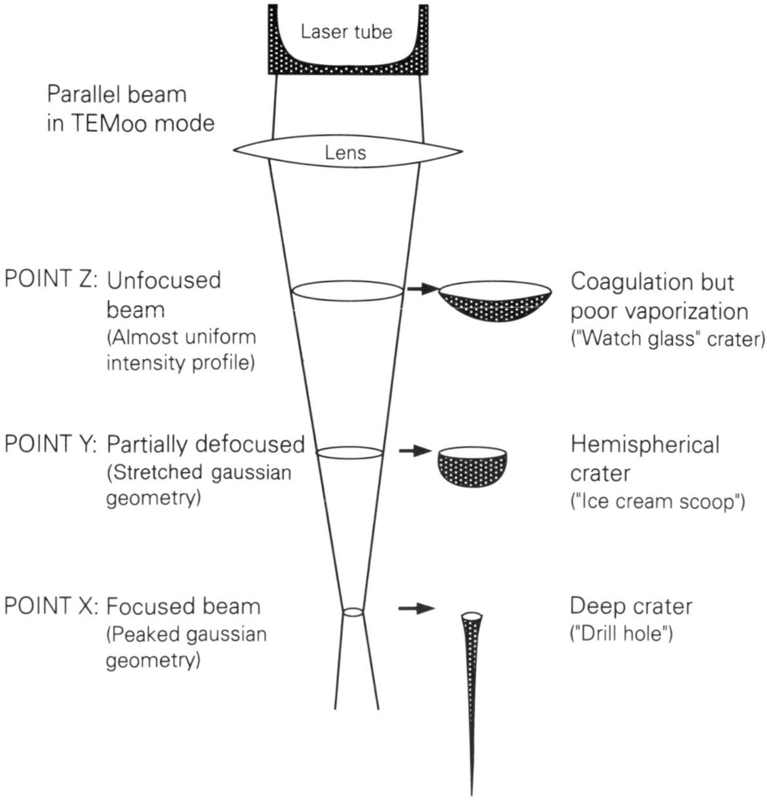

(a)

Figure 12.4 (a) The effect of defocusing on beam geometry. Whereas incisions are best made with a tightly focused beam (point X), surface ablation should always be done at a point of partial defocus (point Y). Fully defocused beams cause extensive char, with negligible penetration (point Z), and therefore have no surgical applications. (Redrawn from Reid *et al.*, 1985.) (b) A modern microslad (the device that couples the articulated arm to the operating microscope, to allow the surgeon to produce progressively greater degrees of laser beam defocus).

this concept of beam geometry is the most important, but also the most neglected aspect of surgical control.

For a laser operating in the Gaussian spatial mode, a sharply focused beam will have a narrow spot diameter and a high amplitude, producing an impact crater like a drill hole (Figure 12.4a). Enlarging spot diameter by partially defocusing the beam will reduce the central amplitude, thereby 'flattening' the geometric shape of the intensity profile. By trial and error, the surgeon can progressively defocus the beam until a point is found at which the impact crater becomes approximately

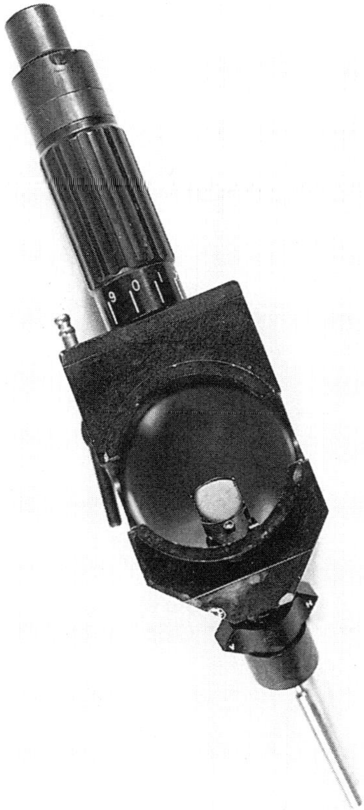

(b)

Figure 12.4 *cont'd*

hemispheric. Hence, beam geometry must be chosen to suit specific surgical objectives, incisions being performed with sharply focused beams and ablations with partially defocused spots. Such fine control over beam geometry depends upon the availability of a modern microslad (a device which allows incremental defocus of the laser beam without disrupting the visual focus of the operating microscope) (Figure 12.4b). Unfortunately, any laser that is not equipped with such a microslad is completely unsuitable for shallow photovaporization of vulvar disease.

(c) Shuttered pulsing techniques

In delicate surgical situations, it is especially hazardous to turn the power down, because the increased thermal damage attending slow rates of energy delivery and low irradiance levels will nullify any

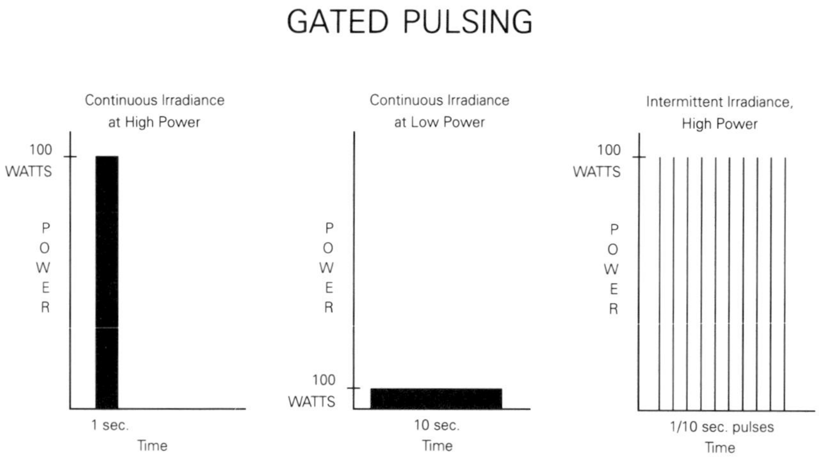

Figure 12.5 The value of intermittent pulses as a means of maintaining surgical control in delicate situations. (a) 100 J delivered by irradiating with 100 W for 1 s satisfies the requirement of rapid energy delivery, but may be hard to control. (b) 100 J delivered as 10 W for 10 s will cause too much conduction burn. (c) 100 J delivered by 10 gated pulses of a 100 W beam, each pulse lasing about 1/10 s, satisfies both requirements (rapid energy delivery and easy control). (From Reid, 1987, with permission.)

potential advantage provided by the laser. Instead, optimal laser setting should be retained, and the beam should be delivered in a series of 1/10 or 1/20 s bursts (either by setting a mechanical timer on the laser console or by adroit control of the foot pedal) (Figure 12.5). This strategy allows ample surgical reaction time between each burst, thereby facilitating the use of high power outputs and high power densities for even the most intricate part of the operation.

12.2.3 SURGICAL STRATEGIES ESSENTIAL TO LASER USAGE

As in other forms of surgery, good results with the laser depend upon both sound theoretic principles and skilled operative technique. Besides selecting optimal physical parameters for each operation, the surgeon must also employ specific surgical strategies that will allow dexterous beam delivery, minimize heat injury to adjacent tissues, ensure haemostasis, facilitate exposure, delineate treatment margins, and confine the depth of thermal denaturation to the desired level. The application of these principles to CO_2 laser surgery within the lower genital tract is fully discussed in much more detailed reviews by Reid (1987) and Reid and Dorsey (1990a). This chapter will discuss only the techniques of depth control.

12.3 Depth control during vulvar laser surgery

Based upon measurements of the average depth of the cervical crypts, most gynaecologists destroy the transformation zone to a depth of 7 mm. The cylindrical nature of the resulting defect and the relatively large dimensions of the intended crater make it quite easy to control the depth of cervical ablation by actual measurement. Satisfactory healing of vulvar wounds depends upon the preservation of the skin appendages, a task that is too delicate to trust to crude measurement. Instead, the surgeon must learn to control depth according to the visual characteristics at the sites of impact.

From the surgical viewpoint, tissue destruction occurs through two distinct mechanisms: immediate photovaporization and delayed coagulation necrosis. The depth of the photovaporization crater is controlled by hand–eye co-ordination. In contrast, the thickness of the zone of coagulation necrosis is quite variable, depending upon laser settings. Surgeons who use suboptimal settings are using the laser as a thermal (rather than an optical) instrument (Walsh *et al.*, 1986). Much of the normal appearing tissue on the wound surface will have suffered coagulation necrosis, and will separate as an eschar after activation of the host inflammatory response. That is to say, if surgery is done with low powered continuous wave, any structures visible within the crater base are already thermally denatured, and will be sloughed off by the succeeding week. In contrast, with optimal laser settings, the extent of laser destruction conforms to optical (rather than thermal) principles. Under these circumstances, crater depth will now conform closely to the actual depth of destruction (Walsh *et al.*, 1986).

Hence, the art of expert CO_2 laser surgery is to ensure that visual appearances correspond to the intended depth of penetration. Surgical orientation is preserved by continuously wiping away the surface char, depth of destruction being inferred from anatomic landmarks in the crater base (Reid *et al.*, 1985). By means of this technique, four characteristic surgical planes are identifiable (Table 12.1) (Reid, 1985b).

12.3.1 THE FIRST SURGICAL PLANE

Destruction to the first plane removes only the surface epithelium, to the level of the basement membrane. This plane is reached by limiting

Table 12.1 Summary of the salient features of the three principal surgical planes

Surgical plane		
First	*Second*	*Third*
Surface epithelium	Dermal papillae	Pilosebaceous ducts
Proliferating layer of epidermis	Superficial papillary dermis	Upper reticular dermis
Basement membrane	Deep papillary	Midreticular
Rapid and cosmetic	Rapid and cosmetic	Slower but usually cosmetic
Opalescent epidermis debris (shiny pink after wiping)	Yellowish and non-reflectant (chamois cloth)	Stark white with arcuate vessels and fibrous 'grain'

Modified from Reid (1985b), with permission.

the penetration of the laser crater to the prickle cell layer, and is accomplished by rapid oscillation of the micromanipulator. When done correctly, the helium–neon spot will describe a roughly parallel series of lines, each pass of the beam revealing bubbles of silver opalescence beneath the charred surface squames (Figure 12.6a). This manoeuvre should be accompanied by a distinctive crackling sound, due to the explosion of the individual epithelial cells. Inadvertent penetration of the basement membrane is signalled by the loss of these two characteristic signs.

Lasing to the prickle cell layer shears the basal cells from the basement membrane, thereby producing a plane of cleavage. These detached basal cells are easily removed by wiping with moistened gauze, thus exposing the smooth, intact surface of the papillary dermis (Figure 12.6b). With optimal techniques, such wounds heal completely within 6–7 days. Cosmetic appearances and functional qualities of the healed wound are entirely indistinguishable from normal vulvar skin.

12.3.2 THE SECOND SURGICAL PLANE

Destruction to the second surgical plane will also remove the papillary dermis (the loose network of fine collagen and elastin fibres lying between the dermal papillae). This plane is reached by a similar set of rapid oscillations, moving the beam so quickly that the laser scorches (rather than craters) the exposed corium. When done correctly, the scorched surface should show a finely roughened contour and a yel-

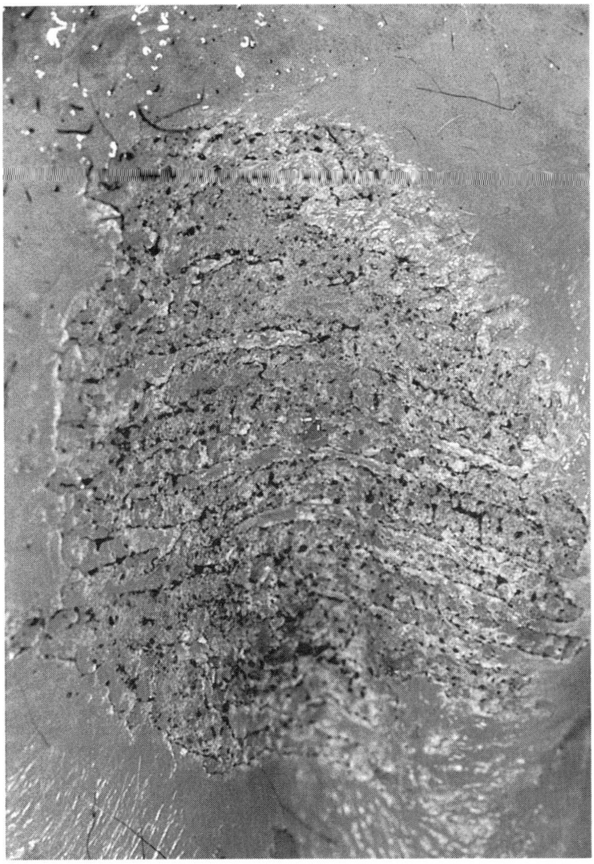

(a)

Figure 12.6 (a) The first surgical plane. (a) A view through the operating microscope after initial 'brushing' with the laser. Beneath the charred remnants of the surface squames can be seen the refractile remnants of plump keratinocytes within the proliferating zone of the epidermis. (b) The first plane, after wiping. The underlying dermal papillae are now exposed, appearing as shiny pink 'bumps'. (From Reid *et al.*, 1987, with permission.)

lowish colour, somewhat reminiscent of a chamois cloth (Figure 12.7a). This clinical appearance indicates that the zone of coagulation necrosis will lie within the papillary dermis, with negligible thermal injury to the underlying reticular dermis (Figure 12.7b). The second plane is the preferred level of ablation for extensive condylomas. Such wounds heal almost as rapidly as destruction to the first plane, yielding an end result that is also indistinguishable from normal skin.

(b) 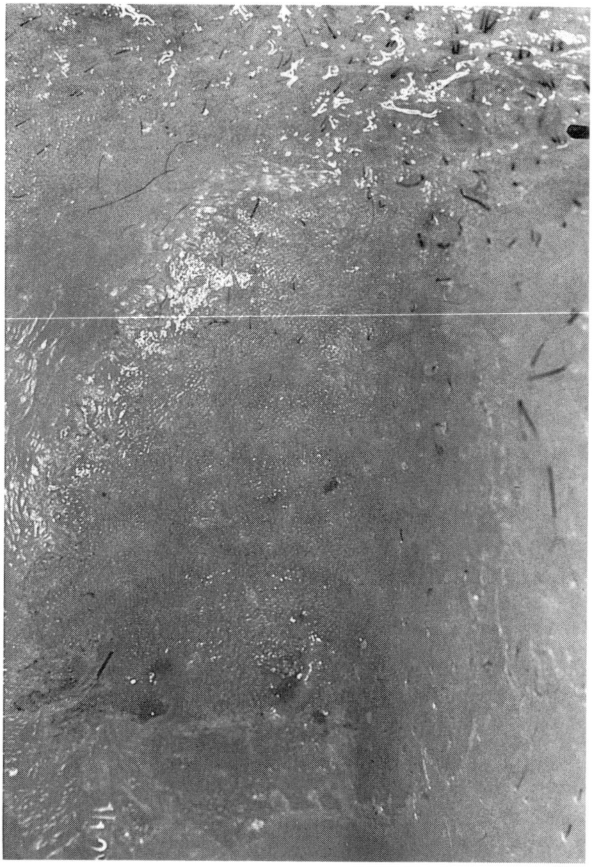

Figure 12.6 *cont.*

12.3.3 THE THIRD SURGICAL PLANE

Vulvar intra-epithelial neoplasia often extends into the pilosebaceous ducts (Figure 12.8a). Involvement is generally limited to the superficial portions of the ducts, making laser ablation to the mid-reticular level (the third surgical plane) an ideal treatment in most instances. Nonetheless, intended depth of destruction should be individualized by examining representative histologic sections. Foci of deep pilar extension are rare; however, any areas of deep pilar extension must be managed by surgical excision, reserving the laser for the ablation of the adjoining superficial disease.

Destruction of the third surgical plane removes the epidermis, the upper portions of the pilosebaceous ducts, and a part of the reticular dermis. Ablation to the mid-reticular layer uncovers coarse collagen

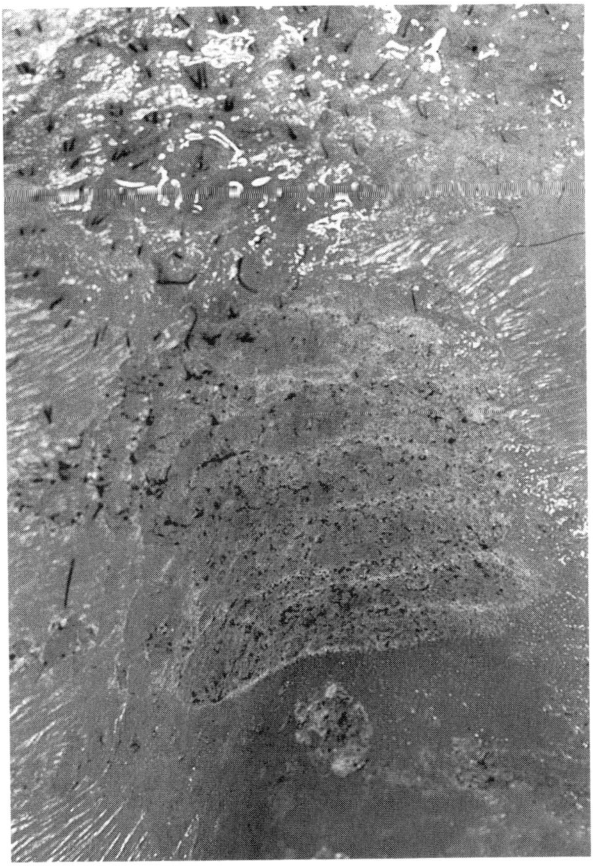

(a)

Figure 12.7 The second surgical plane. (a) In the middle of this photograph, the exposed papillary dermis has been gently released, sufficient to scorch (but not cut) the dermal surface, being seen as a yellow, chamois-like change. Above, there is an area of penetration to the third plane. Below, we can still see the intact dermal papillae of the first plane. (b) The papillary dermis shows coagulation necrosis (top), but the reticular dermis is unaffected (bottom). (From Reid *et al.*, 1987.)

bundles that can be seen through the operating microscope as grey–white fibres resembling water-logged cotton threads (Figure 12.8b). Wiping away the surface char will then reveal a pattern of starkly white collagen plates, interspersed by a horizontally orientated network of deep dermal vessels (Figure 12.8c).

The third plane is reached by lasing the exposed corium with slow, deliberate movements of the beam. The speed of the cut is co-ordinated to the visual recognition of collagen bundles within the

(b)

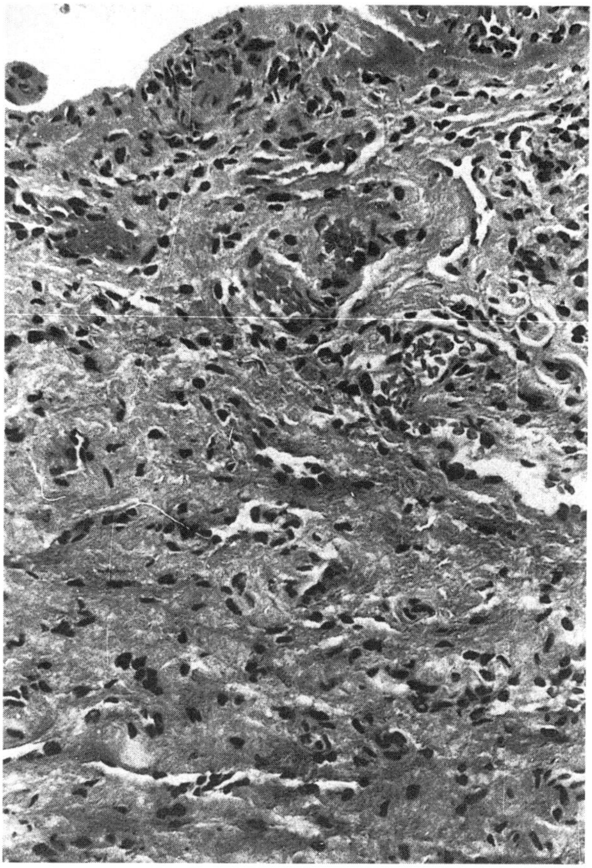

Figure 12.7 *cont.*

crater base. Moving the beam too rapidly will not expose these fibres, and moving the beam too slowly will uncover skin appendages within the deep reticular dermis.

Such hair follicles and sweat glands are readily visible through the operating microscope, being seen as tiny refractile granules that resemble grains of sand. The rationale for limiting destruction to the third surgical plane is to allow the epithelium to regenerate from the keratinocytes within these skin appendages. Exposing the actual hair follicles within the crater base signals that a third-degree burn will be created in this area. Hence, the third surgical plane represents the deepest level from which optimal healing will occur.

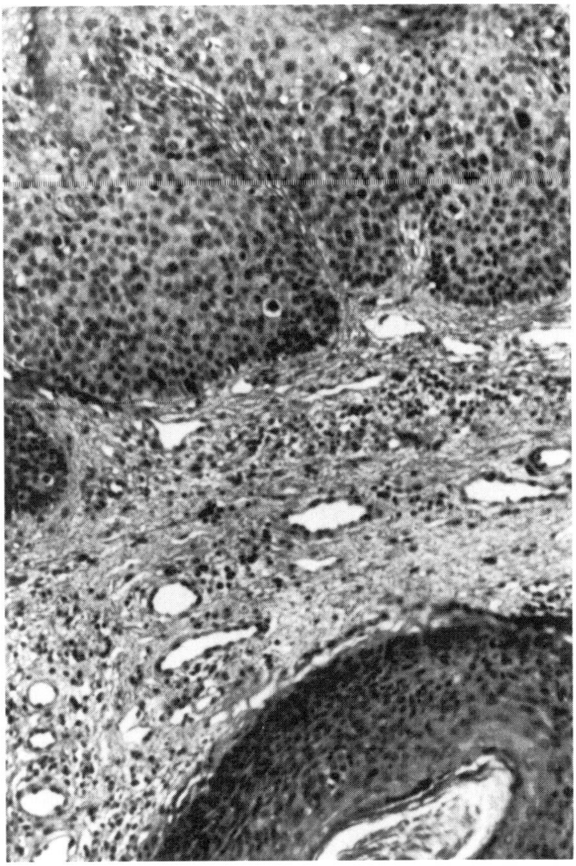

(a)

Figure 12.8 (a) Extension of VIN 3 into the upper half of a pilosebaceous duct. (b) The third surgical plane. A slower, more deliberate movement of the laser beam has vaporized the upper half of the dermis, revealing a vertical pattern of fibres (the coarse collagen bundles of the reticular dermis). (c) The third surgical plane. The arcuate blood vessels of the basal dermis seen against the background of starkly white collagen plates.

12.4 The role of extended laser ablation

Despite the unique physical properties of the CO_2 laser, using such a complex and expensive instrument for the management of the vast majority of patients with HPV-associated vulvar disease is clearly unnecessary. Rather, aggressiveness of treatment must be counterbalanced against the degree of disease expression in the individual

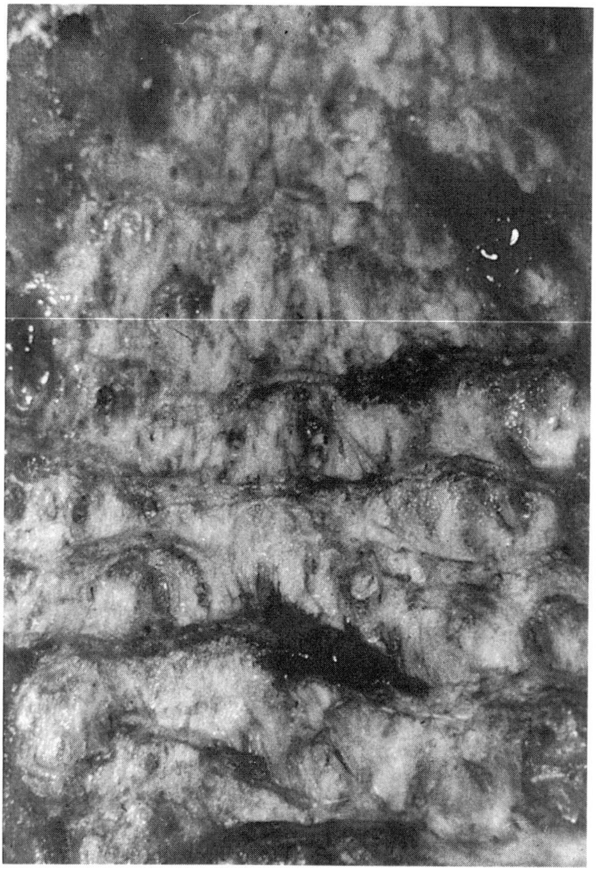

(b)

Figure 12.8 *cont.*

patient. As many as 20% of vulvar condylomas will undergo spontaneous regression, and the great majority of the remainder are easily controlled by office methods. Hence, operative intervention should be limited to specific indications.

12.4.1 INDICATIONS FOR EXTENDED LASER ABLATION

(a) Very extensive condyloma formation

In patients with coalescent lesions occupying 30% of the vulvar surface, the concept of 'spot welding' becomes self-defeating. Under these circumstances, superficial photovaporization of a wider area is preferable to deep destruction of the isolated condylomas. Hence, when confronted with a very large disease volume, the preferred tactic is to

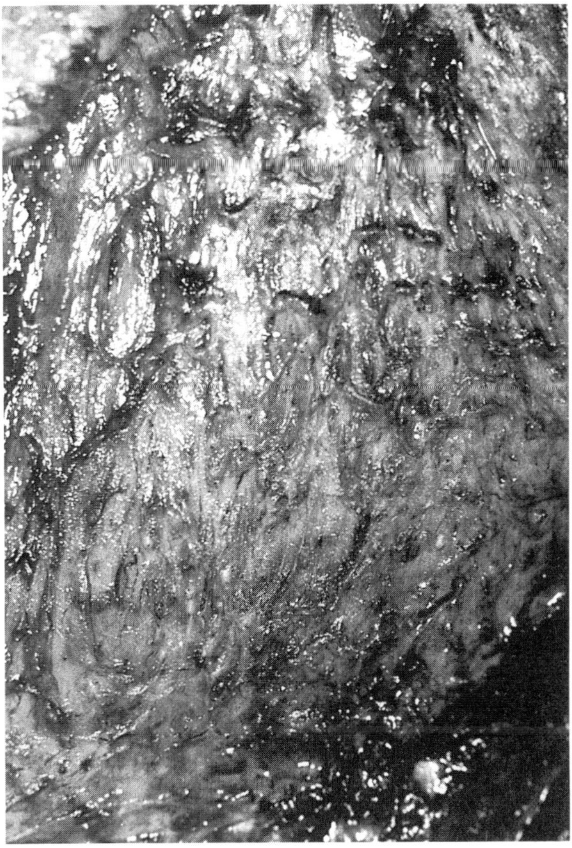

(c)

Figure 12.8 *cont.*

remove the entire field of colposcopically abnormal epithelium, rather than to 'spot weld' to the point of absurdity.

(b) Refractory benign condylomas

Most individuals will mount an effective immune response against continued active expression of any HPV infection, generally within the first 9 months of the initial papilloma formation (Reid, 1989b). Hence, the phase of active growth is counterbalanced by a phase of host containment. However, patients who continue to form new condylomas for 10 months or longer represent an unfavourable subset of the population (Duus *et al.*, 1985). Although comprised of basically healthy women with overtly normal B- and T-cell function, these patients are behaving clinically as though anergic to continued HPV expression.

Whether such suboptimal host defense reflects a failure of immune recognition, the presence of viral-blocking antibodies or some other immune compromise is presently unknown. However, experience has shown that eradication of the 'viral load' within the adjacent field of subclinical papillomavirus infection will be followed by a higher primary success rate than just the repeated destruction of visible papillomas.

(c) Vulvar intra-epithelial neoplasia, grades 2 and 3

The modal age of vulvar intra-epithelial neoplasia (VIN) has fallen by approximately four decades since the Second World War. In the cohorts of women born during the 'baby boom' of the 1940s and 1950s, vulvar neoplasia tends to be multifocal, with a pronounced proclivity to serial recurrence. Hence, it is rational to destroy all visible areas of active viral expression at the time of initial therapy for VIN 2–3. In my experience, this philosophy has generally forestalled the pattern of multifocal recurrence over successive years (Reid, 1989b).

12.4.2 POST-OPERATIVE CARE

To prevent early post-operative pain, the treated areas are infiltrated with 0.25% bupivacaine in 1:100 000 adrenalin. Following the empiric observation that urinary diversion will prevent most of the anticipated post-operative discomfort, patients who require large areas of ablation within the vestibule are offered a suprapubic catheter. Such patients wear a leg bag for 1–2 weeks, malodour being prevented by the daily instillation of 1 oz of white vinegar into the collecting bag. Safeguards against urinary infection include the prescription of prophylactic antibiotics and the daily cleansing of the collection system with household detergents. The catheter is removed at an office visit, when healing is well advanced.

Except in pregnant patients, treatments are performed as out-patient operations. Before discharge, patients must also receive a prescription for a codeine or oxycodone narcotic, a complete set of post-operative instructions, a demonstration of how to care for the catheter and an appointment for office follow-up in 1 week.

The most important part of the post-operative nursing regimen is to apply silver sulphadiazine or nitrofurazone cream, as prophylaxis against labial conglutination. To prevent superinfection, the previous application of cream must be washed off with a Sitz bath, at least three times per day. Except for prophylaxis against urinary infection, post-operative antibiotic therapy is not helpful. However, pre-operative reduction of the vaginal flora by means of a course of vaginal suppositories (oxytetracycline 100 mg bid, clindamycin 200 mg in 2 g of cocoa butter q.h.s. or metronidazole 2 g in cocoa butter q.h.s.) will help safeguard against post-operative infection.

Patients must be seen weekly for 3 weeks, to correct any early coaptation of adjacent raw surfaces. Healing should be virtually complete within 7–14 days. Thereafter, women with refractory condylomas should return every 2–4 weeks for the next 3 months, so that any focal recurrences can be controlled by caustic agents. Because women with vulvar neoplasia or papillomaviral infections are at high risk for developing squamous neoplasia at other sites within the genital tract, surveillance by annual Papanicolaou smears is mandatory (Reid, 1989b).

12.4.3 RESULTS OF EXTENDED LASER ABLATION

Of 160 patients, selected from 1000 consecutive referrals for HPV-associated vulvar disease, 107 (67%) were controlled by a single laser ablation, and another 43 (27%) were controlled by either repeating this surgery or the use of therapeutic levels of topical 5-fluorouracil as soon as recurrence appeared inevitable (Figure 12.9a). Treatment of the remaining 10 (6%) women required deep laser destruction with skin grafting (prior to 1986), or the use of adjuvant alpha interferon (after 1986). Even so, three patients (2%) have never achieved lasting clinical remission (Reid *et al.*, 1990).

Kaplan–Meier cumulative survival analysis shows that recurrences continued for up to 1½ years (Figure 12.9b). Thereafter, the tail of the survival curve becomes quite flat, indicating that these patients are in stable clinical control. It is emphasized that these results refer to long-term freedom from clinical recurrence. In our opinion, the question of whether latent HPV DNA remains at the treatment site is of no practical relevance. Our primary control rate of 67% refers to both the strength and weakness of the CO_2 laser. The strength is that, used skilfully, the laser can remove any volume of diseased tissue under fine control, with the assurance of rapid healing without scarring. However, the weakness is that the laser cannot prevent reactivation of the latent viral reservoir within surrounding areas of surface skin, and perhaps within the skin appendages themselves. Hence, the availability of an effective adjuvant would be a natural complement.

12.5 Adjuvant regimens

12.5.1 NON-CYTOTOXIC DOSES OF 5-FLUOROURACIL

Although a 5- to 10-day course of topical 5-fluorouracil (5-FU) will slough cutaneous lesions, such high dose regimens have been abandoned because they are inefficient, poorly controllable, and extremely

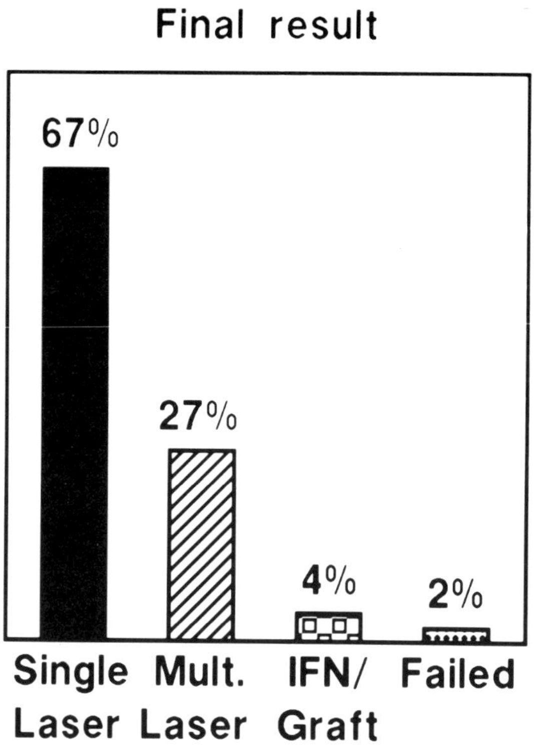

(a)

Figure 12.9 (a) A bar chart showing final outcome following 204 extended laser ablations among 160 women with extensive, refractory or neoplastic vulvar disease. Two-thirds (67%) were controlled by a single laser procedure. Among the one-third of patients in whom the initial laser surgery failed, the majority (27%) were controlled either by a subsequent extended ablation (the strategy prior to 1986), or by pushing topical 5-FU to the limits of patient tolerance (the strategy after 1986). Of the 6% of patients who failed repeated superficial laser ablation, 4% were eventually controlled by deep laser ablation and skin grafting (prior to 1986), or by high dose systemic alpha interferon (after 1986). Three patients (2%) have failed all therapies to this point. (From Reid *et al.*, 1990, with permission.) (b) A Kaplan–Meier survival curve, showing the curability of clinical control obtained by the initial laser ablation in these 160 women. Fifty per cent of failures occurred within 3 months and 95% within 18 months. The lower curve represents just the patients who had no significant recurrences following their first surgery ('immediate successes'), while the upper curve ('eventual successes') represents both immediate successes plus those 'rescued' from a repeat laser ablation by various office therapies. These initial failures were recycled for repeat laser ablation, resulting in the eventual control of all but three women. (From Reid *et al.*, 1990, with permission.)

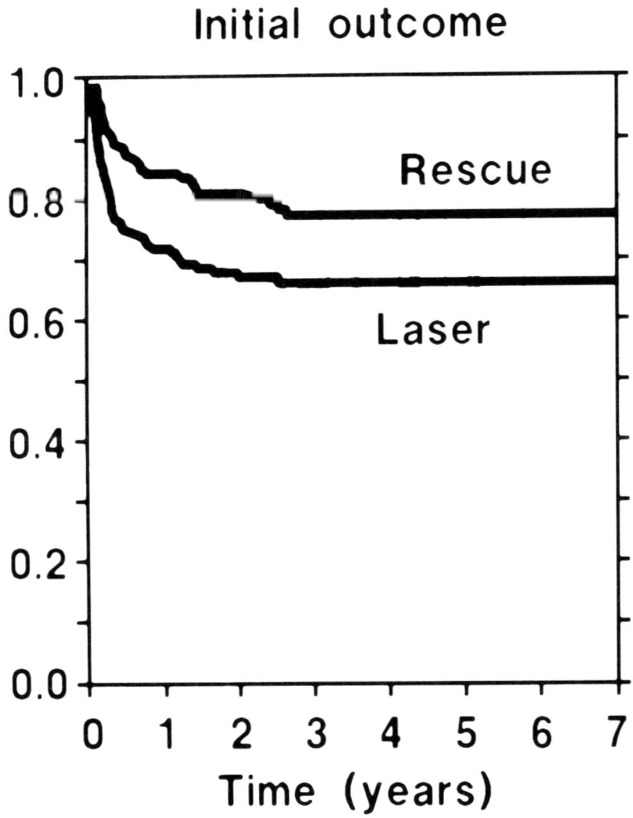

(b)

Figure 12.9 *cont'd*

painful. In contrast, Sillman and Sedlis (1987) have shown that, in patients with renal allografts or other immune deficiencies, the use of lifelong low dose 5-FU is a prerequisite to disease control. Krebs (1986) extended this concept to the treatment of immunologically competent women, reporting improved success (87 vs 62%) in the group randomized to use bi-weekly topical 5-FU for 6 months. However, among the 160 women treated by extended laser ablation, adjuvant once-weekly 5-FU was only helpful among 76 women with two or more adverse prognostic factors (Reid *et al.*, 1990).

12.5.2 THE ROLE OF INTERFERON THERAPY

Interferons are a group of immunomodulatory proteins, produced by all mammalian species, which possess antiviral and antiproliferative properties. Alpha and gamma interferons both have documented effect against HPV infection (Gall, Hughes, and Trofatter, 1985; Kirby *et al.*,

1988). However, even when used in high doses by intramuscular injection, systemic interferons have proven to be disappointing primary therapies for significant HPV infections.

In particular, the recently advocated regimen of intralesional injections appears to offer little to the practical gynaecologist (Eron et al., 1986). Intralesional injections require two or three office visits per week over a several week course, produce substantial pain at the injection sites, and can only be expected to clear the lesions that are actually infiltrated (Friedman-Kien *et al.*, 1988). Even for patients with only three to five warts (the maximum which can be injected in a course), such trivial disease should be readily amenable to simpler therapy.

In contrast, alpha interferon used in a low dose adjuvant regimen significantly reduced the recurrence rate within an open label, randomized study (Reid *et al.*, submitted). Although these results are promising, two or more large-scale, placebo-controlled, multicentric studies will be needed before this regimen can be licensed for routine clinical use.

12.6 Conclusion

The modern gynaecologist is confronted by a burgeoning epidemic of human HPV-associated vulvar diseases. Estimating the true extent of this epidemic is paradoxical. On the one hand, HPV infections are seen as sexually transmitted pathogens, to which only a minority of the population is ever exposed. On the other hand, there is increasing evidence that viral exposure may approach ubiquitous proportions within the population. Whatever the case, it is clear that most HPV-exposed individuals do not progress to papilloma formation.

Before deciding to treat, clinicians must first weigh the evidence as to whether the patient has bona fide disease. Treatment is indicated only in the presence of active viral expression characterized by benign condyloma at one end of the scale, and premalignancy or invasive cancer at the other end. In contrast, chronic latent HPV infections should simply be followed.

For vaginal, vulvar and anal lesions, one should try to use the simplest methods possible; namely, chemical destruction with 85% trichloracetic acid, or physical destruction by electrocautery, cryosurgery or focal photovaporization. However, in problematic patients, attempting to control the disease by destruction of just the individual condylomas will push the strategy of 'spot welding' to the point of absurdity. In the face of such a large disease volume, removing the entire field of HPV-infected epithelium (both clinically apparent and subclinical) to a shallow depth will produce superior results. Done skilfully, extended laser ablation will produce no more morbidity than the use of this instrument as an extensive 'spot welder', since healing occurs from the unaffected keratinocytes within the underlying skin appendages (rather than by epithelial ingrowth from the wound edges).

References

Duus, B. R., Philipsen, T., Christensen, J. D., Lunduam, F. and Sondergaard, J. (1985), Refractory condyloma acuminata: a controlled clinical trial of carbon dioxide laser versus conventional surgical treatment. *Genitourin. Med.*, **61**, 59–61.

Eron, L., Judson, D., Tucker, J., Prawer, S., Mills, J., Murphy, K., Hickey, M., Rogers, M., Flannigan, S., Hien, N., Katz, H. I., Goldman, S., Gottlieb, A., Adams, K., Burton, P., Tanner, D., Taylor, E. and Peets, E. (1986), Interferon therapy for condylomata acuminata. *N. Engl. J. Med.*, **315**, 1059–64.

Ferenczy, A., Mitao, M., Nagai, N. *et al.* (1985), Latent papillomavirus and recurring genital wart. *N. Engl. J. Med.*, **313**, 784–8.

Friedman-Kien, A. E., Eron, L. J., Conant, M. *et al.* (1988), Natural interferon alpha for transmission of condylomata acuminata. *J. Am. Med. Assoc.*, **259**, 533–8.

Gall, S. A., Hughes, C. E. and Trofatter, K. (1985), Interferon for the therapy of condyloma acuminatum. *Am. J. Obstet. Gynecol*, **153**, 157–63.

Kirby, P., Kiviat, N., Beckman, A., Wells, D., Sherwin, S. and Corey, L. (1988), Tolerance and efficacy of recombinant human interferon gamma in the treatment of refractory genital warts. *Am. J. Med.*, **85**, 183–8.

Krebs, H. B. (1986), Prophylactic topical 5 fluorouracil following treatment of human papillomavirus-associated lesions of the vulva and vagina. *Obstet. Gynecol.*, **68**, 837–41.

Lorincz, A. T. and Reid, R. (1989), Association of human papillomavirus with gynecologic cancer. *Curr. Op. Oncol.*, **1**, 123–32.

Reid, R. (1985a), Superficial laser vulvectomy. I. The efficacy of extended superficial ablation for refractory and very extensive condylomas. *Am. J. Obstet. Gynecol.*, **151**, 1047–52.

Reid, R. (1985b), Superficial laser vulvectomy. III. A new surgical technique for appendage-conserving ablation of refractory condylomas and vulvar intraepithelial neoplasia. *Am. J. Obstet. Gynecol.*, **151**, 504–9.

Reid, R. (1987), Physical and surgical principles governing expertise with the carbon dioxide laser. *Obstet. Gynecol. Clinics N. Am.*, **14**, 513–35.

Reid, R. (1989a), Preinvasive disease. In *Practical Gynecologic Oncology* (eds J. S. Berek and N. F. Hacker), Williams & Wilkins, Baltimore, pp. 195–239.

Reid, R. (1989b), Laser therapy of human papillomavirus infections. In *Laser Surgery in Gynecology and Obstetrics* (ed. W. Keye), Yearbook Publishers, Chicago, pp. 46–99.

Reid, R. and Campion, M. J. (1988), The biology and significance of human papilloma-virus infections in the genital tract. *Yale J. Biol. Med.*, **61**, 307–25.

Reid, R. and Dorsey, J. H. (1990), Laser therapy for vulva and vaginal intraepithelial neoplasia. In *Gynecologic Oncology. Fundamental Principles and*

Clinical Practice, 2nd edn (ed. M. Coppleson), Churchill Livingstone, Edinburgh.

Reid, R., Elfont, E. A., Zirkin, R. M. *et al.* (1985), Superficial laser vulvectomy. II. The anatomic and biophysical principles permitting accurate control over the depth of dermal destruction with the carbon dioxide laser. *Am. J. Obstet. Gynecol.*, **152**, 261–71.

Reid, R., Elson, L. and Absten, G. (1986), A practical guide to laser safety. *Colp. Gynecol. Laser Surg.*, **2**, 121–32.

Reid, R., Greenberg, M., Daoud, Y. *et al.* (submitted), Superficial laser vulvectomy. IV. Extended laser vaporization and adjuvant 5 fluorouracil therapy of human papillomavirus associated vulvar diseases. *Am. J. Obstet. Gynecol.*

Reid, R., Greenberg, M. Jenson, A. B. *et al.* (1987), Sexually transmitted papillomaviral infections. I. The anatomic distribution and pathologic grade of neoplastic lesions associated with different viral types. *Am. J. Obstet. Gynecol.*, **156**, 212–22.

Reid, R. and Muller, S. (1980), Tattoo removal by CO_2 laser dermabrasion. *Plast. Reconstr. Surg.*, **65**, 717–28. Reviewed in *Yearbook of Plastic Surgery*.

Schwartz, D. B., Greenberg, M. D., Daoud, Y. and Reid, R. (1987), The management of genital condylomas in pregnant women. *Obstet. Gynecol. Clinics N. Am.*, **14**, 589–599.

Sillman, F. H. and Sedis, A. (1987) Anogenital papillomavirus infection and neoplasia in immunodeficient women. *Obstet. Gynecol. Clin. N. Am.*, **14**, 537–58.

Walsh, J., Morelli, J. and Parrish, J. A. (1986), Laser-tissue interactions and their clinical applications. *Curr. Probl. Dermatol.*, **15**, 94–110.

13 *Laser safety: hazards and precautions*

E. J. KERSHAW and M. J. VAN BOVEN

13.1 Laser safety

The introduction of the laser into medical practice has led to the requirement for a set of rules and regulations to be laid down governing the use of lasers, in order to protect patients and staff from injury (Guidance on the safe use of lasers in medical practice: HMSO, 1984).

The hazards arising from the use of laser energy are a result of the thermal and/or acoustic injury caused by the narrow beam of light. The damage is related to the absorption characteristics of each individual tissue which in turn are affected by the nature of the tissue and its blood supply, and to the form of laser energy imparted to the tissue. The continuous wave lasers tend to produce a thermal injury with resultant protein denaturation, whereas the pulsed beams, which have a much greater peak power, cause damage by acoustic shock waves which result in tissue shearing.

The main danger to the operator, theatre personnel and the patient comes from speculated laser energy reflected off instruments and equipment within the laser controlled area. The main organs that can be damaged are the skin, which suffers premature ageing, increased pigmentation, and pigment darkening, as well as acute thermal injury, and the eye, where macular damage can lead to permanent blindness. Damage to the cornea and anterior chamber may result in corneal burns and cataract formation. The effects of repeated exposure to inadvertent laser energy is cumulative and the injuries are independent of the type of laser used.

13.1.1 HAZARDS AND PRECAUTIONS

The therapeutic advantage that has been created as a result of the use of lasers must be tempered by respect for the risks and hazards incurred by its use. It is imperative that the laser be operated under strictly controlled conditions and that safety should be the watchword.

As the use of laser treatment increases it is advisable that these pieces of equipment be operated by an authorized user of lasers, having undergone specialist training, and that the use of the equipment and its environment be supervised by a qualified laser safety officer. There are no specific educational requirements for qualification as a laser user, but it is accepted that observation followed by supervised hands-on experience with an authorized laser operator on several cases is the minimum experience required.

Because a laser beam is a collimated energy source, the power of which does not diminish appreciably with distance travelled, and because some laser beams (e.g. CO_2) are invisible, it is necessary to prevent accidental entry to the operating theatre or laser controlled area. A warning sign indicating the presence of an active laser should be placed on all doors, and the doors should be lockable from within. A facility for covering all windows should also be available, particularly when using a wavelength not absorbed by glass. All personnel present should be aware of the risks of laser radiation and the precautions necessary to protect themselves and the patient.

Because laser radiation can permanently damage the cornea and/or retina of the eye, all personnel present in the operating theatre should wear protective eyewear, appropriate for the type of laser being used. Generally speaking the filtering glasses should protect against the specific wavelength of the laser in action, and these have coloured lenses, green for Nd-YAG, amber for argon or KTP, and clear for CO_2. The coloured lenses do cause problems for both the surgeon and the anaesthetist but it is important that the particular lens recommended by the manufacturer is adhered to.

The CO_2 laser causes damage to the cornea of the eye resulting in opacification, while the Nd-YAG and KTP lasers focus on the retina and can cause total blindness due to destruction of the macula. It is a consideration that the patient's eyes should also be covered.

A further hazard encountered by surgeons using fibre transmitted lasers down the laparoscope is backscatter. Whilst the CO_2 laser energy is absorbed by the instrument optics, that of the Nd-YAG and the KTP is not, and a special shuttering system is required to protect the surgeon's eyes. The shuttering system should be such that it incorporates a fail-safe device.

13.2 Anaesthetic hazards

Anaesthesia for laser surgery to the airway is an extremely hazardous procedure about which many guidelines have been laid down (Rontal *et al.*, 1986; Anand *et al.*, 1987; Borland and Reilly, 1987; Cork, 1987;

Cohen *et al.*, 1988; Ellis *et al.*, 1988; Keon, 1988; Mayne *et al.*, 1988; Moghissi and Budd, 1988; Schiffman *et al.*, 1988; Sosis, 1989; Weisberger and Miner, 1988). However, now that the laser is being applied to other surgical disciplines, it is important to consider how its use can affect anaesthetic management of the patient, and how anaesthetic management may facilitate surgery and influence its outcome.

In gynaecology the laser is applied to the patient's lesions via three different routes, the colposcope, the hysteroscope, and the laparoscope. Each of these procedures carries with it risks which are of importance to both the surgeon and the anaesthetist.

13.2.1 COLPOSCOPY

The laser most frequently used for treating lesions of the vulva, vagina, and the cervix is the CO_2 laser. The light from a CO_2 laser has a wavelength of 10.6 μm, in the infra-red spectrum, and is absorbed by water. This absorption, especially by cellular water, causes boiling and disruption of the cell with subsequent vaporization of the tissue. Because of this method of action the temperature of the operative site remains at about 100°C and so thermal injury to the surrounding tissues is minimal. It is for this reason that the CO_2 laser has become so popular (Wainwright, 1987). However, the CO_2 laser beam is invisible and loses very little power as it is transmitted through the air between the colposcope and the lesion to be treated. It follows that if the laser beam were to be misdirected then anything or any person in its path would sustain an injury.

The CO_2 laser is capable of heating rubber and plastics at a rate of several thousand degrees centigrade per second and can cause instantaneous combustion of anaesthetic gas carrying equipment. This combustion is supported by a mixture of nitrous oxide and oxygen to an even greater extent than 100% O_2 (Leonard *et al.*, 1975; Hirshman *et al.*, 1980; Chilcoat *et al.*, 1983). It is obvious that the use of inflammable anaesthetic agents such as diethyl ether or cyclopropane is absolutely contra-indicated under these circumstances.

The use of the laser to remove vulval lesions has proved to be very painful for patients post-operatively, and we have found that the local application of lignocaine gel is advantageous in the provision of post-operative pain relief (Sutton and Kershaw, personal communication).

13.2.2 HYSTEROSCOPY

It is useful when considering hysteroscopy to differentiate between diagnostic and operative procedures. The major problems that concern the anaesthetist stem from the media used to distend the uterine cavity to enable the operator to see and to manipulate his/her instruments.

13.2.3 DIAGNOSTIC HYSTEROSCOPY

Where hysteroscopy involves no surgical intervention then CO_2 gas may be used as a distending medium and this provides excellent visualization of the uterine cavity. Unfortunately, from our experience both in this country and in Belgium, the risk of gas embolism is high when CO_2 is used during hysteroscopic surgery and so its use is limited to the diagnostic procedure. The mechanism of action of this problem appears to relate to the opening of venous channels in the endometrium whilst gas is being delivered down the endoscope under pressure. The machines designed to supply this gas do so at low pressure, but during surgery the risk is still present.

13.2.4 OPERATIVE HYSTEROSCOPY

When endoscopic laser surgery is performed, there is always a risk of cutting through blood vessels thus allowing intravenous access by the distending medium whether it is gas or fluid. The side effects of fluid entering the circulation are neither so sudden nor so dramatic as with gas but all the various fluids used today have individual side effects on the human body beside the problem of vascular fluid overload.

Several liquid agents are used to separate the uterine walls. The most frequently used are dextran 70 solutions and low viscosity fluids such as dextrose in water or normal saline. The experience of the urologists in endoscopic surgery has led to the introduction of 1.5% glycine solution.

Beside the risk of introducing endometrial tissue into the peritoneal cavity, it was initially thought that an important part of the distending fluid passed through the open Fallopian tubes and collected in the abdominal cavity.

To prevent large amounts of irrigating solution from entering the peritoneal cavity during the procedure, tubal closure was first proposed. It seems that very little fluid is transmitted up the Fallopian tubes during operative hysteroscopic surgery even if the fluid is applied under quite high pressure. Sterilization before the procedure is no longer systematically performed (Goldrath *et al.*, 1981; Loffer, 1987; Lomano, 1988; Loffer, 1988).

The large raw surface of the endometrium is probably the most important factor influencing fluid absorption (Goldrath *et al.*, 1981; Loffer, 1987). Because of the thickness of the endometrial lining, laser hysteroscopic procedures should best be avoided at mid-cycle or in the secretory phase due to excessive endometrial vascularization (Valle 1978). Inducing an artificial menopause by pre-treatment with danazol or gonadotrophin releasing hormone contributes not only to diminishing the uterine volume but also diminishes the endometrial vascularity (Loffer, 1987; Matta *et al.*, 1988).

(a) Dextran solutions

In 1970, Edstrom and Fernstrom successfully utilized a highly viscous dextran solution (32% dextran 70 in dextrose 10%: Hyskon, for uterine distension (Taylor and Cumming, 1979). Dextran is a collective name for a series of polysaccharides with a high degree of dextro-rotation. It is an antigenic sugar product prepared by bacterial synthesis (Isbister *et al.*, 1987). Thirty-two per cent high molecular weight dextran in 10% dextrose is an optically clear mixture with a high refractory index and high viscosity. This electrolyte-free solution is immiscible with blood, non-toxic and biodegradable and it provides excellent optical properties (Valle and Sciarra, 1979). However, comparing dextran 70 with CO_2, Taylor *et al.* (1987) concluded that many of the apparent adhesions and polyps detected during the use of dextran for hysteroscopy were artefacts.

Severe anaphylactic reactions can also occur with its use. A 10-year study in Sweden reported a 0.025% incidence of dextran-induced anaphylactoid reactions (DIAR) for dextran 70 (Ljungstrom, 1983; Berstein *et al.*, 1987). Reactions occurred with as little as 0.5–1.10 ml of dextran. The clinical picture of DIAR ranges from innocuous skin lesions to circulatory shock, sometimes fatal (Ljungstrom, 1983). Fatal DIAR occurred in 0.0004% of patients receiving dextran in the Swedish series. Severe DIAR is thought to be caused by immune complexes formed by dextran-reactive antibodies predominantly of the IgG class (Renck *et al.*, 1983). These antibodies develop by exposure to dextran contaminates of sugar and cross-reactivity with bacteria in dental plaque (Bailey *et al.*, 1967; Ring, 1984; Isbister *et al.*, 1987). The infusion of clinically available dextran (70 or 40) into a predisposed person with a high titre of dextran-reactive antibodies may lead to a release of vaso-active mediators causing the symptoms of anaphylactic shock (Ljungstrom, 1983).

Because of its optical properties dextran is widely used for hysteroscopic diagnosis. Unfortunately, it seems unsuitable for endoscopic laser surgery because it crystallizes around the laser fibre and the hysteroscope (Loffer, 1988).

It has been known for many years that the dextrans have unique effects on the body's clotting system which may cause significant haemostatic failure if excessive amounts are infused (Alexander, 1978). This factor must be considered if more than 1.5 g/kg body weight is used. Beside the possibility of pulmonary oedema due to fluid overload, several cases of non-cardiogenic pulmonary oedema have been reported (Zbella *et al.*, 1985).

(b) Glycine solutions

Glycine solution was introduced in 1948 by Nesbit as an irrigating medium during transurethral resection of the prostate (Nesbit and Gluckman, 1948). It has been used successfully as a distending medium during hysteroscopic laser surgery. It is an electrolyte-free solution and because of its transparency affords good optical conditions even in the presence of bleeding (Casey *et al.*, 1988). From a surgical point of view it does not crystallize on instruments, laser fibres or gloves (Norlen, 1985). Unfortunately it produces haemodilution effects when absorbed in large volumes. These include decreases in serum sodium, albumin and haemoglobin. In addition to this glycine 1.5% produces a reduction in plasma osmolality (Hoekstra, 1983; Osborn *et al.*, 1984; Norlen, 1985; Sinclair *et al.*, 1985).

Glycine is a non-essential aminoacid. It readily crosses the blood–brain barrier where it functions as an inhibitory neurotransmitter. Glycine is metabolized in the body to ammonia, lactate, pyruvate, alanine and serine (Casey *et al.*, 1988). Large infusions of glycine have been shown to cause toxicity in the human being (Doolan *et al.*, 1956). After absorption of large quantities of glycine solution, hypovolaemia and haemodilution with hyponatraemia have been described as the transurethral resection (T.U.R.) syndrome. The signs and symptoms of acute hyponatraemia with water overload in the central nervous system are apprehension, restlessness, headache, nausea, vomiting, confusion, transient blindness, coma, convulsions and paralysis. These are all masked by general anaesthesia and so the cardio-respiratory signs, severe hypertension, cyanosis and increased amplitude of the QRS complex with T-wave inversion on the ECG, are the most important indicators. It has been suggested that hypovolaemia and haemodilution were the only explanations for the T.U.R. syndrome. From recent data, however, the direct toxicity of glycine or its metabolites has been questioned (Fitzpatrick *et al.*, 1981; Ovassapian *et al.*, 1982; Roesh *et al.*, 1983; Bowman *et al.*, 1986; Vila *et al.*, 1987; Casey *et al.*, 1988).

(c) Other solutions

Several other low viscosity fluids may be used to separate the uterine walls. These include 5 or 10% dextrose in water, 0.9% sodium chloride, 5% dextrose in 0.9% sodium chloride and Ringer's lactate solution. One of the main disadvantages of these solutions is that the technique using 5% dextrose in water or saline does not allow for major uterine dissections since bleeding may obscure vision (Guerrero *et al.*, 1972; Sciarra and Valle, 1977; Valle and Sciarra, 1979; Goldrath *et al.*, 1981). Moreover, beside the fluid overload and electrolyte dilution after massive absorption of 5% dextrose, hyperglycaemia has been reported.

It is fashionable to combine laser hysteroscopic surgery with the use of diathermy during selective endometrial ablation. It would be pointless having an electrolyte solution during the application of diathermy as this would cause a dissipation of the current and render it ineffectual.

Liquid absorption should be carefully monitored by measuring the inflow and outflow fluid balance, especially in patients with poor cardiac function, and intravenous fluids should be restricted during the procedure. When significant fluid absorption with an electrolyte-free solution is suspected, post-operative electrolyte monitoring is necessary.

The major surgical problem encountered during operative hysteroscopy is bleeding, and its effect upon the operator's view. There are two ways to overcome this. It is possible to increase the intra-uterine pressure until the bleeding is actively prevented. This is relatively easy to achieve but has a number of disadvantages, including increased fluid absorption and the increased risk of vaso-vagal attack. The other alternative is to increase the flow of fluid through the uterus at low pressure and employ outflow suction via a continuous flow operating hysteroscope.

Our experience with hysteroscopic endometrial ablation has shown that the patients may experience severe pain in the immediate post-operative period. For this reason as well as the fact that peroperative symptoms of water intoxication may be masked by general anaesthesia, regional anaesthesia could be considered as a viable alternative especially if a prolonged procedure is anticipated.

13.2.5 LAPAROSCOPY

Laparoscopic laser surgery is being used with increasing frequency. Because the laser is contained within the optical systems of the surgical equipment until it is aimed at the lesions inside the abdominal cavity, it would appear that the protection of the eyes of theatre personnel is of lesser importance. This is certainly the case with the CO_2 laser which with its long wavelength has by necessity to be transmitted along rigid optical pathways. However, the Nd-YAG laser produces light of a much shorter wavelength which can be transmitted along flexible fibre-optic cables. It is the fragility of these cables and the possibility of damage to or fracture of them that create the necessity, even during laparoscopy, for the eyes of operating department personnel and patients to be protected. In the case of the Nd-YAG laser the eye glasses have green lenses which would render the anaesthetist unable to assess the skin colour of his/her patient. It is, therefore, mandatory that the patient should be connected to a pulse oximeter at all times during the use of this laser in order that peripheral oxygen saturation may be monitored continuously.

Although in some centres it is accepted that during anaesthesia for laparoscopy it is not essential to intubate the trachea and ventilate the patient to prevent hypercapnia or acidosis (Kenefick, 1987), and that by not doing so, the incidence of post-operative side effects is reduced and the speed of recovery is enhanced (Herbert *et al.*, 1983; Kurer *et al.*, 1984, Kenefick, 1987), it is this author's preference to employ intubation and ventilation particularly during laser laparoscopy. Whilst non-laser and out-patient laparoscopy may be of short duration this is certainly not always the case when laser laparoscopy is performed.

There are a number of respiratory physiological problems which are compounded by the use of this technique. During laparoscopy the abdominal cavity is insufflated with CO_2 in order to create a space for the operator to see and operate within. The machines used to provide the CO_2 have automatic pressure and volume-limiting devices to prevent intra-abdominal pressure from rising high enough to embarrass the ventilation of the patient. During laparoscopic laser surgery, due to the action of the laser vaporizing tissue, a considerable amount of 'smoke' is produced which rapidly obscures the surgical field of view. In order to facilitate continuous surgery, it is necessary to evacuate the 'smoke' whilst at the same time maintaining the insufflation of the abdominal cavity with fresh CO_2 gas. This involves a high-flow gas extraction system coupled with a high-flow fresh gas supply. It is apparent that these two should be accurately balanced in order that, on the one hand, the abdominal cavity does not collapse thus preventing surgery, and on the other hand, that the abdomen does not overinflate preventing adequate ventilatory support for the patient.

(a) Physiology

Functional residual capacity (F.R.C.) and closing capacity (C.C.).

The patient undergoing laparoscopy is in a position that would defy the normal laws of respiratory physiology. There are two fundamental measurements of interest to the anaesthetist here. These are the functional residual capacity (F.R.C.) and the closing capacity

Table 13.1 Factors reducing functional residual capacity (F.R.C.)

1. Increasing age
2. Obesity
3. Anaesthesia (general)
4. Abdominal and thoracic surgery
5. Pulmonary interstitial disease
6. Abdominal distension
7. Thoracic injury and distortion
8. Reduced muscle tone
9. Posture – supine
   – Trendelenberg
   – lithotomy

(C.C). The F.R.C. is the volume remaining in the lungs at the end of a normal expiration and the closing capacity is the volume at which airway collapse occurs during expiration. The F.R.C. is determined by the balance between the inward elastic recoil of the lung and the outward pull of the thoracic wall. It is altered by various intrinsic and extrinsic factors. In the normal upright lung the C.C. is a small proportion of the F.R.C. but the F.R.C can be considerably reduced by increasing age, obesity and certain pathological lung conditions which cause a reduction in lung compliance (Table 13.1). Extrinsically, F.R.C. is reduced by the supine position, the Trendelenberg position, the lithotomy position and abdominal distension causing diaphragmatic splinting. All of these conditions may and often do occur during laparoscopy and when compounded by possible overdistension of the abdomen it can be seen that the closing volume may eventually exceed a much reduced F.R.C. with the result being airway collapse and hypoxaemia. This can occur both during anaesthesia and in the recovery period and is made worse by the administration of opioid analgesia (Hanning, 1989).

Ventilation/perfusion ratio.

In the upright lung the flow of blood through the alveolar walls varies from apex to base, being virtually zero at the apex and maximal at the base. It is not surprising that the alveolar volume is greatest at the base, as it is here that the majority of gas exchange occurs. If the situation were to be reversed whereby the apices of the lungs became dependent and received the greater blood supply, then the bases would be relatively starved of de-oxygenated blood from the right ventricle. It has already been shown that the patient in typical laparoscopy position has a relatively immovable diaphragm thus preventing adequate ventilation of the lung bases. Reduced ventilation coupled with reduced perfusion at these bases will result in hypoxaemia.

As a result of these physiological forces it is important to be meticulous in balancing the inflow and outflow of insufflating gas through the laparoscope.

With regard to the scavenging of gas containing vaporized tissue, it has been our experience that the operating department atmosphere rapidly becomes an unpleasant working environment and a special filtration system for the evacuated gas is necessary. In addition to the quality of the atmosphere, there is also the potential hazard of personnel inspiring vaporized tissue which may contain virus particles. The significance of this is as yet unknown.

References

Alexander, B. (1978), Effects of plasma expanders on coagulation and hemostasis: dextran hydroxyethyl starch, and other macromolecules revisited. Blood substitutes and plasma expanders. *Prog. Clin. Biol. Res.*, **19**, 292.

Anand, V. K. *et al.* (1987), Safe anaesthesia for endoscopic laryngeal laser surgery. *Lasers Surg. Med.*, **7** 275–7.

Bailey, G. *et al.* (1967), Dextran-induced anaphylaxis. *J. Am. Med. Assoc.*, **200**, 185–7.

Berstein, R. L. *et al.* (1987), A severe reaction to dextran despite hapten inhibition. *Anesthesiology*, **67**, 567–9.

Borland, L. M. and Reilly, J. S. (1987), Jet ventilation for laser laryngeal surgery in children. Modification of the Saunders jet ventilation technique. *Int. J. Paed. Otorhinolaryngol.*, **14**, 65–71.

Bowman, T. M. *et al.* (1986), Glycine induced ammonia toxicity following transurethral resection of the prostate. *Anesth. Rev.* **XIII**, 39–42.

Casey, W. F. *et al.* (1988), Visual evoked potentials and changes in serum glycine concentration during transurethral resection of the prostate. *Br. J. Anaesth.*, **60**, 525–9.

Cohen, S. R. *et al.* (1988), Anaesthetic management of microlaryngeal laser surgery in children: apnoeic technique anaesthesia. *Laryngoscope*, **98**, 347–8.

Cork, R. C. (1987), Anaesthesia for otolaryngologic surgery involving use of a laser. *Contemp. Anaes. Pract.*, **9**, 127–40.

Chilcoat, R. T. *et al.* (1983), The hazards of nitrous oxide during laser endoscopic surgery. *Anesthesiology*, **59**, 258.

Doolan, P. D. *et al.* (1956) The renal tubular response to amino-acid loading. *J. Clin. Invest.* **35**, 888–96.

Ellis, D. J. *et al.* (1988), Anesthesia for laser resection of a tracheal tumour in a woman pregnant with twins. *Anesthesiology*, **68**, 629–31.

Fitzpatrick, J. M. *et al.* (1981), Hyperoxaliuria following glycine irrigation for transurethral prostatectomy. *Br. J. Urol.*, **53**, 250–2.

Goldrath, H. M. *et al.* (1981), Laser photovaporization of the endometrium for the treatment of menorrhagia. *Am. J. Obstet. Gynecol.*, **140**, 14–19.

Guerrero, R. Q. *et al.* (1972), Tubal catheterization: applications of a new technique. *Am. J. Obstet. Gynecol.*, **114**, 674–8.

Hanning, C. D. (1989), *Anaesthesia*, Vol. 1 (Eds W. S. Nimmo and G. Smith), Blackwell Scientific Publications, pp. 162–90.

Herbert, M. *et al.* (1983), Profile of recovery after general anaesthesia. *Br. Med. J.*, **286**, 1539–42.

Hirshman, C. A. *et al.* (1980), Indirect ignition of the endotracheal tube during carbon dioxide laser surgery. *Arch. Otolaryngol.*, **106**, 639–41.

Hoekstra, P. T. (1983), Transurethral prostatic resection syndrome – a new perspective: encephalopathy with associated hyperammonaemia. *J. Urol.*, **130**, 704–7.

Isbister, J. P. *et al.* (1987), Adverse effects of plasma volume expanders. *Anaesth. Int. Care*, **8**, 145–51.

Kenefick, J. P. (1987), Laparoscopy: Blood gas values and minor sequelae associated with three techniques based on isoflurane. *Br. J. Med. Assoc.*, **59**, 189–94.

Keon, T. P. (1988), Anesthetic considerations for laser surgery. *Int. Anesthesiol. Clin.*, **26**, 50–3.

Kurer, F. L. *et al.* (1984), Gynaecological laparoscopy: Clinical experiences of two anaesthetic techniques. *Br. J. Med. Assoc.*, **56**, 1207–12.

Leonard, P. F. *et al.* (1975), Lower limits of flammability of halothane, enflurane and isoflurane. *Anesth. Analg.*, **54**, 238–40.

Ljungstrom, K. G. (1983a), Prevention of dextran induced anaphylactic reactions by hapten inhibition. *Acta Chir. Scand.*, **149**, 341–8.

Ljungstrom, K. G. (1983b), Prophylaxis of postoperative thromboembolism with dextran 70. *Acta Chir. Scand.*, Suppl. 514.

Ljungstrom, K. G. *et al.* (1983), Adverse reactions to dextran in Sweden 1970–1979. *Acta Chir. Scand.*, **149**, 253–62.

Loffer, F. D. (1987), Hysteroscopic endometrial ablation with the Nd-YAG laser using a nontouch technique. *Obstet. Gynecol.*, **69**, 679–82.

Loffer, F. D. (1988), Laser ablation of the endometrium. *Obstet. Gynecol. Clin. N. Am.*, **15**, 82.

Lomano, J. (1988), Dragging technique versus blanching technique for endometrial ablation with the Nd-YAG laser in the treatment of chronic menorrhagia. *Am. J. Obstet. Gynecol.*, **59**, 152–5.

Matta, W. H. M. *et al.* (1988), Doppler assessment of uterine blood flow changes in patients with fibroids receiving gonadotrophin-releasing hormone agonist Buserelin. *Fertil. Steril.*, **49**(6), 1083–5.

Mayne, A. *et al.* (1988), Intravenous infusion of propofol for induction and maintenance of anaesthesia during endoscopic carbon dioxide laser ENT procedures with high frequency jet ventilation. *Anaesthesia*, **43**, Suppl. 97–100.

Moghissi, K. and Budd, A. (1988), Laser treatment for tracheobronchial tumours: Local and general anaesthesia? (letter). *Thorax*, **43**, 218.

Nesbit, R. M. and Glickman, S. I. (1948), The use of glycine solution as an irrigating medium during transurethral resection. *J. Urol.*, **59**, 1212–16.

Norlen, H. (1985), Isotonic solutions of mannitol, sorbitol and glycine in

distilled water as irrigating fluids during transurethral resection of the prostate and calculation of irrigating fluid influx. *Scand. J. Urol. Nephrol.*, Suppl. 96.
Osborn, D. E. *et al.* (1984), Fluid absorption during transurethral resection. *Br. Med. J.*, **281**, 1549–50.
Ovassapian, A. *et al.* (1982), Visual disturbances: an unusual symptom of transurethral prostatic resection. *Anesthesiology*, **57**, 332–4.
Renck, H. *et al.* (1983), Prevention of dextran induced anaphylactic reactions by hapten inhibition. *Acta Chir. Scand.*, **149**, 355–60.
Ring, J. (1984), Colloids. *Clin. Anesthesiol.*, **2**, 619–41.
Roesh, R. P. *et al.* (1983), Ammonia toxicity resulting from glycine absorption during transurethral resection of the prostate. *Anesthesiology*, **58**, 577–9.
Rontal, M. *et al.* (1986), Anesthetic management for tracheo-bronchial surgery. *Ann. Otol. Rhinol. Laryngol.*, **95**, 556–60.
Schiffman, P. L. *et al.* (1988), Arterial oxygen saturation during Nd-YAG laser photoresection of endobronchial tumours under local anaesthesia. Use of intermittent supplemental oxygen with pulse oximetry guidance. *Chest*, **94**, 1300–1.
Sciarra, J. J. and Valle, R. F. (1977), Hysteroscopy: an experience with 320 patients. *Am. J. Obstet. Gynecol.*, **127**, 340–8.
Sinclair, J. F. *et al.* (1985), Absorption of 1.5% glycine after percutaneous ultrasonic lithotripsy for renal stone disease. *Br. Med. J.*, **291**, 691–2.
Sosis, M. B. (1989), Evaluation of five metallic tapes for protection of endotracheal tubes during CO_2 laser surgery. *Anesth. Analg.*, **68**, 392–3.
Taylor, P. J. and Cumming, D. C. (1979), Hysteroscopy in 100 patients. *Fertil. Steril.*, **31**, 301–14.
Taylor, P. J. *et al.* (1987), A comparison of dextran 70 with carbon dioxide as the distending medium for hysteroscopy in patients with infertility or requesting reversal of a prior tubal sterilization. *Fertil. Steril.*, **47**, 861–3.
Valle, R. F. (1978), Hysteroscopy, diagnostic and therapeutic applications. *J. Reprod. Med.*, **20**, 115–19.
Valle, R. F. and Sciarra, J. J. (1979), Current status of hysteroscopy in gynecologic practice. *Fertil. Steril.*, **32**, 619–32.
Vial, R. *et al.* (1987), Resection endoscopique sous irrigation de glycine. *Ann. Fr. Anaesth. Reanim.*, **6**, 48–9.
Wainwright, A. C. (1987), Anaesthesia and laser surgery. *Anaesth. Rev.* (4) (ed. L. Kaufmann), pp. 159–65.
Weisberger, E. C. and Miner, J. D. (1988), Apneic anesthesia for improved endoscopic removal of laryngeal papillomata. *Laryngoscope*, **98**, 693–7.
Zbella, E. A. *et al.* (1985), Noncardiogenic pulmonary edema secondary to intrauterine instillation of 32% dextran 70. *Fertil. Steril.*, **43**, 479–80.

14 *Education and credentialling in gynaecologic laser surgery*

JAMES H. DORSEY

14.1 Introduction

In 1917, Albert Einstein described the basic theory of stimulated emission of radiation (Einstein, 1917), however it was not until 1953 that Charles Townes and co-workers produced the progenitor of the modern laser, the 'maser', which amplified microwaves, by the mechanism of stimulated emission (Schawlow and Townes, 1958). Theodore Maiman actually constructed the first laser in 1960 and a few years later the CO_2 laser was developed by Patel (Patel *et al.*, 1964). It was with the CO_2 laser wavelength that laser surgery in gynaecology began in 1974 when several gynaecological clinicians in widely separated localities first used laser energy to ablate infected cervical tissue.

During the next few years, pioneering gynaecologists recognized the unique properties and benefits of laser as a surgical tool. Although the lower reproductive tract remained the target of the gynaecological laser surgeon for several years, by 1978 intra-abdominal laser surgery and, in particular, laser laparoscopy had begun.

14.2 Education and training

Early laser surgeons were, by necessity, self-taught. However, during the 1970s in the United States and elsewhere, concern about the adequacy of post-graduate education was growing. In most states, laws were enacted which required proof of a specific number of hours spent each year in formal medical education in order to maintain licensure. This concern was fuelled by the increasing number of medico-legal suits filed against practising physicians, the great progress being made in medical technology and the mounting emphasis on the use of this new technology for conservative surgery. The use of lasers in all aspects of

Table 14.1 Laser course topics

1. Laser physics
2. Laser energy and tissue reaction
3. Laser safety
4. Laser energy delivery systems
5. Laser surgical theory and technique
6. Surgical technique with specific wavelengths
7. Laser laboratory

medicine and surgery serves as an excellent example of technological advance which has promoted conservatism.

Surgical technique is, of course, initially learned by the gynaecologist during the residency training years. Even now residency programmes seldom include laser surgery as a part of their curriculum. In order to educate gynaecologists interested in performing laser surgery, postgraduate courses dedicated to gynaecological surgery were introduced in 1978. As laser surgery grew in scope and credibility, the number of course participants increased. Within a very short time it was obvious that a didactic presentation about laser surgery was not sufficient to prepare the gynaecologic surgeon to perform the laser procedures in the operating room. Laboratory experience and actual 'hands-on' practice was a necessity. Various different scientific committees on both sides of the Atlantic have influenced the format of these courses (Sharp and Jordan, 1986). Table 14.1 outlines the general subject matter of the typical university sponsored laser course for gynaecological surgeons. This type of course is often used by gynaecologists to justify requests for credentialling in laser surgery.

14.3 Specific credentialling procedures

Early in the 1980s there were several landmark medico-legal decisions in United States courts which led to the development of the process referred to as 'specific credentialling' and the 'delineation of privileges'. Prior to this time, surgeons who had trained in approved residency programmes simply requested the privilege of performing 'gynaecological surgery' in general without specifically indicating which of the many possible surgical procedures were within their capabilities. In an effort to ensure better patient care, proper physician training and to reduce medico-legal risk, a much more careful approach has been taken by all specialties. Table 14.2 lists the credentialling criteria used at our hospital for gynaecological laser surgery.

Table 14.2 Credentialling criteria for gynaecological laser surgery

1. Thorough knowledge of the disease or abnormality to be treated by laser
2. Thorough knowledge of the conventional methods of treating the disease process
3. Participation in a formal laser course which presents physics, safety, techniques and theory of gynaecological laser surgery
4. Hands-on laboratory experience with different surgical laser systems
5. Hands-on training with patients
6. Maintenance of skills by continued practice

Credentialling is the process by which a hospital grants permission to a physician to perform surgery. The specific listing of surgical and other special procedures which the surgeon is allowed to perform in the hospital is referred to as the 'Delineation of privileges'. Although the ultimate responsibility for credentialling rests with the governing board of this institution, often this board is not composed of physicians and the credentialling responsibility is relegated to a medical staff committee. Thus the credentialling decisions are made by a jury of peers.

In the case of laser surgery, credentialling becomes somewhat involved. Not only are specific procedures of great variety performed with the aid of the laser but there are four different wavelengths which are currently available for use in our specialty. 'Delineation of privileges' forms should mention specific laser wavelengths which the surgeon wishes to use since the tissue effects produced by different lasers are not the same. Table 14.3 presents an example of a 'Delineation of privileges' form that could be used for specific credentialling requests.

14.4 Criteria for evaluating laser surgery

To the enthusiastic laser surgeon, many of the benefits of laser surgery seem quite obvious. Precision, accuracy, lessened surgical procedure and rapid recovery time all are suggested as advantages of laser usage. Much of this optimism seems justified. However, enthusiasm for a new modality may sometimes cloud the judgement of the surgeon unless objective criteria are applied in the effort to identify indications, contra-indications and the true worth of the laser procedure. In every instance, before the laser can be said to offer superior advantage over the conventional method, that definite benefit must be scientifically justified. In some instances laser operations have offered an entirely

Table 14.3 Delineation of laser surgical privileges

Wavelengths to be used
CO_2
Argon
KTP-532
Nd-YAG
Other (specify)
Delivery system
Micromanipulator
Laser handpiece
Laparoscope
Hysteroscopy
Other (specify)
Type of surgery
Lower reproductive tract
Laparotomy
Endoscopy
Procedures
Lower reproductive tract laser surgery
Cervix
Vagina
Vulva
Laparotomy
Use in all open abdominal procedures
Laparoscopy
Lysis of adhesions

new approach to surgical management of a disease. For example, combination cervical conization and peripheral vaporization is a procedure which provides a diagnostic (and hopefully therapeutic) specimen for pathological examination while destroying proven peripheral intraepithelial neoplasia. There is no other method which offers such a conservative approach to large fields of epithelial dysplasia, particularly if the vagina is involved since removal of normal tissue is reduced to a bare minimum. In other instances, the laser has been used simply as an instrument to replace a scalpel, cautery or cryo-probe. In any event, to be academically convincing, the specific benefits of the laser must be documented by carefully designed clinical trials.

There is now a relatively large body of scientific opinion which seems to support the argument that laser surgery for lower reproductive tract intraepithelial neoplasia is often the procedure of choice.

Most studies have compared indications, ease of the procedure, complications and results of laser vs conventional instrumentation, but most have been retrospective and non-randomized. Consequently, discussion concerning the validity of the conclusions of some of the investigators still persists. Although intra-abdominal laser started in 1978 the procedures are so varied, and meaningful randomized comparative series so few, that controversy about the value of the laser is even more prevalent. The difficulty in making a valid judgement is compounded by the fact that some of the so-called 'conventional' procedures used to replace an older type of operation are of unproven benefit themselves, and the laser has now been added as an additional variable. For example, the laparoscopic treatment of certain stages of endometriosis is still a controversial topic whether electrosurgery and scissors or laser energy is used.

The fact that certain benefits of the laser in gynaecology are not conclusively proven is not an argument against laser usage but simply points to the need for more controlled studies. Many surgeons have developed great expertise and competence in the application of laser. Obviously, the more comfortable the surgeon becomes with any modality or technique, the better the surgical result is likely to be.

14.5 Endoscopic laser surgery

Within the last decade, there has been growing interest in advanced operative laparoscopic surgery. The actual definition of this approach has included the statement that it is designed to replace laparotomy for benign gynaecological conditions since it offers a more conservative procedure that is economically more acceptable to the patient and the third-party payer. During the 1970s, Semm described many ingenious ways in which conventional methods of excision and haemostasis could be applied with laparoscopic techniques. This type of surgery is certainly an exciting new alternative to open abdominal surgery and already has demonstrated, in some areas, significant advantage. The laser is a part of the new technology which makes operative laparoscopy so attractive. The development of magnificent fibreoptic telescopes, effective and rapid methods of abdominal insufflation and additional operative instrumentation to fit through relatively small trocar sheaths have added to the ability of the surgeon to perform these complicated surgical procedures which previously required laparotomy.

Since the early reports of Bruhat and Tadir on CO_2 laser laparoscopy first appeared (Bruhat, Mages, Manhes, 1900; Tadhir, *et al.*, 1981) there have been many papers and patient series published concerning the use of evolving laser laparoscopic techniques. However, the majority of the reports have been supplied by a relatively small number of laparoscopic surgeons. Critics of the method have suggested that perhaps the surgical manoeuvres are too difficult for the average surgeon to master, and further, that the laser adds little to a procedure which can be accomplished equally as well by using bipolar cautery or Semm's 'pelviscopic' techniques. We feel that our experience at the Greater Baltimore Medical Center provides some answers to these questions.

In our clinic, laser laparoscopy began in 1982 with the CO_2 operative laparoscope. Though laser laparoscopy was initially used by the author alone, within the following 2 years, efforts to both educate and properly credential other interested staff members were well under way. Our programme has also included the training of residents in advanced laparoscopic techniques. At the present time, approximately 1000 advanced laparoscopic procedures are done each year at our institution and the vast majority of these surgical operations include the use of the laser. Seventeen laparoscopic surgeons have been credentialled.

Analysis of our programme serves to emphasize two important points: firstly, advanced endoscopic techniques may be taught and careful credentialling can be applied to the majority of gynaecologists who are willing to spend the necessary time to learn the procedures. Secondly, laser adds new dimensions to standard operative laparoscopy in terms of the speed and ease with which the procedure can be accomplished.

It is necessary to emphasize that in our experience only about 25% of the attending staff indicated the desire to learn advanced operative laparoscopy. The credentialling requirements demand the expenditure of effort, time and money. A significant number of gynaecological surgeons (albeit a minority of those eligible) were willing to pay the price. It should come as no surprise that the hand-eye co-ordination necessary to perform a complicated surgical manoeuvre while watching a video monitor is within the capability of most surgeons. This was particularly obvious for those of us who watched our resident's progress in the field. The point is also demonstrated in other specialties such as orthopaedics where residents learn to perform similar techniques during arthroscopy performed with the video monitor as the main method of visualization.

In our experience, careful analysis of operating times and inspection of countless video tapes indicates that the use of the laser speeded the operative procedure. Certainly the obvious advantages of haemostatic laser incisions and the rapid vaporization of smaller endometriotic implants seem to be validated in our large series.

At the Greater Baltimore Medical Center, four laser wavelengths are currently in use for laser laparoscopy, i.e. CO_2, Nd-YAG, KTP-532 and argon. Only three laparoscopists are credentialled to use all wavelengths. However, there does not appear to be a definite overall advantage to any specific laser type. Surgeons certainly have individual preferences but the end results seem to be similar no matter what laser is used. Our conclusion must be that the general laser advantages to laparoscopic laser surgery hold true for each wavelength and that the competence and confidence of the surgeon with a specific laser are the most important factors for a successful outcome. There have been no major mishaps or complications in a series of over 1500 laser laparoscopies.

14.6 Conclusion

The laser is a tool which is used by the knowledgeable surgeon to achieve as satisfactory an end result as possible. In many instances, he/she is able to perform a given surgical task more rapidly and accurately than by using the conventional approach with knife, scissors or another ablative method such as endocoagulation or electrocautery. The benefits of lower reproductive tract laser surgery seem to be more easily documented and 'proven' than do those of intra-abdominal surgery. However, there are still those who remain unconvinced even about the superiority of laser in the former area.

Replacement of an older, successful surgical technique by one which involves use of a new modality should be justified by application of a rational set of criteria. Comparisons between surgical procedures are difficult because of the variations in the skills of different surgeons, the differences in the degree of abnormalities produced by a disease and the lack of objective criteria to effectively judge results. Until more data have been accumulated, it may prove difficult to claim superiority for 'laser surgery' in some procedures over the conventional approach. However, it is difficult to argue with the surgeon who maintains that the laser provides a simple, fast method of accomplishing a task which is tedious or more complicated when performed by another surgical method. Surgeons must understand and know how to use all of the tools which are utilized in the modern armamentarium. Lasers are now an integral component of our instrumentation. There should be no 'mystique' concerning their use. A conservative prediction foresees the laser as the accepted tool of future surgery.

Operative laparoscopy has been suggested as a substitute for open abdominal procedures done for benign disease. One of the criticisms of advanced laparoscopic surgery has been that it is difficult to teach to the general obstetrician and gynaecologist. This has not been our experience. Residents who are enrolled in an accredited programme demonstrate satisfactory abilities in laparoscopic surgery at the conclusion of a programme as long as it contains sufficient numbers of this type of surgical procedure.

The limits of laser surgery have not been defined and each year technology is added to both endoscopy and to lasers which makes their use easier and broadens their applications. Certainly, the future will continue to produce exciting innovations in these fields.

References

Bruhat, M., Mages, C. and Manhes, H. (1979), Use of CO_2 laser via laparoscopy. In *Laser Surgery III. Proceedings of the Third Congress of the International Society for Laser Surgery* (ed. I. Kaplan), Tel Aviv: International Society for Laser Surgery, pp. 275–6.

Einstein, A. (1917), Zur quantentheorie der strahlung. *Physio Z.*, **18**, 121–8.

Maiman, T. H. (1960), Stimulated optical radiation in ruby masers. *Nature*, **187**, 493–4.

Patel, C. K. N., McFarlane, R. A. and Faust, W. L. (1964), Selective excitation through vibration energy transfer and optical maser action in nitrogen – carbon dioxide. *Physiol. Rev.*, **8**, 470–3.

Schawlow, A. L. and Townes, C. H. (1958), Infrared and optical masers. *Physiol. Rev.*, **112**, 1940–56.

Sharp, F. and Jordan, J. (1986), *Gynaecological Laser Surgery. Proceedings of the Fifteenth Study Group of the Royal College of Obstetricians and Gynaecologists.* Perinatology Press. Ithaca, New York.

Tadir, Y., Kaplan I. and Zuckerman, Z. (1981), A second puncture probe for laser laparoscopy. In *Laser Surgery IV. Proceedings of the Fourth Congress of the International Society for Laser Surgery* (eds K. Atsumi and N. Nimsakul), pp. 25–6.

15 *The future of laser surgery*

WILLIAM R. KEYE

15.1 Introduction

Despite claims from critics that lasers offer little advantage to the gynaecologist, lasers will continue to play a major role in gynaecology in the future. When introduced in the 1970s, lasers were a novelty with a still undefined role. Many reproductive surgeons were sceptical about the laser and rejected its use in gynaecology due to the unsupported and exaggerated claims of some early laser users. However, in the early 1980s cooler heads prevailed, and serious attempts were made to study the interaction of lasers and the female reproductive tract in a formal and more scientific way. Simultaneously, new wavelengths appeared and new delivery systems were developed. As a result, lasers began to gain respectability, and many of the world's foremost reproductive surgeons began to test the laser in their practices and laboratories.

Finally, in the early 1990s, the laser has become a common modality in the armamentarium of the gynaecologist, often making it possible to perform surgical procedures with greater ease and less morbidity than with traditional techniques. However, with only one exception (the coagulation of placental vessels by the Nd-YAG laser at fetoscopy in the twin transfusion syndrome), the laser has not made it possible to perform any gynaecologic operation that cannot be done using other techniques. Thus, although the laser may simplify a given technique, it clearly has not replaced any standard technique nor is it the absolute standard of care for any gynaecologic disease.

However, as we develop second- and third-generation lasers, new wavelengths and delivery systems, and new means of sensitizing diseased tissue to laser light, I predict that the laser will expand our current capabilities and will enable us to perform old procedures with far better results. This chapter looks into the future and predicts some of the developments and applications of the next decade.

15.2 Current status and future needs

In 1990 gynaecologists were using lasers for their photothermal effects and their ability to cut or coagulate tissue. In this respect the laser is very similar to diathermy. However, there are several unique features of the laser. They include:

1. The ability to transmit the laser beam across space, so eliminating the need for the laser device or delivery system to touch or contact the tissue. Additionally, some laser beams can be reflected off surgical mirrors, allowing tissue to be more easily treated in areas of the pelvis that otherwise are hard to access.
2. The ability of some lasers (argon and KTP-532) to selectively coagulate tissue because of its colour. This allows pigmented endometriotic implants to be coagulated with very low power densities that results in minimal effect on surrounding and relatively unpigmented tissues.
3. The ability to control and accurately predict the volume of tissue damage. The CO_2 laser used in the superpulse mode and the synthetic sapphire tips applied to the Nd-YAG laser provide an extraordinary degree of control, making it possible to coagulate or cut tissue juxtaposed to critical organs such as the bladder, ureter, major blood vessels, or Fallopian tubes.

Despite these unique and advantageous features, several claims have not been substantiated by currently available laser technologies. First, the claim that laser dissection is followed by fewer reparative adhesions than dissection with scalpel, scissors, or diathermy has not been proven. In fact, animal studies show no benefits from the laser. Second, the claim that blood loss is reduced when performing gynaecological surgical procedures with the laser has rarely been tested or proven. In fact, because of the rapidity with which the laser can vaporize tissue, unnecessary bleeding may occasionally occur when used by an inexperienced, poorly trained, or careless laser surgeon.

In my opinion, the real value of the laser in gynaecology in the early 1990s is its simplification of some surgical procedures for some surgeons. It extends the surgeon's ability to perform procedures at endoscopy that typically are performed at laparotomy. While the clinical results may not be any better, the savings in terms of money; the reduced time required for hospitalization, convalescence, and caretaking; less time lost from work; and less pain clearly justify the use of the laser, particularly at laparoscopy and hysteroscopy.

What then are our needs and how will lasers of the future help meet these needs? The first and probably greatest need is to develop a technique for cutting or vaporizing tissue, particularly at endoscopy, with little or no thermal or acoustic damage, with the greater precision, and without the creation of smoke and carbon formation. Secondly, we need smaller delivery systems in order to deliver laser energy into the Fallopian tube or ovary for the truly microsurgical dissection or ablation of disease. Thirdly, we need improved techniques to identify and destroy infectious agents, microscopic foci of endometriosis, and non-invasive malignancies of the genital tract. Fourthly, we need the ability to treat diseases such as endometriosis, ovarian carcinoma, or dysfunctional endometrium completely without damaging the surrounding and adjacent normal uninvolved tissue. Finally, we need smaller, more efficient, and less costly lasers. From projections based on current research it appears that the lasers of the future may meet these needs.

15.3 Development of new delivery systems

The initial enthusiasm following the introduction of the CO_2 laser in gynaecologic surgery was soon replaced by frustration with the bulky and delicate articulating arm that limited its use at laparoscopy. The frustration with the CO_2 delivery systems led to the development of a flexible fibreoptic delivery system for the argon laser for use at laparoscopy and greatly simplified the treatment of pelvic diseases. Soon thereafter, the Nd-YAG laser was used through an optical fibre at laparoscopy and hysteroscopy. Unfortunately, the characteristics of the Nd-YAG laser-tissue interaction limited its use in the pelvis. Thereafter, a sapphire probe was developed which, when coupled to the Nd-YAG laser, made it possible for the surgeon to actually touch the tissue with the fibre. This allowed a surgeon to produce a limited, safe, and predictable pattern of thermal damage, including vaporization and coagulation. Later, the KTP-532 laser was also used at laparoscopy through a flexible fibre.

While initial attempts to develop a flexible fibre for the delivery of the CO_2 laser at laparoscopy were unsuccessful, there have been two recent developments that have simplified the endoscopic delivery of the CO_2 laser. The first was the development of a rigid waveguide, which, when introduced through the operating channel of the single-puncture laparoscope, simplified the focusing of the beam through the laparoscope and improved the efficiency of the laparoscopic delivery of the CO_2 laser (Infraguide, Haraeus Lasersonics, Inc. Santa Clara, California).

The most recent development has been a flexible fibre for delivery of the CO_2 laser by Fuller Research, Detroit, Michigan. The fibre, which measures 1 mm outside diameter, is non-toxic and capable of delivering argon, Nd-YAG, and CO_2 laser energy. It can bend in a very small radius, is reusable, and is projected to be very reasonable in cost. Hopefully, the fibre will be commercially available in the near future.

Just as there have been a number of changes in delivery systems during the last 10 years, there will be advances in delivery systems during the next decade. The delivery systems of the future will be designed for specific surgical procedures. For example, specialized fibreoptic tips may be specially designed to simultaneously ablate large areas of the endometrium. Others may give off circumferential (360°) beams or a 180° beam that will uniformly destroy the walls of ovarian cysts, the core of uterine myomas, or malignant pelvic nodules. Other delivery systems may facilitate tissue welding of vessels, Fallopian tubes, or the surface of the uterus or ovary to decrease adhesion formation.

Finally, an important advance in the delivery of laser energy will be the development of micromanipulators capable of creating spot sizes of 5–10 μm or smaller. With these small spot sizes, lasers may be used to drill the zona pellucida of human oocytes to facilitate sperm penetration or to dissect a blastomere from a blastocyst for biochemical or genetic analysis.

15.4 Controlled tissue destruction

The ability to vaporize or incise tissue more cleanly and with little or no thermal damage will depend upon the development of more powerful lasers and unexplored wavelengths of light.

During the last 10 years medical lasers have become more powerful. Through the development of the superpulse, CO_2 lasers can now deliver peak powers of several hundred watts, and the KTP-532 and argon lasers can deliver powers of more than 15 W. However, the experimental free-electron laser (FEL) will allow laser scientists to investigate average powers of several hundred watts and peak powers in the gigawatt range during pulses as short as 500 femtoseconds. Because of these properties, the FEL, developed by John Madey at Stanford University in the 1970s, has captured the imagination of basic science and medical scientists. It is driven by a linear accelerator, which generates a beam of electrons that are passed between rows of powerful magnets called wigglers. As the polarity and strength of the magnets are varied, a large and variable range of wavelengths of laser energy can be produced and finely tuned. Because of its tunability over a wide range of wavelengths and its ability to deliver energy of high powers for very short periods of time, the FEL will make it possible to study the non-thermal effects of laser energy on biological tissues. Although not likely to be clinically available because of cost ($5 million), size, and complexity, this laser is and will be an excellent tool for screening new wavelengths and parameters of higher power and shorter duration. For example, using low powers of a laser beam with a wavelength near 3 μm, we have been able to cut through bone and gallstones without gross mechanical or thermal damage to the surrounding bone. The ability to deliver laser energy in high-powered, short bursts may make it possible to dissect and ablate gynaecologic tissues with greater precision and with less unintended thermal injury to surrounding tissues than is currently possible.

While most gynaecologists are familiar with the CO_2, Nd-YAG, argon, and frequency-doubled Nd-YAG laser, several other wavelengths are currently being investigated for their gynaecologic applications. Recent reports suggest possible roles in medicine and gynaecology for mid-infrared and heavy metal vapour lasers such as the erbium-YAG laser, the gold vapour laser, the copper vapour laser, the argon-pumped dye laser, and the helium holmium chromium-YAG laser.

The process of exploring new wavelengths is complicated by the cost and difficulties of developing individual lasers to study each wavelength of interest. The more practical approach may involve a tunable laser, such as the FEL, which can be tuned continuously from 4 to 300 μm. Using the FEL laser, it may be possible with a single machine to explore many wavelengths and their unique biological effects [i.e. to influence cellular (fibroblast migration and collagen deposition) and subcellular processes (rate of cell division or protein production)]. One might also envisage that the exposure of human gametes or preembryos may enhance the success rates of *in vitro* fertilization or cryopreservation.

15.5 Techniques for development of tissue sensitization to laser energy (photodynamic therapy)

15.5.1 BIOLOGY OF PHOTODYNAMIC THERAPY

In photodynamic therapy (PDT), light or other forms of electromagnetic radiation are absorbed by an exogenous photosensitive chemical that is retained in a target tissue such as a neoplasm. A commonly used photosensitizer, haematoporphyrin derivative (HPD), absorbs light energy between 400 and 800 nm and initiates photophysical and photochemical changes that lead to selective tissue destruction.

In PDT light is absorbed by HPD, the energy absorbed is then transferred to molecular oxygen or tissue biomolecules, and oxidation of the biomolecules in the target tissues takes place. Mild thermal effects (a rise in temperature of 1–10°C) and chemical reactions of the sensitizer with biomolecules may also take place. This process involves the formation of a reactive oxygen molecule called 'singlet' oxygen, although free electron radicals may also be formed. Both lead to the photodynamic destruction of tumours or other tissue containing HDP.

The photochemical and photobiological effects are readily produced by low-energy photons of light at relatively low irradiances using lasers that generate continuous wave (CW) light such as the argon-pumped dye laser. Pulsed lasers, such as the gold or copper laser (metal vapour lasers) with low-energy, high-repetition rate (8 kHz) pulses, are also effective.

The various photobiological and physiological effects that are seen in PDT depend on where the photosensitizer is located in the biological target (organ, tissue, cell type, membrane, cytoplasm, mitochondria, nuclei) and on which biomolecule(s) is damaged.

The properties of photosensitizers that are important to PDT include (1) their solubility in blood; (2) the capacity to localize and be retained in selective tissues; (3) the ability to absorb light efficiently; and (4) the ability to produce necrosis of tumour tissue upon exposure to light and to fluoresce. Porphyrins such as HPD were among the first naturally occurring compounds shown to photosensitize tissues to visible light. Porphyrins are unique photosensitizers that can be useful in both the detection and photochemotherapy of selected tissues because of their retention and fluorescence in tumour tissue and their ability to produce necrosis in tumour tissue upon exposure to light.

There are other photodynamic sensitizers that have been shown to destroy tumours photodynamically *in vivo*. These include the dyes rhodamine 123, merocyanine 540, and the cyanine dyes. These sensitizers appear to be retained in tumours and to produce a phototoxic reaction by a different mechanism than HPD.

The active components of HPD are aggregates of monomers, dimers, and polymers derived from haematoporphyrin. These aggregates compete with the binding of endogenous porphyrins to tumour tissue proteins. This aggregation may play a key role in the uptake and retention of fluorescent and photoreactive dyes in tumour tissue. Aggregated photosensitizers including the porphyrins may circulate in blood with very weak protein binding and be deposited via altered capillary permeability in tumour tissue. It has been suggested that the localization of HPD in tumours and other tissues with altered vascular permeability such as inflammation and wound healing is due to the relatively high influx and the inefficient removal and trapping of the colloidal or the protein-bound components of HPD. In addition to tumour cells, the capillary endothelial cells and cellular and extracellular components of microvascular septae are important binding sites for photosensitizers and may be targets for photodynamic action. As a result of the photo-oxidation reactions occurring within these cellular components, especially within the vascular compartment, the photosensitized tissue is destroyed by ischaemia.

Other factors may also play a role in the selective binding and retention of porphyrins, such as metal chelation, covalent binding, pH, phagocytosis, and lipoprotein receptor binding. The relative importance of these factors is unknown.

Porphyrins may localize in either the cell membrane or in subcellular compartments. Studies show that cell membranes are the major targets of photodynamic action when cells in culture are exposed to HPD and are irradiated. The photo-oxidation reactions manifest themselves as membrane blebbing, lysis, enzyme inactivation, and protein cross-linking. They may also occur at the mitochondrial, microsomal, and lysosomal membranes, and perhaps at the nuclear membrane. Damage to the DNA appears to be minimal. Several investigators have suggested that damage to the vascular supply of a tumour may be of major importance in tumour destruction.

15.5.2 GYNAECOLOGIC APPLICATIONS OF PHOTODYNAMIC DIAGNOSIS AND THERAPY

Since an early report by Mack *et al.* (1957), who treated 24 patients with cancer of the cervix with a combination of haematoporphyrin and radiation therapy, we have known that porphyrins would accumulate in these lesions and serve as a fluorescent diagnostic marker.

Lipson *et al.* (1964), also have shown that HPD accumulates in malignant tissue in the cervix and that its fluorescence can be helpful in the detection of these neoplasms. They studied the use of HPD fluorescence in a study of neoplastic lesions of the cervix. Recently, Fioretti, Facchini and Gadducci (1984), noted a greater uptake and retention of HMD in cervical cancer than in normal surrounding tissues.

McCaughan, Scellhashf and Lomano (1985) treated five patients with gynaecological neoplasms using HPD and light from an argon dye laser. One patient with squamous cell cancer of the vagina was free of disease 15 months after her PDT. In another patient there was no evidence of tumour on the surface of the vagina at autopsy performed 9 months after PDT. Even metastatic disease to the reproductive tract has responded to PDT. Vaginal bleeding from breast cancer metastatic to the endometrium was controlled by a single treatment. Metastatic adenocarcinoma to the vaginal cuff showed partial response to PDT.

There are several other reports in the literature of the treatment of gynaecological cancers with PDT. These include a study by Ward, Forbes and Cowled (1982), who treated five patients with gynaecological cancers with PDT. They reported no evidence of recurrence of one tumour at 12 months, another patient free of tumour at 10 months, and varying degrees of response in three other patients.

Kennedy (1983) also reported a marked response with vaginal cancer using a tunable dye laser and a slide-projector as a source of light and a solid lucite cone to deliver the light to the tissue.

Soma and Nutahara (1983) reported treating five patients with cancer of the vagina and the vulva, five patients with carcinoma *in situ* of the uterine cervix, and three patients with cancer metastatic to the vagina using a tunable dye laser system and a colposcope.

15.5.3 FUTURE DEVELOPMENTS FOR LASER PHOTOCHEMOTHERAPY

The future development of (1) new laser systems for generating light at many wavelengths with a wide range of pulse characteristics, (2) photosensitizing drugs and drug delivery systems that can be used to selectively target tissue components, and (3) optical fibres and devices to irradiate and treat a biological target almost anywhere in the body are providing exciting new therapeutic and diagnostic tools for surgery and medicine. For example, viral lesions and infections may be treated by laser PDT. Preliminary studies suggest that the herpes virus is more sensitive than human cells to HPD photochemotherapy. The treatment of herpes lesions by laser HPD photochemotherapy may become a useful clinical procedure.

In addition, there is evidence from *in vitro* studies that papilloma virus (HPV) lesions are sensitive to PDT (Abramson, Shikowitz and Steinberg, 1986). If animal studies are equally successful, PDT treatment of viral papillomas in humans may be possible.

Microbial and fungal infections can also be treated by photochemotherapy. For example, *Staphylococcus aureus* has been inactivated *in vitro* and *in vivo* animal models by HPD-sensitized PDT (Martinett *et al.*, 1985). In addition, mycoplasma cells have also been killed by HPD-sensitized photodynamic action (Bertoloni *et al.*, 1985). Eukaryotic micro-organisms, including yeast cells (*Saccharomyces cervisiae*), are killed on exposure to light in the presence of HPD (Kvello-Stenstrom *et al.*, 1980). Further animal and clinical studies are needed to determine the clinical utility of PDT in these indications.

Recently, the visible and occult lesions of *endometriosis* in both a rabbit and a rhesus monkey model have been shown to take up HPD. The lesions were treated with argon laser light and PDT was demonstrated. These preliminary unpublished studies were carried out at the University of Adelaide and by the Utah Laser Institute in collaboration with the Oregon Primate Research Center. Further studies are under way to determine whether successful treatment of occult endometrial lesions is possible.

Finally, Schneider *et al.* (1988) at the University of Cincinnati and the Jewish Hospital Laser Laboratory have demonstrated the rapid uptake of dihaematoporphyrin derivative and selective tissue necrosis by the endometrium of the rat after exposure to the gold vapour laser. These preliminary animal studies suggest that PDT may be of use in the ablation of the endometrium in women with menorrhagia. The technique, using a quartz rod passed into the uterine cavity through the cervix, would be simpler than the current technique using the hysteroscope and the Nd-YAG laser and could possibly be performed in the office without anaesthesia.

15.6 Diagnostic techniques using lasers

The ability of tissues to fluoresce when exposed to certain dyes and wavelengths of light may aid in the earlier detection of microscopic areas of pre-invasive malignancy, infection, and benign conditions such as endometriosis. For example, we have demonstrated that experimental endometriosis selectively retains HPD and fluoresces when exposed to ultraviolet light (unpublished data). Conceivably, the pelvis of a woman undergoing laparoscopy could be lavaged with a dilute solution of HPD and within minutes illuminated with ultraviolet light, thus identifying microscopic and otherwise invisible implants of endometriosis. These microscopic implants could then be destroyed using a laser selectively absorbed by the HPD. By this means, the recurrence or persistence of endometriosis after standard surgical treatment might be reduced or even eliminated. What is especially exciting about this approach is that foci of endometriosis below the peritoneal surface could be treated as effectively as superficial implants.

Another potential use of lasers for diagnosis involves endoholography or endoscopic holography. In endoholography, a special contact endoscope is fitted to a special laser such as the krypton ion laser. The endoscope is advanced into the cavity to be examined and applied to the surface of the tissue (endometrium, endosalpinx, ovarian cyst wall); then with the aid of the laser a three-dimensional holographic picture is taken. The film is rapidly developed, and the photograph yields a view of the tissue similar to that seen through a microscope. Using this technique, one may examine the histologic features of tissues without destroying, sampling, or removing the tissue. Theoretically, this could make it possible to evaluate ovarian cysts at endoscopy. Additionally, the nature of the endometrium could be examined at the time of embryo implantation without disturbing the endometrium or the pregnancy.

Holographic interferometry is a procedure utilizing a laser-generated signal (such as from the double-pulsed ruby laser) to measure dynamic events such as ciliary beating of the endosalpinx. One can picture the gynaecologist of the future threading a special endoscope through the cornual ostium of the Fallopian tube to measure tubal motility, peristalsis, and ciliary action in order to assess the functional and structural integrity and health of the tube.

15.7 Miniaturization of laser systems

The most recent development in laser technology has been the reduced laser size and decreased energy requirements. Portable, hand-held CO_2 and Nd-YAG lasers are now capable of generating powers sufficient for many gynaecologic applications. In addition, diode lasers of the future will aid in the miniaturization of lasers to an even greater degree. Hopefully, the cost of manufacturing and purchasing these lasers will drop as the size decreases. Certainly, the cost of providing space, power, and water for cooling will also decrease as the lasers become smaller and more efficient.

15.8 Conclusion

In addition to the development of new lasers and laser accessories, in the future the role of lasers in gynaecology will also change. To date, the major role for the intra-abdominal use of lasers has been the treatment of infertility. The laser and its accessory equipment have been adapted to lyse adhesions, to treat polycystic ovaries, to open up obstructed Fallopian tubes, and to destroy endometriosis. However, as the success of the assisted reproductive technologies (*in vitro* fertilization, gamete intrafallopian transfer, zygote intrafallopian transfer, and cryopreservation) improve, the role of the laser in infertility surgery probably will change. Instead of performing a neosalpingostomy with the laser to achieve a 5–20% pregnancy rate, women may choose *in vitro* fertilization with a pregnancy rate of 25–40%.

Finally, as the laser assumes its place among the traditional and standard surgical instruments and devices that we have used for decades, the mystique of the laser will disappear and it will become an adjunct to more traditional devices. Free-standing laser units will cease to exist as they become incorporated into standard hospital or outpatient surgical administrative units. Training in lasers will become a standard part of residency training, and the demand for postgraduate education and the need for certification will level off. Hopefully, the extraordinary claims, the blatant examples of self-promotion, and the occasional unjustified fees that have accompanied the introduction of lasers in gynaecology will also cease.

Non-laser technologies, such as electrocautery and ultrasonography, will be modified to accomplish many of the tissue effects now achieved with lasers at a fraction of the cost of lasers. For example, electrosurgical probes will be introduced to coagulate and incise tissue with the same degree of precision and greater safety than with the laser. As a result, the use of lasers in gynaecology to merely coagulate and vaporize may decline while the use of new techniques such as PDT increases.

While the use of lasers in gynaecology has grown rapidly during the last decade, the developments of the next decade will be even more dramatic and rapid. It behoves gynaecologists to become familiar with the current generation of lasers and laser procedures so that they will be well positioned to take advantage of the next generation of lasers and their applications.

References

Abramson, A. L., Shikowitz, M. and Steinberg, B. (1986), The effects of hematoporphyrin derivative-photodynamic therapy on experimental viral papilloma. *The First International Conference on the Clinical Applications of Photosensitization for Diagnosis and Treatment*, Tokyo, p. 59.

Bertoloni, G., Viel, A., Grossato, A. *et al.* (1985), The photosensitizing activity of haematoporphyrin on mollicates. *J. Gen. Microbiol.*, **131**, 2217–23.

Fioretti, P., Facchini, V. and Gadducci, A. (1984), Monitoring of hematoporphyrin injected in humans and clinical prospects of its use in gynecologic oncology. *Med. Biol. Environ.*, **12**, 355–61.

Kennedy, J. (1983), HPD photoirradiation therapy for cancer at Kingston and Hamilton. In *Porphyrin and Photosensitization* (eds D., Kessel and T. J. Doherty), Plenum Publishing Co., New York, p. 53.

Kvello-Stenstrom, A. G., Moan, J., Brunborg, G. *et al.* (1980), Photodynamic inactivation of yeast cells sensitized by hematoporphyrin. *Photochem. Photobiol.*, **32**, 349–52.

Lipson, R. L., Pratt, J. H., Baldes, E. J. *et al.* (1964), Hematoporphyrin derivative for the detection of cervical cancer. *Obstet. Gynecol.*, **24**, 78–84.

Mack, H. P., Diehl, W. K., Tek, G. C. *et al.* (1957), Evaluation of the combined effects of hematoporphyrin in radiation. I. Treatment of carcinoma of the cervix. *Cancer*, **10**, 529–39.

Martinett, P., Gariglio, M., Pancani, I. *et al.* (1985), *Photodynamic Therapy of Tumors and Other Diseases*. Edizioni Liberia Progetto, Padova, Italy, pp. 367–70.

McCaughan, J. R., Scellhashf, J. S. and Lomano, J. (1985), Photodynamic therapy of gynecologic neoplasms after presensitization with hematoporphyrin derivative. *Laser Surg. Med.*, **5**, 491–8.

Schneider, D. F., Schellhas, H. F., Wesseler, T. A., Chen, I. W., and Moulton, B. C. (1988), Hematoporphyrin derivative uptake in uteris of estrogen-treated ovariectomized rats. *Colpos. Gynecol. Laser Surg.*, **4**, 67–71.

Soma, H. and Nutahara, S. (1983), Cancer of the female genitalia. In *Lasers and Hematoporphyrin Derivative in Cancer* (eds Y. Hyata and T. J. Doherty), Igaku-Shoin Ltd., Tokyo, pp. 97–109.

Ward, V. G., Forbes, K. G. and Cowled, T. A. (1982), The treatment of vaginal recurrences of gynecologic malignancy with phototherapy following hematoporphyrin derivative pre-treatment. *Am. J. Obstet. Gynecol.*, **142**, 356–61.

Index

Numbers in italic represent tables, those in bold represent figures

Abdominal pain,
 and adhesions 98–9
 laparoscopic adhesiolysis *100–101*
Adhesiolysis 33, 35–8, **80**
 for abdominal pain *100–101*
 adjuvant therapy 109–12
 clinical techniques 36–8
 laparoscopic 65–6, 95–117
 laser advantages 35–6
 Nd-YAG laser therapy for synechiae 189
 performance 103–9
 pregnancy rates after treatment *62*
 visible light laser energy 133–4
Adhesion Barrier Group Study 112
Adhesions,
 abdominal pain 98–9
 adjuvant therapy and formation 110
 clinical implications 98
 formation,
  167–8, 169
  mechanism 95–8
 and infertility 102
 pathogenesis **97**
 pre- and post-CO_2 laser adhesiolysis *110*
 tubo-ovarian 102
Adhesions Study Group 111
Adjuvant therapy,
 in adhesiolysis 109–12
 for vulvar laser ablation 231–4
Adnexal structures, removal with laparoscopic laser 135
American Fertility Society 42, 86, 152
Amplitude, light wave 4
Ampullary disease 38–9
Anaesthetic hazards 238–46
Anaphylactic reactions 241
Aquapurators 56
Argon *10*–11
Argon laser,
 comparative long-term results *192*
 development 119
 for ectopic pregnancy 162
 physics and tissue interaction 120
 tissue absorption **18**
Asherman's syndrome 175–6, 183–4
Aspiration, ectopic pregnancy 160

Basov, N. 2
Beam geometry
 adjustment 217–19
 defocussing effect **218**
Beam splitter 125
Bernard-Soulier syndrome 179
Beta-human chorionic gonadotrophin values after linear salpingotomy **170**
Bruhat technique 129
Bupivicaine hydrochloride 178
Buserelin **85–9**, 91

Carbon dioxide (CO_2) *10*–**12**
Carbon dioxide (CO_2) laser,
 anaesthetic hazards 239, 243–4
 for cervix 201
 CIN 206
 condylomata 213
 contact probe 143, 146–8
 ectopic pregnancy 161
 'endometriotic' adhesions **79–80**
 equipment 74
 flexible delivery fibre 259–60

laparoscopic adhesiolysis for abdominal pain *100–101*, 105–6
laparoscopy in endometriosis 73–93
metroplasty **49–51**
microsurgery 25–53
myectomy **48–9**
ovarian cystectomy 46
ovarian wedge resection 45
physics mistakes 19, 21
salpingostomy **45**
suction probe 123
tissue absorption **18**
vs diathermy 108–9
Carboxymethyl cellulose (CMC) 112
Carcinoma *in situ* 196–7
Cervical intraepithelial neoplasia (CIN),
conservative management 198–9
historical aspects 195–8
laser therapy 195–205
Cervix,
laser vaporization 201
premalignant disease 197
Chondroitin sulphate 112
Chopped wave laser pulse 214
CIN, *see* Cervical intraepithelial neoplasia
Clomidiphene 128
Clomiphene 46–7, 126, 152
Clotting disorders 179
Cold coagulation 201
Cold knife excisional cone biopsy 202
Collimation **9**
Colon, endometriosis 31–2
Colposcopy 199, 202
anaesthetic hazards 239
laser service, organization 206–7
Conception, assisted, by laparoscopy 131–2
Condyloma,
benign, laser ablation 229–30
colpophotograph **212**
extensive, laser ablation 228–9
Cone biopsy,
cold knife 202
laser 202–3
Continuous wave (CW) 15–16
Continuous wave (CW) light 262
Cornual obstruction 39
Cornual polyps 43–4
Corticosteroids and adhesions 111
Cryocoagulation 176
Cryotherapy for CIN 199–200

Danazol 85, **87–9**, 152, 176, 178, 180, 240
Danocrine 28–9, 176
Depo-Provera 179
Dextran solutions 241–2
Dextran-induced anaphylactic reactions (DIAR) 241
Direct current (DC) excitation 12
Doyle procedure 63
Dysmenorrhoea,
LUNA treatment *135–6*
Nd-YAG laser therapy *188–9*

5-Fluorouracil 231, 233

Gas cartridge for probe cooling **148**
Gestrinone 85–7, **89**
GIFT procedure 131–2
Glycine solutions, toxicity 242
GnRH **85–6**, **90**, 152
Goldrath's technique 184–5

Haematometra 180, 193
Haematoporphyrin derivative (HPD) 261–5
diagnostic 263
Haemostasis, laser 21
Heat conduction, limitation 213–16
Heparin and adhesions 111
High power outputs **215–16**
Holographic interferometry 266
Human papilloma virus (HPV),
oncogenic 211
vulvar diseases 234–5
Hydrosalpinx **41–2**
laser treatment 128–9
Hyskon 111, 177, 185, 241
Hysterectomy for CIN 203–4
Hysterosalpingography 39, 43, 166
Hysteroscope, flexible 185
Hysteroscopy,
anaesthetic hazards 239

diagnostic, hazards 240
laser surgery 183–94
complications and side effects 192–3
Nd-YAG laser 175–81
methods 176–8

Infertility,
and adhesions 102
hysteroscopic therapy results *191*
Nd-YAG laser therapy 190
Interceed 112
Interferon 233–4
Intermittent pulses **220**
Interstitial isthmic anastomosis 42
Interstitial obstruction 39–**40**
Intraabdominal CO_2 Laser Adhesion Study Group 66
Isthmic disease 38–9

Jones procedure **50**

Kaplan-Meier survival curve **232**
Koebner phenomenon 212
Krypton *10*–11
KTP laser **106–8**
development 119–20
for ectopic pregnancy 162
physics and tissue interaction 120

Laparoscope, double-puncture **75–6**
Laparoscopic surgery,
instruments **158**
technical aspects for ectopic pregnancy 158–63
Laparoscopic uterosacral nerve ablation (LUNA), KTP laser results *135–6*
Laparoscopy,
for adhesiolysis 103–8
advanced operative 119–40
anaesthetic hazards 243–6
CO_2 laser 22
coagulation *57–8*
delivery techniques 122–5
efficacy 65–6
in endometriosis 73–93
fibreoptic laser **159**
haemostasis *58*–9
incisional instruments *56–7*
indications *82*
probe placement 123
procedures 59, 63
safety 17–8
single-puncture **71–5**
surgery result assessment 55–71
technology and instrumentation advances *56*
video use **124**–*5*
with visible light laser **122**
vs laparotomy 109
Laparotomy, for adhesiolysis 103
Large loop excision of transformation zone 203
Laser,
course topics *250*
delivery system development 259–60
diagnostic techniques 265–6
for ectopic pregnancy 157
experimental and clinical studies 163–4
energy pulsing *15*
excisional cone 205
handles 147
handpiece 26–7
hazards and precautions 237–8
mechanisms 1
nonlinear effects 15–16
photochemotherapy 264–5
physics 1–23
safety 237–48
sealed tube 11–13
free space 12
surgical control 14–15
systems comparison *146*
systems miniaturization 266
vaporization cone 204
wave differences *215*
Laser ablation,
extended 227–8
indications 228–30
vulvar, results **231–3**
Laser chamber, diagram **8**
Laser excisional cone biopsy 202–3

Laser light 1
  absorption **17–18**
  characteristic wavelengths *10*
  coherence 8–9
  reflection **17–18**
  scattering **17–18**
  special properties 8–11
  transmission **17–18**
Laser light, *see* Light
Laser medium 11–13
Laser surgery,
  comparative results **192**
  control strategies 217–20
  credentialling procedures *250–1*
  education and training 249–50
  effective 213–21
  endoscopic 53–5
  essential strategies 220–1
  evaluation criteria 251–3
  planes **221**–**7**
    first 221–2, **223**
    second 222–3, **225**–**6**
    summary of features *222*
  privilege delineation *252*
LHRH analogues 88–9
Light,
  coherent 5
  physics 1–23
Light Amplification by Stimulated Emission of Radiation, *see* Laser
Light emission **5**–**7**, 8
  stimulated 6, **8**
Light lasers, history of development 119–20
Light waves 2–5
  properties **3**
Lung,
  compliance reduction *245*
  physiology 244–6
Lupron 28–9
Lynestrenol 86–7, **89**

Maillard Effect 185
Maiman, T. 2, 249
Marcaine 178
Menorrhagia,
  Nd-YAG laser therapy 183–4
  treatment 175–6

Mesotubarium ovarica (MTO) 102
Metroplasty 49–51
Microcolpohysteroscope 202
Microelectrosurgery, adhesions 35
Micromanipulator 27
  development 260
Microslad **218**–19
Microsurgery,
  CO_2 laser 25–53
  instrumentation 26–8
Mirrors 27–8
Mode-locking 16
Monochromaticity 9–11
Multiple second puncture probes 55–6
Myomectomy **47**–**9**
  with YAG laser 153

Nd-YAG *10*–11
Nd-YAG laser,
  anaesthetic hazards 243–4
  basic science 141–2
  coagulation 21
  coagulative effect 57
  contact probe, tissue effect 143, **145**
  dysfunctional uterine bleeding 183–4
    recurrence treatment **189**
    results *188*
  dysmenorrhoea infertility 188–9
  for ectopic pregnancy 162
  endometrial ablation 185–7
  haemostatic properties 143, **145**
  hysteroscopy 175–81
  infertility results 190
  intra-uterine septae and synechiae 189–90
  laparoscopy 141–54
    for endometriosis 151–2
  technique description 151–2
  tissue absorption **18**
  see also YAG laser
Neosalpingostomy 40–2
  laparoscopic *130*

Oocyte recovery 66
Out-patient surgery, benefits *139*
Ovariolysis 79

Ovary,
  cystectomy 46
  cysts,
    evaluation 67
    hormonal modifications **89**
  endometriosis **30**–**1**
  laser for endometriosis **78**–9
  wedge resection 45
    laparoscopic YAG laser 152

Patency test **166**–**7**
Peritoneum,
  effect of damage 96–8
  endometriosis **29**–**30**
  reduced fibrinolytic activity 97–8
Phase, light wave **4**–**5**
Photochemotherapy 264–5
Photocoagulation 177
Photodynamic diagnosis and therapy 263–4
Photodynamic therapy (PDT) 11, 261–5, 267
Photons 2–3, 6, 8
Photovaporization 177
Pilosebaceous ducts, neoplasia **224**–**7**
Pitressin 42–4, 48, 50
Plasminogen activator activity (PAA) 97–8
Polycystic ovarian syndrome **46**–7
  laparoscopic treatment 64–5
  YAG laser use 152
Polycystic ovaries, laser treatment 126, 128
Popcorn effect 216
Porphyrins as photosensitizers 262–3
Potassium titanyl phosphate laser, *see* KTP laser
Power density,
  choice 217
  maintenance **216**
Power output 217
Pregnancy rates,
  after adhesiolysis *62*, 80
  after ectopic pregnancy *60*, 170
  after endometriosis *61*, *82*, *84*–5, 87–8
  after laparoscopic neosalpingostomy *130*
  after laser surgery 32, 35, 41, *60*–*2*
  after Nd-YAG laser therapy for endometriosis 152
  after vaporization of polycystic ovaries *127*
Probe placement for laparoscopy 123
Probes **75**–**6**
  cooling **147**–**8**
Progestin 152
Prokhorov, A. 2
Prostaglandin synthetase inhibitors (PGSIs) 183
Pulmonary oedema, after hysteroscopy 179
Pulsing concepts 15–16

Q-switching 16
Quinacrine 183

Radio-frequency waveguides 12–13
Radiofrequency (RF) 11
Recombinant plasminogen activator (rt-PA) 98
  and adhesion 111–12
Reproduction technology, assisted, alternatives 66
Rhodium mirror vaporization **36**–**7**

Salpingectomy 153
  segmental 155–6, 159–60, **161**
Salpingitis isthmica nodosum (SIN) 26
Salpingo-ovariolysis, laparoscopic, results *105*
Salpingolysis 79
  pregnancy results *104*
    by microsurgery *104*
Salpingoophorectomy 153
Salpingoscopy 68
Salpingostomy,
  for ectopic pregnancy **44**–**5**
  linear 44
Salpingotomy,
  adhesion formation **168**
  laparoscopic 158–9
  linear 153, 155, 157, **160**
    animal experiments **163**–**5**, **166**
Sandwich technique 191
Sapphire endoprobes **163**

Sapphire probe 142–3
  contact **143–4**
  geometry **142–3**
  tissue interaction 19
Schawlow, A. 2
Scissors for adhesiolysis 104–5
Semm's 'pelviscopic' techniques 254
Sensitizers, photodynamic 262–3
Shuttered pulsing techniques 219–20
Singlet oxygen 262
SLT liquid for probe cooling **148**
SLT unit **146–7**
Smoke reduction **143–4**
Spot brightness 14
Squamocolumnar junction (SCJ) 195, 200, 202
Staphylococcus aureus, photochemotherapy 264
Storage-pool disease 179
Suction probe 123
Superpulse 16
  rapid 213–14

Tissue,
  biophysical interaction 16–22
  controlled destruction 260–1
  laser effects *17*, 19–22
  sensitization to laser energy 261–5
Titanium rods 28
Tompkins unification **51**
Townes, C. 2, 249
Transition energy (TE) 5
Trophoblastic tissue, persistent, after tubal pregnancy **169–70**
Tubo-ovarian adhesions 102
Twin transfusion syndrome 257

Uterine nerve, laparoscopic ablation 63–4
Uterosacral ablation with laser energy 135–6
Uterosacral ligament separation 135–6

Vaginal intraepithelial neoplasia (VAIN) 205–6
Vaporization,
  cervical 201
  cone techniques 204–5
  ovarian biopsy **83**
  peritoneal biopsy **81**
  speed 217
  tissue **19–20**
  tissue removal 246
Velocity, light wave 4
Ventilation/perfusion ratio 245–6
Video, in laser laparoscopy **124**–*5*
Visible light laser 106–7
  laparoscopy,
    advantages 120–2
    possibilities 137
Visible light laser energy,
  for adhesiolysis 133–4
  for ectopic pregnancy 129
  for endometriosis 132–3
Vulva,
  HPV-associated diseases 234–5
  intra-epithelial neoplasia (VIN), laser ablation 230–1
  laser ablation,
    adjuvant regimens 231–4
    results 231
  laser surgery 211–36
    depth control 221–7

Warfarin 179
Wavelength 3–4

YAG laser,
  clinical applications 150
  contact probe vs CO_2 laser 143, 146–8
  frequency-doubled, *see* KTP laser
  laboratory experiments **148–50**
Yoon rings 185